A NEW KIND OF DOCTOR

A NEW KIND OF DOCTOR

The General Practitioner's Part
in the Health of the Community

Julian Tudor Hart

MB BChir DCH FRCGP FRCP

London
Merlin Press

First published in 1988
by The Merlin Press Ltd.,
78 Lawn Road,
London NW3 2XB

© Julian Tudor Hart 1988

Printed in Great Britain by
Whitstable Litho,
Whitstable, Kent
Text typesetting by
Heather Hems
Tower House, Gillingham, Dorset

British Library Catalogue-in Publication Data

Hart, Julian Tudor
    A New Kind of Doctor: The General Practitioner's
    Part in the Health of the Community
    1. Great Britain. General Practice
    I. Title
    362.1'72'0941

ISBN 0 85036 299 7

CONTENTS

AUTHOR'S FOREWORD

In 1977 the World Health Assembly of the United Nations agreed that

> The main social target of governments and WHO in the coming decades should be the attainment by all the citizens of the world by the year 2000 of a level of health that will permit them to lead a socially and economically productive life.

This was further elaborated at the WHO Alma Ata conference in 1978, with a declaration endorsed by the British government, which spelled out that this ambitious target could never be achieved by medical action alone, centred on hospitals. It depended on adoption of health-oriented policies on incomes, housing, transport, nutrition, education and sport, but above all on development of primary health care as the foundation and principal focus of future health services.

The British government later endorsed the 38 regional targets set by WHO Europe to implement the Alma Ata declaration. Despite all the rhetoric no British government has yet made any substantial changes in health policy to translate the slogan of Health For All into a reality. Government welcomed the implied de-emphasis on hospital services, because they are expensive; but the emphasis on environmental and social improvement was first ignored, and finally opposed. As for primary care, British governments have assumed that this simply means the work of general practitioners, plus some dentists, chemists and opticians as a peripheral afterthought. As all of these are in Britain still private entrepreneurs, albeit in loose contract with government to provide public services, their work is unplannable and the government has no plan. The central actors are the GPs; they occupy the stage, and without their consent, the play can't proceed.

The medical profession has until recently insisted on its unique responsibility for maintaining the health of nations. There are of course many other ways, often much more important, in which health can be either damaged or conserved, but so long as doctors retain this unique role, other people who want to take effective action on health are prevented from doing so, and governments are provided with a credible excuse for inaction. One solution, much written about but not as yet put into practice anywhere, is to bypass the doctors and construct primary care systems without them. A curious feature of this strategy is that none, so far as I know, who have advocated it for other people, have ever accepted it for themselves. Another, the one advocated in this book, is so to change the clinical and social orientation of the medical profession that it can accept teamwork in primary care as a central and obligatory rather than peripheral and optional role.

Indignant descriptions of what's wrong with society, and the doctors' role in it, are increasingly superfluous and irrelevant; few of us need convincing that there are more and more reasons for despair, not only about our own society, but about the future of mankind. Somehow we have to find rational, historically credible foundations for renewed optimism, convincingly supported by evidence, with positive programmes for something better, which do not depend on defensive faiths in obsolete solutions. There is now a large medical literature of denunciation listing the major errors of medical professionalism, but because nearly all of it comes from observers in academic community medicine rather than from clinicians in the field, it often lacks realism. Though a transformation of the social direction and mode of thought of medical professionalism is certainly necessary, this does not mean that all our problems will disappear, only that we

shall face a new but still very difficult agenda, hopefully
more relevant to health than the one we have now, but
demanding even more work by more people. We need a more
positive critical literature which draws more from the many
examples of work already going on in primary care, which
give us the first working models of a new approach. These are
of much greater value than schematic approaches which try
to build new worlds from political drawing boards, deriving
what is useful and possible from first principles often held
with a fierceness and indifference to real experience, suggesting religion rather than science. One of the most hopeful
features of medical science is its combination of theory with
practice, particularly in primary care, where if it is not also
streetwise it might as well not exist; we need a critical
literature that reflects this very positive feature, and respects
everyone who, however mistakenly, actually works in the
health service.

Though I have used many examples of clinical evidence to
support my argument, I have tried to make their presentation
simple; anyone who can read this rather unexciting foreword
should be able to manage the rest, and also find it a lot more
interesting because it is more concrete. The book is aimed at
students, doctors, other health workers, and non-medical
people interested in the National Health Service (NHS),
regardless of their political affiliations. Though the different
social assumptions from which people begin in trying to
make sense of their work are important, more important are
their attitudes to the work itself. Doctors, other health
workers, patients, and their caring relatives, who loyally slog
away day after day, night after night, month after month,
year after year doing the best they can in usually difficult
circumstances, are the audience I want; I have tried not to
make my argument inaccessible to them by assuming that
their social and political points of departure are the same as
my own. This has not been easy, because central to my
argument is the view that medical care has always been a
highly political subject, though only recently has this begun
to be generally recognized, and I cannot pretend to believe
in other than socialist solutions of some kind. However, just

as I have learned as much from non-socialists and even anti-socialists as I have from people who share my beliefs, so it is possible that readers who are not socialists will find material which helps them to work out other solutions.

General practitioners dominate primary care by right of inherited tradition, because they are there. This situation won't last; if doctors are to retain a leading role in the future, they'll have to earn it, and if some other kind of health worker can do better in terms of measured health outcomes, good luck to them. The present dominance of doctors is a fact, but this in no way excuses the failure of so-called general reviews of primary care, as for example the government's Green and White papers on primary care have purported to be, to take account of other primary care workers. That problem has been dealt with excellently by Linda Marks in her King's Fund paper,[1] but my book is not intended to cover that ground except incidentally. I have set out to examine the way that doctors, and particularly doctors in primary care, have come to regard their relation to society, and how society has come to regard the function of doctors; once this matter is settled, it will, I hope, be easier to sort out the functions of the many other kinds of primary health workers, many of them as yet scarcely born or thought of, who are needed for effective maintenance of health in whole populations.

I have relatively little to say about hospital specialists, because I don't believe a solution to the crisis in the NHS and in medical professionalism can depend on change at this level. Any effective hospital specialist service must rest upon general practice, because its efficient function depends on appropriate selection of cases and adequate continuing care before and after episodes of hospital care. General practice is both the largest and the most obsolete part of the NHS, and is probably also the most susceptible to fundamental reform.

My argument is based on general practice and its historical development: because in Britain general practice has been the often creaky foundation on which all the rest of the NHS has been built; because general practice is both its main present weakness and main potential strength; because it is the most credible means of renewal of the NHS, of medical professionalism, and of medical science; and perhaps most of all because general practice is what I know, having practiced it for over 30 years in my own country and observed it in 17 others.

I have also concentrated on the development and problems of general practice in urban and industrial areas, because it's here that problems are most serious and solutions most difficult, and again because this is what I know: the South Wales mining valleys are the inner-city of Wales, the Appalachia of Britain, the nearest we come to the problems of the Third World.

As the book went to press a government White Paper on primary care at last appeared, together with the announcement of what purports to be a major Bill to be put into law in the 1987–8 session of parliament. More people need to know and think about primary care and about general practice than at any time since the NHS began in 1948. My impression is that few either of the public whose lives will be affected by this legislation, or of the politicians who have devised or will criticize it, are well-informed about developments in British general practice over the past 30 years and the large discussion and research literature it has built up. For most people most of the time, above all for most politicians, the NHS has been the hospital service.

I have not aimed to describe British general practitioners as people, a task done very well by Jonathan Gathorne-Hardy,[2] but to explain the nature of their work, how it came to be as it is (different in many ways from general practice in other countries) and how change in this work could alter the whole of medical practice, in hospitals as well as in the community, so that it might become feasible fully to apply continued advance in medical science to the whole population; and how change in medical practice might contribute to profound and positive changes in the whole of our society. It is no secret that I am unable to conceive of a society in which medical science is fully applied, which would not be some form of socialism. People who share Mrs Thatcher's belief that socialist ideas of any kind are now un-British as

well as un-American, an alien infection to be purged from
clean minds, will find this book irritating. Everyone else,
whether or not they agree with my solutions, may nevertheless find my definition of our problems helpful in devising
alternatives of their own. If we are permitted to have it,
time will tell.

Julian Tudor Hart   December, 1987

The Queens
Glyncorrwg
West Glamorgan
Wales SA13 3BL

NOTES

1. Marks, L., *Primary health care on the agenda? A discussion document.*
   Primary Health Care Group, King's Fund Centre for Health Services
   Development, 125 Albert Street, London NW1 7NF, 1987.
2. Gathorne-Hardy, J., *Doctors: the lives and work of GPs.* London:
   Weidenfeld & Nicolson, 1984.

ACKNOWLEDGEMENTS

Many allies and opponents, some now dead, have contributed to ideas developed over the past forty years, and finally expressed here. I am particularly indebted to Hazel Ackery, Dr Henry Blaker, Prof. Archie Cochrane, Drs John and Jean Coope, Dr Alastair Donald, Prof. Michael Drury, Dr Hugh Faulkner, Prof. Ron Frankenberg, Dr John and Julie Frey, Dr John Fry, Dr Hugh Gainsborough, Dr Kate Gardner, Sir George Godber, Dr Steve Iliffe, Tal Jones, Dr John Horder, Prof. Harry Keen, Dr Bruce Lervy, Dr Irvine Loudon, Prof. Jerry Morris, Dr Guy Mouyen, Bert Pearce, Dr Dennis Pereira Gray, Annie and Trevor Powell, Dr Hugh Price, Prof. Geoffrey Rose, Dr Reg Saxton, Dr Conrad Seipp, Dr Cyril Taylor, Prof. Milton Terris, Prof. Sir Peter Tizard, Dr Cuys Van den Dool, and Dr Alastair and Olive Wilson. I have had generous and loyal support from Dr Tom Meade at the Medical Research Council's Epidemiology Unit at the Clinical Research Centre, Northwick Park since 1973, and from my own practice and research staff, notably Betty Ackery, Mair Boast, Anita Davies, Dr Ann Delahunty, Susie Dixon, Cath Edwards, Prof. Andy Haines, Dr Adrian Hastings, Dr Cerys Humphreys, Janet Jones, Margaret Jones, Dr Alex Mills, Dr John Robson, Dr Ian Scott, Jaqueline Sexton, Evelyn Thomas, Margaret Thomas, Dr Martin Walsh, Pam Walton, Dr Graham Watt, Dr Bob Williams, Dr Richard Williams and Dr Marek Wojciechowski. I am particularly grateful to my partner Dr Brian Gibbons, Dr Bryn John, and Joy Townsend for reading the final draft and giving helpful criticism. The librarians at the Royal College of General Practitioners and the BMA Nuffield library have taken trouble to find and photocopy references. Martin Eve at Merlin Press has been encouraging and tolerant throughout. Finally, my wife Mary has led our research team since 1973 with warm flexibility and strict professionalism, run a home, raised a family, and yet made time and space for me to write books; I hope this book will eventually be as effective as she is.

To my parents

Dr Alison Nicol Macbeth, 1897–1951, MB BS London 1923, University College Hospital and Lausanne, South London Hospital for Women, Queens Hospital for Children Bethnal Green, Brompton Hospital for Diseases of the Chest, the Maudsley Hospital, and Organon Laboratories,

and

Dr Alexander Ethan Tudor Hart, 1901–, MRCS LRCP, St. Thomas' Hospital, Major Spanish Republican Army 1937–8, Captain RAMC 1940–45, Booth Hall Children's Hospital, St. Mary Abbott's Hospital, Hampstead General Hospital, general practitioner Llanelli, Brixton and Colliers Wood,

who failed to deter me from becoming a doctor.

Chapter 1
POINTS OF DEPARTURE

The National Health Service (NHS) Act was promised in the Labour landslide election of 1945, passed into law in 1946, and the service itself launched in 1948: a non-contributory comprehensive service making all forms of medical, dental and nursing care, in hospitals or in the community, available free to the whole population, paid entirely from central government funding. I qualified from St. George's Hospital in London four years later, and will retire from full-time clinical practice in 1988; the NHS allowed me to do my own work and refer my patients to the full range of specialist services during an entire working lifetime, without ever having to collect a fee. Several generations of British doctors have followed, with essentially the same historically novel experience.

We have come a long way since then; there have been huge changes in the work and effectiveness of medical care, and exponential growth in medical science which will require even bigger changes in the future. If advances in medical science are to be available for all of the people, the principles on which the NHS was founded must be both restored from their present shorn condition, and extended in entirely new directions. The NHS is under attack as never before, its enemies confident that medical care can again become a commodity on the market, many of its former friends confused and capitulating. The whole world has entered a dangerous time, perhaps most dangerous of all in our own destabilizing society.

Some Illustrative Autobiography

All history must be selective, and therefore judgmental. Its contemporary actors, by living through one set of experiences, are denied others. Like everyone else, my assumptions derive from my own background, experience, the books that I read and the books I avoided, and my readers deserve to be warned what these were.

I was what Americans call a 'red diaper child', my mother in the Labour Party, my father in the Communist Party, our home among other things a transit camp for anti-Fascist refugees from Austria, Germany and Italy. Both my parents were doctors, my father a GP recruited by the South Wales Miners' Federation to help them in a dispute with general practitioners in Llanelli (a redleg?) who later went off to Spain as a surgeon for the International Brigades. Unlike most medical students in 1947, I knew exactly what I wanted to do before I left school; to become a general practitioner in a coal-mining community, because to me that was the highest possible ambition. Like others of that immediately post-war generation, I also felt unjustly spared. My survival was, quite possibly, accidental. Had I been born one year sooner, I might have died in the war, and therefore felt permanently bound not merely to enjoy the peace, but to win and defend it; and not just any peace, but precisely the peace that was won at that time, against Fascism and for a new era of the Common Man, as we still said in those days.

After qualifying in 1952 and disenchanted with teaching hospitals, I sought 'real life' as a House Physician at Kettering General Hospital in the East Midlands, just as general practitioner (GP) surgeons in provincial hospitals were beginning to be replaced by professionals. All routine and much emergency surgery in Kettering had always been done by GPs, helped once a week by a part-time consultant who travelled 100 miles by rail from London. About six months previously, one of the GP-surgeons had been presented with a young woman with acute intestinal obstruction, a condition easily reversed by early surgery but otherwise rapidly fatal. He opened the abdomen, to find multiple obstructions by scarring from Crohn's disease. He excised four or five segments at several points along the seven metres of small intestine, leaving the loose ends to be reconnected. Then his troubles began; which end belonged to which? Never having met this unusual condition before, he had waded into the macaroni without planning his return. In those days emergency surgery was still regarded by patients as a gamble with death. If he had confidently reconnected the tubes as best he could, praying he hadn't created any collisions, dead ends, or inner circles, he would probably have been acclaimed whatever the outcome. Being a man of integrity, he persuaded his GP-anaesthetist colleague to keep the patient unconscious for what turned out to be four hours with a small coppice of metal clamps splayed out from the incision, telephoned the London consultant, and waited for him to come up by the next train to sort it all out. Remarkably, the patient survived. It was the last anecdote of a closing era of GP surgery; the professionals put an end to all that, and not before time.

The General Hospital served two distinct catchment areas: on one hand, the pleasant market towns of Kettering and Wellingborough and their surrounding countryside, with deeply rooted populations of middling provincial gentlefolk and workers in farms, breweries, railways, shops and light industry; on the other, the steel manufacturing town of Corby, with a population largely imported from Glasgow. From Kettering we had people generally at an early stage of illness, with helpful, informative letters from their GPs, who often visited the wards or at least telephoned to see how their patients were getting on, and made use of the x-ray department and laboratory to investigate patients themselves before referral. From Corby we received patients with gross end-stage disease, and hastily scribbled notes from their GPs:

Dear doctor,
    Billy Briggs, 22 Tipslag Terrace, Corby ? acute abdomen (or chest, heart, or whatever), please admit.
    Yrs etc.

Hearts sank when requests for admission came from Corby. They were usually about some medical crisis, often avoidable by earlier diagnosis and appropriate action. The Corby and Kettering GPs seemed to work, as their patients lived, in different worlds. It was my first introduction to the divisions of medicine corresponding to the two nations of British society.

My boss was a bachelor who ran an Austin-Healey sports car, and endlessly complained to his junior staff about his poverty and sufferings under the NHS. I earned £250 a year looking after 20 men, 20 women and 16 children on acute medical wards, on call 24 hours a day, without right to any evenings or weekends off for six months except those personally wheedled from the boss. We differed about the NHS: he believed it would end enterprise and reward sloth, I thought it was the best thing that could have happened for the future of medicine. When he went off for the weekend he would fix me with his pale blue eye: 'Hart: when I come back on Monday I don't want to find the beds filled with rubbish. Old men with chronic bronchitis belong in Local Authority Part III accommodation, not this hospital.' Some old man living alone with advanced smoker's lung was sure to tip into pneumonia, and his GP, rightly acting as advocate, would press for admission. Though squalid dormitory geriatric accommodation did exist under Part III of the Insurance Act in what had been the Kettering workhouse, it was not bad enough to deter a queue to get in. The real choices were between solitary death at home, or a hospital bed with warm nursing, antibiotics (all requiring injection in 1952), and a good chance of recovery. That was my introduction to contradictions between what doctors were interested in and what mattered to patients.

I asked for a reference at the end of my six months, which read as follows: 'Dr Hart has performed his duties as a House Physician adequately during the past six months.' At the time this seemed faint praise, but only later did I realise it conveyed the same lethal message to any experienced medical employer as Hamlet's note on his journey with Rosencrantz and Guildenstern; my introduction to the 18th Century structure of servility and patronage endured by all doctors for some of their lives, and by many for all of their lives.

My junior hospital career was therefore on course for self-destruct, postponed for a few more months by a consultant chest physician who persuaded me to work for him as registrar at the Watford Chest Clinic on the outskirts of London, dealing almost entirely with tuberculosis, then still a common cause of death. I was not properly trained for such responsibility, but the previous man in the job was an alcoholic with drug problems, and no other applicant could be found. The clinic was responsible for tuberculosis patients on the wards of a local hospital which had been a workhouse until 1948. The workhouse master and matron still lived in an elegant residence within the walls, waited on by high-grade mentally defective or so-called morally defective inmates. The barrack-complex contained geriatric and chest wards for sick people, as well as dormitory accommodation for the workhouse inmates who, though liberated by repeal of the Poor Law and advent of the Welfare State, had nowhere else to go. Men lived at one end of the building, women at the other. Most were old people without either money or relatives able to look after them, but there were also mentally or physically handicapped younger people, and several young homeless families. Young or old, married, widowed, or single, males over seven years of age were separated from females except at strictly enforced visiting times. The work was interesting but uncomfortable, not because of the Dickensian surroundings but because I knew I was under-trained. Sink or swim, I learned as I went along; I swam, patients sank.

Just before the lethal reference could catch up with me, I was saved and diverted prematurely into general practice in the wrong place. At the end of 1952 I was chatting to an old Irish GP, Dr Henry Blaker, in a corner dairy in North Kensington. He had retired from a lifetime of work for the Indian Medical Service in Calcutta, to buy a practice from an old colleague, Dr Sweeney, in the slums of North Kensington, with about 2,000 registered patients. His sight was failing from cataracts and he was no longer able to drive, doing his home visits on foot or on the underground. On hearing I was a Cambridge graduate, a fact which impressed him more than me, he asked me to join him as an equal partner starting tomorrow. Only later did I realize how exceptionally just he was; then even more than now entry into general practice, or into almost any other medical job, was difficult, and many established GPs took full advantage of this to exploit their younger colleagues with grossly unequal partnership contracts. Postgraduate experience before starting practice was still an optional extra generally reserved for entry into 'practices of the better type'. North Kensington was Corby not Kettering country, and even the scanty hospital experience I had seemed much more than my local colleagues expected. Under personal pressures which are irrelevant here, I took the job.

Urban Industrial General Practice in the 1950s

The surgery was in what had been a large corner pub in Clarendon Road, off Holland Park. The area is now gentrified beyond recognition, full of media persons and croupiers at the Stock Exchange, but then it was the edge of one of the worst slums in London, stretching from the bottom of Notting Hill in the south, to Harrow Road and the Grand Union Canal in the north. The pub was all elaborately decorated plaster cornices, frosted glass, and engraved mirrors still advertising various ales, stouts, porters and whiskys. Dr Blaker's surgery was in the saloon bar, the waiting room in a narrow adjoining room previously used for off-licence sales. It was nearly always full of people waiting to get in, often with more standing in the street, sometimes in the rain. Patients entered the consulting room at one corner, stepped down from the raised area previously behind the bar counter, and sat in front of an enormous oak desk covered with wooden boxes, books, urine test glassware, and unopened copies of the British Medical Journal. When I eventually sorted this out, I found one of the boxes contained a full set of equipment for post-mortem examination, with bone saws and knives of every size and description. A small working area of desk was cleared in front of the doctor's swivel chair. Behind him was a threadbare printed fabric screen, folded and apparently rarely used. Behind this again was a low divan couch covered in American cloth and stuffed with horsehair, much of it bursting out through ulcers and abrasions acquired in forty or fifty years of combat. On the wall to his right was a large white semicircular washbasin with a single brass cold water tap, an amenity added a few months previously; Dr Blaker warned me not to pee in it, as some previous locums had done. Next to this was a metal stand with a china bowl and ewer, now redundant but, like the junk on the desk, kept on standby in case the 19th Century returned, a not unlikely event to any thoughtful observer. This time-warped impression was strengthened by a glass fronted cupboard set in the wall of the waiting room, still full of dusty medicine bottles waiting to be collected by patients whose names could still just be made out on the elegantly scripted labels. Apparently Dr Sweeney had done his own dispensing, and when the practice finally gave up competing with the local pharmacy this cupboard was simply locked and left as it stood.

There was no receptionist, so patients' medical records, the small pocket envelopes devised in 1916 for the Lloyd George Act and still used by nine out of ten English GPs, were housed to the left of the great oak desk in a nest of wooden drawers. Virtually the only entries ever made were of medicines prescribed, but occasionally there would be a brief diagnosis ('asthma', 'fractured femur', 'neurotic') without any of the evidence on which the diagnosis was based. Useful clinical information, if any, was confined to hospital correspondence, folded and pushed into the record envelope in a more or less randomly ordered and increasingly tattered bundle.

Twenty to thirty patients came each morning, about the same number in the evening, and between these two sessions I was supposed to fit in about 15 house calls. There were nearly always two or three visits left to do after the evening session, together with any late calls. I would finish by 7.30 if I was lucky, by 9.00 if I was not. I did all the night work for that first year.

One year to the day after I started, without warning or discussion, I found a note from Dr Blaker on the desk to say he had retired and the practice was mine. I took a partner of

my own age and we built up the practice to about 3,000
when I left in 1957 to resume my interrupted hospital training, this time on the children's wards at Hammersmith
Hospital. Workload steadily fell, reduced by good practice
organization, employing a receptionist and dealing with the
underlying causes of such clinical problems as were soluble,
rather than sidestepping them with symptomatic treatment.
When I left the practice, we often saw only ten or twelve
patients at each session, despite a much larger population
at risk.

South Wales in the 1960s

After another three years of junior hospital posts and some
experience of epidemiological research, first with Richard
Doll and later with Archie Cochrane, in 1961 I finally reached
my original goal, a single-handed general practice in a small
coal-mining community in the Afan Valley in South Wales.
The daily consulting rate in Glyncorrwg was roughly the
same as when I started in London: 20 to 30 patients at the
morning session, the same in the evening, 12 to 15 home
visits, for about the same number of people at risk. The time
available for each consultation was 5 or 6 minutes, slightly
more than was found in a large study of practices in Aberdeen
ten years later,[1] but less than the average 8.25 minutes found
in the most recent survey of GP workload in 1986.[2] Unlike
my London experience, improved practice organization had
little effect on workload; the reserve of unmet need seemed
inexhaustible.

The squalid conditions of industrial working-class practice
I met, first in London and later in South Wales, were
incompatible with the standards of clinical medicine taught
in medical schools, denying self-respect and limiting the
imaginations of GP and patient alike. They were essentially
the same as those pilloried by Collings[3] in his classic report
in 1950 on British general practice. Thirty-four years later
Eric Wilkes,[4] professor of general practice in Sheffield,
described the same squalor in 1984 in a despairing paper
entitled 'Is good general practice possible?'. British general

practice has changed in my lifetime, but very unevenly and very incompletely. It has changed least of all in the old areas of heavy industry, where the real wealth of this country was originally made, and where poverty and unemployment are now most miserably endured.

Genᵉral Practitioner and Referred Care

Having worked a lifetime in general practice, that is the point from which I see the NHS as a whole, and the people it serves; a close underview from where the action begins, rather than an overview from hospital specialism where some of it ends, or from the outer space of a university library.

To an extent unique in Western Europe and North America, the British medical profession is and has for well over 50 years been divided into two easily defined groups, with little overlap: GPs responsible for registered lists of patients, who care for them only in their own homes and communities; and consultant specialists responsible for all hospital work, assisted by young doctors in training (most of whom later become GPs), who only see patients on referral from GPs. GPs therefore remain generalists, whose real specialized skills are based on familiarity with a specific local population. All other levels of the NHS rest on general practice; the quality, efficiency, and effectiveness of specialists are limited not only by the resources made available to them by the State, but also by the quality and completeness of GP care.

The National Health Service created, and was designed to create, a dramatic improvement in both the extent and the quality of care by specialists in hospitals. It also suddenly extended GP care from the minority of male manual workers covered by the old Lloyd George Insurance Act, to the entire population. It vastly increased the accessibility of general practice but did nothing, and was not designed to do anything, to improve its quality. Clinical medicine in British general practice did improve between 1948 and 1967 (the first important structural reform of NHS general practice), but not at anything like its pace of improvement in hospital care. Nor were improvements selective for those social and geographical areas most in need of them. In general, the quality of all medical care, and particularly of GP care, was lowest where the needs of the population were highest; what I later described as the Inverse Care Law.[5] Neighbourhoods with the worst health inherited the worst traditions, expectations and resources, and were least competitive in the market for well-trained, innovative young doctors. General practice remains an area of relatively poor performance, falling short even of its traditional task of meeting the immediate demands of patients for care of symptomatic illness; it is better, much better, than it was, but still far below what it should be. General practice is even now only beginning to accept its huge future potential for effective health conservation, through which its impact on the health of the general population could be greater than anything possible through specialist care in hospitals.

'The Health Service is Hospitals'

Most politicians, media persons, or members of the general public, asked for their mental picture of what is central, important, and effective in the NHS, will describe something going on in a hospital. For most people, hospitals appear to be virtually the only source of effective treatment for life-threatening or seriously disabling conditions; the job of GPs is to sort out major from minor conditions, referring major ones to specialists in hospitals, dealing with minor ones themselves. Planned government investment in hospitals throughout the land, in their staff, equipment, and buildings, with demand from the whole population limited only by the process of GP referral, was the great leap forward which made the NHS such a huge public success.

Until 1967, there was virtually no investment at all in general practitioner services, except what GPs themselves were prepared to spend from their own pockets. The 1966 Package Deal (also known as the GP Charter) brought some indirect public investment in the form of 70% reimbursement of wages to encourage employment of office and nursing staff, 100% reimbursement of rent for suitable buildings, and incentive payments for group practice. Eventually this almost wiped out two common features of industrial general practice; the seedy front-parlour surgery in the GP's own home, and the squalid shop on the high street with a half-painted glass front, staffed only by a harassed GP's wife. It reduced the proportion of GPs working single-handed from 43% in 1952, to only 14% by 1980. This did not always improve access for patients, but did encourage sharing of staff and equipment, and placed some limit on the idiosyncratic behaviour of GPs.

Even this investment was not fully taken up. GPs are now entitled to claim 70% reimbursement of office and nursing staff wages up to two Whole-Time-Equivalent (WTE) staff for each GP. For the past ten years the actual number employed has stuck around 1.1–1.2 WTE per GP, and only about 15% employ their full entitlement;[6] most GPs evidently don't think they need a larger team.

The most important feature of public investment in general practice, however, is that it is neither planned nor plannable. Though GPs now accept some public investment, they are not publicly accountable, except in the narrow and negative sense that they are answerable for complaints. General practice has for seldom-considered historical reasons become a public service privately administered. GPs are independent contractors with government, to provide a public service on their own initiative, with little public control, all of it negative. Even within the narrow limits set by the maximum resources available through the present GP contract, quality of service depends on autonomous decisions by GPs.

Imagine the state of our national road network, if it were financed by a multitude of turnpikes, the quality of each stretch depending on local owners and local expectations; a few miles of motorway, suddenly replaced by a three-lane A road, then a narrow, rutted, unpaved lane, then another mile of motorway, and so on, each depending on the interest and integrity of its owner. It would be an inherently corrupt situation, since whatever he spent on his stretch of road he would be unable to spend on himself or his family. It would be cheap, and occasionally charming, but ineffective as a transport system. For the same reasons, general practice is also cheap, occasionally charming, and, if its task is so far as possible to maintain the health of the whole population, ineffective.

1935–1970: An Age of Optimism

Aneurin Bevan's bold nationalization and expansion of hospitals coincided with a worldwide wave of optimism about the effectiveness of medical science, and the feasibility of delivering it to all of the people.

The 35 years from the discovery of sulphonamides in 1935, the first antibiotics suitable for mass use by non-specialist doctors, were a golden age of uncritical faith in the social value of applied medical science. This began to collapse around 1970, with a general mood of radical criticism among young people, together with the beginnings of doubt and retreat from the commitments of the Welfare State and the social contract built on the double victory of 1945, the war and the Labour landslide election. Criticism of medical activity at all levels, focused particularly on high technology care in hospitals, has persisted ever since, both from 'Left' and from 'Right' perspectives.

There is little doubt about the starting date for this era, which more than most historic turning points derived from precise technical as well as less easily defined social and political change. Dramatic effects on valid indicators of disease susceptible to sulphonamide treatment are shown in Fig. 1.1 for death-rates of women in childbirth (maternal mortality),[7] and in Fig. 1.2 for death-rates from pneumonia in young men.

Clearly something dramatic happened in the mid-1930s to two common causes of premature death, but it is important to remember that this advance in effective treatment occurred against a background of steady improvement in death rates from all causes, which seems to have started around 1870 (Fig. 1.3), with full industrialization of the British economy, and the beginning of intensive rather than extensive exploitation of industrial workers. This improvement in health was probably caused mainly by improved nutrition, education,

Fig. 1.1 Maternal mortality, death rate per 100,000 total births, 1860–1964, England and Wales.

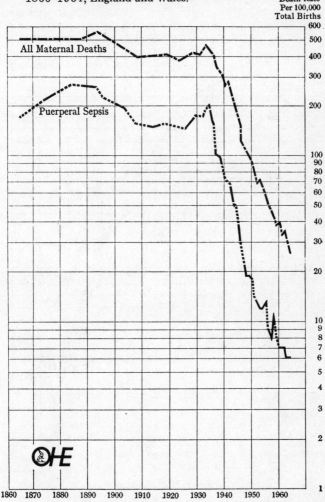

Death Rate
Per 100,000
Total Births

All Maternal Deaths

Puerperal Sepsis

OHE

Note: (1) Ten year averages 1861 to 1890, five year averages 1891 to 1930, annual rates 1931 to 1964.
(2) Logarithmic scale.

Source: Derived from Registrar General's Decennial Supplement, England & Wales 1931, Part III, and Registrar General's Statistical Review of England & Wales, various years. Figure reproduced from 'Disorders which shorten life', OHE 1966, by kind permission of the Office of Health Economics, London.

Fig. 1.2 Pneumonia, death rate per million males living, by age, 1861–1964, England and Wales.

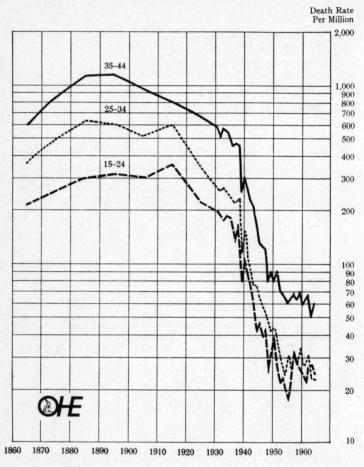

Note: (1) Females rates are similar and in order to facilitate graphic presentation are not shown.
(2) Ten year averages 1861 to 1930, annual rates 1931 to 1964.
(3) Logarithmic scale.

Source: Derived from Registrar General's Decennial Supplement, England & Wales 1931, Part III, and Registrar General's Statistical Review of England & Wales, various years. Figure reproduced from 'Disorders which shorten life', OHE 1966, by kind permission of the Office of Health Economics, London.

Fig. 1.3 Death rates per million living from all causes, by age, 1841-1964, England and Wales.

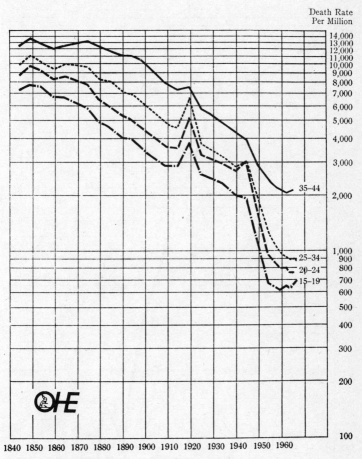

Death Rate
Per Million

Note: (1) Five year averages 1841 to 1960, annual rates 1961 to 1964.
(2) Logarithmic scale.

Source: Registrar General's Statistical review of England & Wales 1964, Part I. Figure reproduced from 'Disorders which shorten life', OHE 1966, by kind permission of the Office of Health Economics, London.

Fig. 1.4 Diphtheria. Child death rates per million; England and Wales 1931-60.

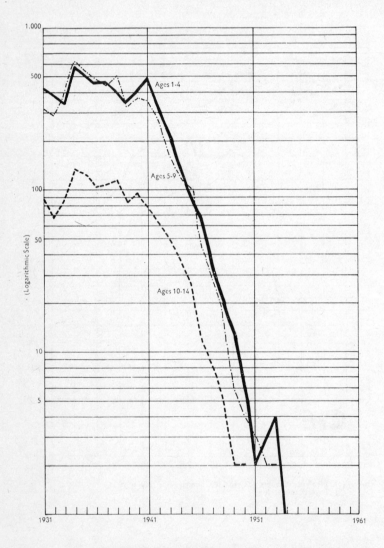

Source: Registrar General's Statistical Review, Part I. Figure reproduced from 'The lives of our children: a study in childhood mortality', OHE 1962, by kind permission of the Office of Health Economics, London.

and housing, and by reduced occupational risks (in that order of importance), all of which have bigger effects on health than personal medical care.[8]

It is equally important to remember that advances in medical science only lead to improvements in health to the extent that they are generally applied; sulphonamides did not save women in childbirth or young men with pneumonia unless doctors prescribed them. On the other hand, sulphonamides were toxic in high dosage, and a lot of damage was done by doctors who used them inappropriately or carelessly. This is obvious, but seems to have been ignored both by pre-war Ministers of Health and by practising doctors. Fig. 1.4 shows deaths of children from diphtheria from 1931 to 1961. Clearly there was a dramatic improvement in 1941; an effective diphtheria vaccine had been commercially available from about 1922, but was not applied as an organized programme for mass immunization to the whole child population until nearly 20 years later.

The NHS is a social construct, whose advance or decline depends on social ideas and competing social pressures. Advances in medical science like the discovery of diphtheria vaccine are not automatically applied to the general population. The age of optimism in medicine was just one part of a general period of post-war liberal illusion, which denied the value or necessity of social struggle, and imagined that a classless society could be painlessly achieved by 'levelling up' in a consumerist, capitalist and corporate nation. That kind of liberal optimism died in Vietnam. It has been replaced by strategies of retreat, the subject of the next chapter.

NOTES

1. Buchan, I.C., Richardson, I.M., 'Time study of consultations in general practice'. *Scottish Health Studies no. 27.* Edinburgh: Scottish Home & Health Department, 1973.
2. 'Survey of GPs' workload', *British Medical Journal 1987*, 294: 1241.
3. Collings, J.S., 'General practice in England today', *Lancet 1950*, i:555-85.
4. Wilkes, E., 'Is good general practice possible?', *British Medical Journal 1984*; 289:85-6.

5. Hart, J.T., 'The Inverse Care Law', *Lancet 1971*; i:405–503.
6. Hart, J.T., 'Practice nurses: an under-used resource', *British Medical Journal, 1986*, 290:1162–3.
7. Loudon, I., 'Puerperal fever, the streptococcus, and the sulphonamides, 1911–1945', *British Medical Journal 1987*; 295:485–490.
8. McKeown, T., *The role of medicine*, Oxford: Blackwell, 1979.

Chapter 2
LIBERAL RETREAT

The late 1960s was a time of ideological confusion when the idea of social progress generally lost the association with science it had in the 1930s. The medical age of optimism began to seem an age of credulity. In 1971 Cochrane[1] was the first of a series of authors presenting fundamental criticisms of the theory, practice and profession of contemporary medicine in Britain and North America[2, 3, 4] which were rapidly accepted by an unusually wide range of opinion-formers from both 'Left' and 'Right' traditions. In its most popular form, and with an irresponsible use of evidence setting it apart from the medical pioneers of this trend, it was presented by Ivan Illich in his book *Medical nemesis*,[5] which sold over 3 million copies worldwide. He accused doctors of expropriating the personal right of patients to control their own health, from a combination of greed and intellectual arrogance. He accused the medical profession of being the main danger to public health, as he had pilloried teachers as the main enemies of education in his previous book *Deschooling society*. Illich went to extraordinary lengths in pursuit of his medical enemy; here is a sample:

> Medical civilisation tends to turn pain into a technical matter and thereby deprives suffering of its inherent personal meaning. . . Culture makes pain tolerable by interpreting its necessity; only pain perceived as curable is intolerable.

Like any intellectual fashion achieving wide influence, Illich's argument used some elements of truth, though nearly all his evidence was derived from medical sources, suggesting that medical science was more self-critical than his theory allowed. It still seems extraordinary that so weak an argument was taken so seriously, even in authoritative medical journals like the *British Medical Journal* and the *Lancet*, which devoted pages of self-doubt to an assault which would once have been brushed aside as a trivial impertinence. Ten years later, the *Lancet* still has space for random reflections of Chairman Illich, of a banality too complex and pretentious for analysis either as prose or scientific argument.[6]

The most credible explanation for this seems to be that many intellectual leaders of the profession were already looking for ways to justify their own retreat from the full social implications of making all important advances in medical science available as a human right to the whole population. Assured of sponsorship, doctors still wanted to provide effective skills whatever the cost; but as the State set limits on its sponsorship for innovative medical science, the profession discovered new doubts about its mass application, though medical science itself was unquestionably in better shape than ever before.

Common to all these intellectual critics were the following beliefs:

1. That medical care has contributed little to improvements in health or expectation of life compared with nutrition, education, and conditions of life and work.
2. That doctors and their public have expected too much from attempts to restore health by surgical or biochemical excision or substitution, which now incur increasing and eventually prohibitive costs for diminishing returns.
3. That personal medical care should therefore retreat to a more modest role in curing seldom, relieving often, and comforting always.

This currently dominant set of ideas I shall refer to as the Liberal Critique, since it has all the historic qualities of Liberalism: scholarly backing, humane intentions, appeal to both Left and Right intellectual radicals without embarrassment to either, and ability to interpret defeat as victory. This is a savage description, but anger is justified; not because these three conclusions are untrue, but because of the increasingly obvious social and political context in which only these truths have been proclaimed, while others, less convenient to this scoundrel time, have been forgotten. The Liberal Critique has disarmed professional resistance first to revision, then to destruction of the post-war social settlement of which the NHS was an important part.

Does Medical Care Matter?

The view that medical care contributes less to health than nutrition, education and conditions of life and work is not new or original. It is difficult to think of any important innovator in medical thought who has not held this opinion. If you take a thousand people and lock them up, their first thoughts are of food, not doctors. The more primitive life is, the more important food and shelter become, but a society that is becoming more rather than less civilized gives more not less priority to education and health services, in that order.

Even in specialized hospital medicine, outstanding innovators like Paget, Osler, Albutt, Pickering and Platt always conceded the pre-eminent role of nutrition, education, and living and working conditions, compared with the salvage work they performed. Like pioneers in any field, they may sometimes have expected too much from attempts to restore health by surgical or biochemical excision or substitution, but again this is not new, and the general public, encouraged by press entertainers, has been far more credulous than its doctors. In Britain more than most countries there has been a vigorous tradition of medical scepticism ever since the Second World War, probably because until recently nearly all doctors were in a free public service rather than trade, and therefore had fewer incentives to deceive either themselves or their customers.

The novel feature of the Liberal Critique is not this re-discovery of the dominant importance of environment for health, and our still limited ability to cure illness, but its emphasis on a diminishing role for medical care; not only the alleged pettiness of its actual contribution, but of its potential contribution in the future. The question would have been easier to understand around 1905, when the only major diseases in which medication influenced outcome were syphilis and heart failure, and effective surgery was limited to injuries and a few abdominal and obstetric emergencies. The rate of successful clinical innovation, far from levelling out or diminishing, is increasing every year. Seeds of a vast expansion of innovation in applied medical science were sown with the discovery of the structure of DNA in 1953, 'a revolution in the biological sciences comparable to that in physics earlier this century'.[7] Medicine is applied human biology. It took about 40 years for nuclear physics to find a practical application; 34 years after Crick and Watson we are already beginning to see evidence that 'medical sciences are about to enter the most exciting period of their development'.[7] Undeniably, basic medical science is advancing with accelerating speed. Practical applications in teaching hospitals, though most of them still depend on basic medical sciences of the pre-molecular era, are already arriving faster than we can assimilate them within present staff resources.

There is no real doubt that these new techniques are increasingly effective. Coronary artery bypass grafts (CABG) are a good example. When they began to be widely used in the United States in the early 1970s, thoughtful doctors had mixed feelings. On the one hand, CABG relieved the symptoms of chest pain from coronary heart disease (angina) almost completely in about 70% of cases, and increased survival by about 50% over the first seven years following operation for the minority of patients with angina who have left main coronary artery disease (about 13% of cases), with less than 3% mortality from the operation itself.

CABGs may appear to support the view that effective medical care now incurs increasing and eventually prohibitive costs for diminishing returns, but this is so only if the technique is applied without an overall policy for control of coronary disease. Once-for-all surgical costs for CABG are £2,500–£4,500 at 1983–4 prices, not all that much more than the cost of modern medical care for the expected life-time of angina patients.[8] The difference in cost, around £2,500, is about the same as the cost of one total hip replacement operation. Surgical costs are more than twice as high in marketed, fee-paid care systems such as that in the USA, so in terms of cost-effectiveness, the case for CABG is stronger in a free public service, where surgeons are paid by salary. Like all new surgical treatments for common conditions, the technique becomes cheaper as it becomes perfected and standardized; the more advanced centres are now well into the next generation of surgical procedures for coronary salvage, coronary angioplasty, an essentially simpler procedure which provides a rebore of the original vessel instead of replacing it, an even safer and much cheaper procedure. These techniques are effective and should be generally available without delay to those who need them, a policy which in no way contradicts the need simultaneously to step up health promotion, prevention and anticipatory care.

One of the saddest recent developments in the NHS is the attempt to supplement inadequately funded NHS heart surgery by getting coronary surgery done privately under contract to the NHS, as my own Health Authority in West Glamorgan has recently decided to do. NHS units are still the sole source of training for the very specialized surgical teams which perform these operations, whether they ultimately work in the NHS or the private sector. Farming the work out to private contractors working for profit accelerates the destruction of the training, research and development facilities on which all progress depends.

Though coronary death rates have fallen in USA, Australia, and New Zealand by about one-third over the same period that CABG has been in wide use in these countries, heart surgery has been estimated to contribute only 4–5% of this reduction.[9] It is still not clear why these big falls in coronary mortality have occurred, nor why they appeared first in the USA and Australia, and have hardly occurred at all in Britain and Sweden; on the whole, the most convincing evidence is for a reduction in average blood total cholesterol because of changes in the composition of quantity of fat in common foods, which have occurred in some countries and not others. There is no doubt at all that they do reflect changes in the way people live more than changes in medical care, except insofar as medical advice may accelerate changes in personal behaviour, on a scale sufficient to affect fashion. There has certainly been a stark contrast between the active advocacy of coronary prevention as well as surgical salvage by doctors in the USA, and the passivity of British doctors.[10] There is still much that is unexplained about coronary disease. Big reductions in coronary atheroma in young men preceded any big shifts in adult eating patterns, exercise, smoking or heart surgery by about ten years. They may at least in part have been caused by contrasts between childhood and adult nutrition in the entire cohort of men born between about 1910 and 1940.[11, 12] These questions are important, because molecular biology is going to give us weapons that act upon causal mechanisms in very large numbers of people, rather than the primitive strategy of salvaging advanced disease.

There is no longer any doubt that CABG is a real advantage to patients carefully selected on clinical grounds, or that surgical salvage should have a useful, though relatively small and eventually diminishing part to play in any overall strategy for dealing with coronary disease. This was exactly the (unplanned) sequence followed for rheumatic valvular damage, the principal cause of early death from heart disease before coronary disease began to be common in the 1930s; a rapid but incomplete decline because of changed living conditions, accelerated and completed by surgical salvage. The difference between surgical valve repair or replacement in the 1950s and '60s, and CABG today, is that free access to surgery on the basis of need alone is no longer expanding for the whole population.

Studies in Sweden suggest that the justifiable annual demand for CABG would be around 300 per million population, if all suitable cases were accepted in the age-range 45–54. Reviewing the provision of CABG in Wales in 1983, the Royal College of General Practitioners found the operation was being offered at 7% of this ideal rate in Wales, and 80% of it in the London (SE Thames) region, after subtracting cases 'imported' from other regions,[13] although male death rates in middle age from coronary disease in the South Wales valleys are about one-third higher than in England and Wales as a whole, and nearly twice as high as in the South East.[14] Unlike facilities for open heart surgery for rheumatic valvular disease, regional availability of CABG is unrelated to need. In the absence of an active policy for preferential development in areas of high coronary mortality, there is a large element of social selection because of the lower expectations and therefore lower effective demand of poorer and less well-informed people, even in a system of free care. There is no evidence that any such policy is currently pursued or planned.

Even if coronary surgery were available in proportion to regional need, no matter how successful it might be tactically, it could not be an effective mass strategy. Without organization of anticipatory care and prevention it only offers a personal short-term technological fix to a small high-risk minority, instead of tackling what is essentially a long-term behavioural problem for the whole population. Though molecular biology may give us alternative solutions, even these will probably have to be applied to whole populations at risk rather than to a few with advanced damage.

The truth is that until we have successful prevention, we must have salvage; if we want to remain a civilized country, both strategies must be pursued, and for everyone. I have yet to meet any well-informed person who, having developed angina uncontrollable by stopping smoking, by medication and by minor restrictions in exercise, does not want a skilled surgical opinion. Whatever their views on grand social strategy, the experts all seem to make intelligent and discriminating use of high technology salvage for themselves and their families, and they still do this through the National Health Service whenever they can. In practice, even within the NHS we already have a two-tier system, in which a minority of well-informed people, and those with unusually energetic GPs, gain access to the best high-technology salvage, while the majority go by default.

In an under-funded public service, as more people rightly

make more sophisticated demands, waiting lists lengthen, and more people have to seek treatment privately. This is only beginning with CABGs, of which only 0.1% were done privately in 1981, but it is well established for hip replacement, 26% of which were done in the private sector in the same year. New techniques are either introduced reluctantly and inadequately, as with CABG, or in some regions abandoned almost completely to the private sector, as with vasectomy and termination of pregnancy. Using available data from various years from 1981 to 1984, private market penetration had reached 1% for obstetric care, 1.5% for mental handicap, 2% for chronic mental illness, 4% for acute mental illness, 13% for all elective surgery, 35% for long-stay institutional care of the elderly, and 47% for terminations of pregnancy.

Paying More and More for Less and Less

Of course, believers in the Liberal Critique deplore all this. They would like everyone to enjoy the same quality of care as themselves, but (they argue), Britain in its post-imperial state is becoming a poor country, in which painful choices have to be made; to them it is obvious that with limited resources, the first things to go from a shorn public service should be luxury items like high technology medical care. The argument has even influenced people who consider themselves Marxists. Writing in *Marxism Today*, Dr Steve Iliffe[15] has come to believe that:

> the guiding principles of the National Health Service are no longer workable. . . overall staffing levels should be kept constant. . . budget restraints on health authorities should be maintained. . . principled objections to charges for services should be overruled. . . Medicine is steadily becoming less cost-effective. . . money will come from different directions in different places, ending the pretence of a tidy monolithic institution. If this happens, we will be in debt to the Conservatives for the instability they once inflicted on the biggest institution in Europe outside the Red Army, and also on the traditions of the British Left.

Iliffe gives CABG and total hip replacement as examples of

rising costs with diminishing effectiveness. He can hardly deny that these procedures are effective in making thousands of lives enjoyable rather than miserable. As techniques become standardized, costs fall, particularly if they are organized in a non-profit public service. The proportion of our Gross National Product spent on medical care has risen only from 4% in 1949 to 6% in 1981, is still less than any other country in Europe, and almost half that in the USA. The rate of fall of age-specific mortality has, of course, declined as more people reach a healthy old age, and more deaths result from natural senescence, but effectiveness of medical care in improving the quality of life has enormously improved. There is no evidence that this tendency will diminish; on the contrary, the immense potential benefits of advances in basic biological science have hardly been tapped. It has been estimated that 25-30% of hospital beds, and probably an even higher proportion of all NHS spending, goes on care during the last year of life,[16] either terminal care or more less unsuccessful salvage. In the light of current medical knowledge, this proportion is too high, but that means an increased investment in care in the community at earlier stages of disease, rather than a reduction in care of advanced disease and terminal illness.

Social Causes of Disease

Believers in the Liberal Critique nevertheless maintain that because in an ideal world each pound spent on better food, housing or education in deprived sections of the population would yield greater health benefits than each pound spent on medical care, public spending should follow the same order of priorities. Granted the unlikely premise (an ideal world), this would be true, and the argument is important.

Although death rates at all ages have been falling ever since 1870, the difference between death rates for the rich and the poor has been widening since the 1930s (Fig. 2.1). Mortality differences for women follow the same trends, but are more difficult to interpret because women are classified by their husbands' occupations.

Fig. 2.1 Standardized Mortality Ratios (100 = average mortality across all classes) by social class, 1931–81, men 15–64, England and Wales.

Class	1931	1951	1961*	1971*	1981**
I professional	90	86	76 (75)	77 (75)	66
II managerial	94	92	81	81	76
III skilled manual and non-manual	97	101	100	104	103
IV semi-skilled	102	104	103	114	116
V unskilled	111	118	143 (127)	137 (121)	166

* Figures have been adjusted to classification of occupations used in 1951.

** Men 20–64 years, Great Britain.

Source: Wilkinson, R.G., 'Socio-economic differences in mortality: interpreting the data on their size and trends'. In Wilkinson, R.G., (ed.), *Class and health: research and longitudinal data*, London: Tavistock Publications, 1986.

Fig. 2.2 shows data from follow-up of a 1% sample of the
population of England and Wales, occupationally classified in
the 1971 census, for the periods 1971–5 and 1976–81.[17] It
includes two further social groups, the 'inadequately described'
(including many chronic sick with a high mortality) and the
'unoccupied' (including long-term unemployed whether or
not they are able to claim unemployment benefit). Clearly
there are even higher death rates for these groups than for
Social Class V, the unskilled manual workers. Social class
differences increased for all groups except the 'unoccupied',
which fell from an SMR of 299 in the first period to 213 in
the second. The authors of this study interpret this fall as an
effect of ageing; men selected out of occupational classification by ill-health and who did not die in the first period, were
less unlike those who remained classifiable in the second.

Social and regional distributions of deaths from all causes
differ little from social and regional distributions of death-
rates from major specific causes, particularly premature
deaths from coronary heart disease. Social class differences in
coronary death rates for men in Wales aged 20–64 are shown
in Fig. 2.3.

Data from a recent survey of coronary risk factors in Wales
based on a random sample of the whole population,[18] set
out in Fig. 2.4, confirm that in Wales at least, with very high
rates of unemployment, both fatalism about the possibility
of preventing heart attacks, and the proportion who smoke
the cigarettes responsible for many of the deaths, increase
with descending social class, worst of all in those out of work.

This picture of inequalities in distribution of actual disease,
of informed confidence that disease can be prevented, and of
avoidable precursors of potential disease, is true not only of
coronary heart disease, but of all the main causes of premature death and chronic disability. Worst of all, these
inequalities are increasing. The available evidence was
presented in the Report of Sir Douglas Black's Committee
on Inequalities in Health[19] in 1980, powerfully reinforced
by a wide range of subsequent research reviewed by
Wilkinson, Marmot, Blaxter, Wadsworth and others.[20]

Social inequalities in health are neither just nor inevitable.

Fig. 2.2 Mortality of men aged 15-64 by social class, 1971-75 and 1986-81.

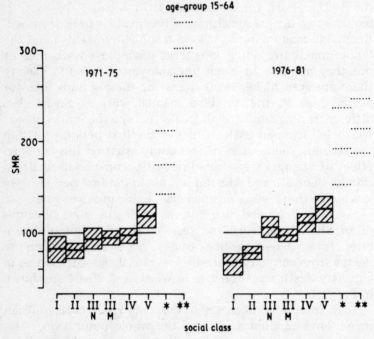

hatched areas represent approximate 95% confidence intervals[19] for SMRs; each SMR is indicated by a horizontal line within the hatched area

* inadequately described

** unoccupied

Source: Fox, A.J., Goldblatt, P.O., Jones, D.R., 'Social class mortality differentials: artefact, selection, or life circumstances?' Fig. 3.1. In Wilkinson, R.G. (ed.), *Class and health: research and longitudinal data*, London: Tavistock Publications, 1986. Reproduced with permission.

Fig. 2.3 Standardized mortality ratios for coronary heart disease in men aged 20-64, Wales, 1979-83.

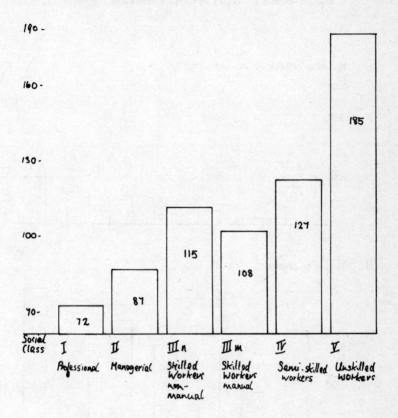

Fig. 2.4 Percentages of Welshmen aged 45–64 who 1) thought it was impossible to reduce the risk of heart attacks; and 2) smoked cigarettes every day; by sex and social class, 1985.

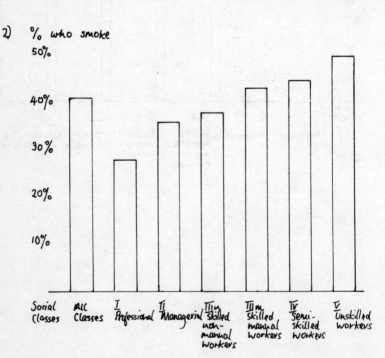

1) % who think risk inevitable

2) % who smoke

They are the result of social and economic policies adopted by governments, which clearly reveal the priorities of the social groups they represent. Fig. 2.5 shows the relation between inequalities of income and expectation of life for 11 developed countries.

The countries grouped on the upper left with relatively high life expectancy and minimal inequality of income, the Netherlands, Norway and Sweden, have strong egalitarian traditions which they still uphold. The countries grouped on the bottom right, with relatively low life expectancy and maximal inequality of incomes, the USA, Germany, Spain and France, have long been strongholds of social Darwinism. The war of every man against every man may be good for business, but certainly not for health.

Paradoxically, the most rapid improvements in life-expectancy this century in Britain were concentrated in the war periods 1911-21 and 1940-51.[21] Though these were years of relative austerity for the middle class, they were years of full employment and full bellies for the poor, with government policies of planned social intervention to create what was later called the 'social wage'; free school meals, maternity and child benefits, sickness benefits, free access to museums, libraries, and parks, cheap municipal housing and public transport, and finally a free and comprehensive health service; the working model for the NHS hospital service in 1948 was the Emergency Medical Service scheme which effectively nationalized hospital resources during the war.

Investment in a shared infrastructure of free services is a political choice, of proven effectiveness. Before the Second World War, infant mortality in Stockholm varied according to socio-economic group from 14 to 49 per 1,000 live births; today it is below 7 per 1,000 live births, with virtually no difference between socio-economic groups.[22] Governments, like our own in 1945 or in Scandinavia today, can choose to increase the social wage relative to personal incomes, or they can revert to sale and purchase of these elements of civilization, piece by piece, every man for himself, as Thatcher Conservatism does today.

Redistributive income policies are another way of

Fig. 2.5 Life expectancy (male and female) and gini coefficients of post-tax income inequality (standardized for household size).

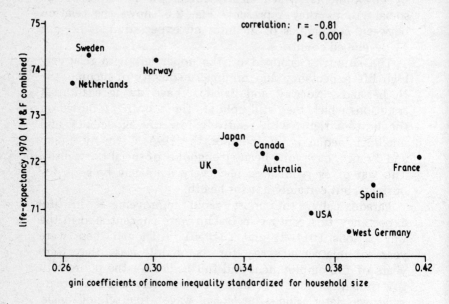

Source: Fig. 6.3 in Wilkinson, R.G. (ed.), *Class and health: research and longitudinal data*, London: Tavistock Publications, 1986. Reproduced with permission.

improving health selectively for least healthy social groups. Fig. 2.6 shows the relation between income and one indicator of health, the standardized mortality ratio.

Wilkinson[23] explains the significance of this curve:

> successive increases in income bring diminishing health returns. The shape of the curve suggests that income transfers from the rich to the poor might be expected to bring substantial health benefits to the poor while having little effect on the health of the rich. Every pound transferred from people earning (in 1970) £60-70 a week to people earning £10-20 would reduce the death rates of recipients by five times as much as it increased those of the donors.

The Black Report was commissioned by the last Labour government, but was completed and published in the early months of Margaret Thatcher's first term as prime minister. In a foretaste of authoritarianism to come, everything administratively possible was done to smother the report at birth, but it quickly achieved the widest sales and press attention given to any similar document since the Beveridge Report. The Black Report is now being implemented in reverse; that is to say, government policies are, virtually without exception, the opposite of those recommended by the Black working party. By every measure of income, education, housing, availability of employment, nutrition, participative sport facilities, nicotine and alcohol dependence, and increasingly by access to sophisticated medical care (curative or preventive), Britain is becoming a more divided and unequal society.

A Strategy for Advance

The first step in devising strategies for more effective, and cost-effective, health services must be to oppose this policy of de-civilization. Scholars seeking solutions within limits set by the de-civilizers deceive themselves, and disarm and confuse what should be, and will become, a previously unimaginable social alliance of professional and public opinion for resumed social progress. Some advocates of the Liberal Critique have had useful things to say, and pro-

Fig. 2.6 Cross-sectional relationship between occupational earnings and standardized mortality ratios, England and Wales.

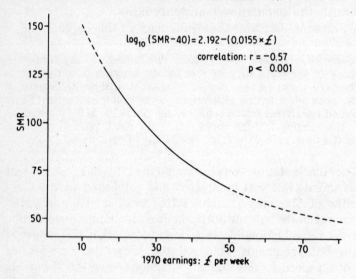

$$\log_{10}(SMR-40) = 2.192 - (0.0155 \times \pounds)$$

correlation: $r = -0.57$

$p < 0.001$

1970 earnings: £ per week

Source: Fig. 6.2 in Wilkinson, R.G. (ed.), *Class and health: research and longitudinal data*, London: Tavistock Publications, 1986. Reproduced with permission.

gressives can learn from them, but the essence of their strategy is retreat; an inglorious abdication from previous beliefs about the potential effectiveness of medical care, the potential value of medical science, the dignity and independence from the market of Medical Professionalism, and the feasibility of real social advance.

Our health services have developed not in an ideal, painless world of armchair social strategies, but in the real, bitter world of injustice consciously and deliberately maintained by real, powerful people who gain from things as they are, in which the distribution of wealth and power is never changed without struggle. Priority investment in social infrastructure, redistributive personal income policies, and higher priority for health service spending rather than preparation for war or reduction in personal income tax, are not rival alternatives. None of them will be pursued by a government which assumes that what is good for the Stock Exchange is good for the nation; all of them would be pursued by a government concerned with the health and happiness of all of the people.

On the other hand, realistic strategies for renewed advance must start from where we are, with the people we have. We cannot devise ideal solutions on a blank page, without regard to where we have come from, or where medical science is going. The content of potentially effective medical care has changed, both because of changes in public health, and because of advances in medical science, requiring big changes in the structure and staffing of care, most of all at primary care level.

We have to consider a set of historical choices, in a way that has not faced doctors since they first began to define their professionalism in the early 19th Century.[24] If we wish to continue the association of Medical Professionalism with Medical Science, we must prepare to accept solutions outside the limits of professionalism as then defined.

NOTES

1. Cochrane, A.L., *Effectiveness and efficiency*, London: Nuffield Provincial Hospitals Trust, 1971.

2. Powles, J., 'On the limitations of modern medicine', *Science, Medicine and Man 1973*; 1:1-30.
3. Fuchs, V.R., *Who shall live?*, New York: Basic Books, 1974.
4. Cochrane, A.L., '1931-1971: a critical review with particular reference to the medical profession'. In, *Medicines for the year 2000*, pp. 1-11. London: Office of Health Economics, 1979.
5. Illich, I., *Medical nemesis: limits to medicine*, London: Marion Boyars, 1976.
6. Illich, I., 'Body history', *Lancet 1986*; ii:1325-7.
7. Weatherall, D., 'Molecular and cell biology in clinical medicine: introduction', *British Medical Journal 1987*; 295:587-9.
8. Williams, A., 'Economics of coronary artery bypass grafting', *British Medical Journal 1985*; 291:326-9.
9. Goldman, L., Cook, E.F., 'The decline in ischemic heart disease mortality rates: an analysis of the comparative effects of medical interventions and changes in lifestyle', *Annals of Internal Medicine 1984*; 101:825-36.
10. Beaglehole, R., 'Medical management and the decline in mortality from coronary heart disease', *British Medical Journal 1986*; 292: 33-5.
11. Marmot, M.G., Shipley, M.J., Rose, G.A., 'Inequalities in death: specific explanations of a general pattern?', *Lancet 1984*; i:10003-6.
12. Forsdahl, A., 'Are poor living conditions in childhood and adolescence an important risk factor for arteriosclerotic heart disease?', *British Journal of Preventive & Social Medicine 1977*; 31:91-5.
13. Report of a Working Party. 'Stitches in time', Welsh Council, Royal College of General Practitioners, 1983.
14. Hart, J.T., 'The marriage of primary care and epidemiology', *Journal of the Royal College of Physicians of London 1974*; 8:299-314.
15. Iliffe, S., 'The painful path to health', *Marxism Today 1986*; 30:34-8.
16. Cartwright, A., Hockey, L., Anderson, J.L., *Life before death*, p. 79. London: Routledge & Kegan Paul, 1973.
17. Fox, A.J., Goldblatt, P.O., Jones, D.R., 'Social class mortality differentials: artefact, selection, or life circumstances?' In Wilkinson, R.G. (ed.), *Class and health: research and longitudinal data*, London: Tavistock Publications, 1986.
18. Nutbeam, D., Catford, J., 'Pulse of Wales: social survey supplement', *Heartbeat report no. 7*, Cardiff: Heartbeat Wales, 1987.
19. Department of Health & Social Security, *Inequalities in health: report of a research working group chaired by Sir Douglas Black*, London: DHSS, 1980.
20. Wilkinson, R.G. (ed.), *Class and health: research and longitudinal data*, London: Tavistock Publications, 1986.
21. Winter, J.M. Quoted in Wilkinson, R.G., ibid., p. 110.
22. Dahlgren, G., Diderichsen, F., 'Strategies for equity in health: report from Sweden', *International Journal of Health Services 1986*; 16:517-37.
23. Wilkinson, R.G., 'Income and mortality', p. 109 in Wilkinson,

R.G. (ed.), *Class and health: research and longitudinal data*,
London: Tavistock Publications, 1986.
24. Loudon, I.S.L., *Medical care and the general practitioner 1750*,
Oxford: Clarendon Press, 1986. Together with Rosemary Stevens'
book, this is the best detailed account of the rise of British medical
professionalism.

Chapter 3
ORIGINS AND LIMITS OF
MEDICAL PROFESSIONALISM

If positive answers to the defeatism of the Liberal Critique can only be found beyond the present limits of professionalism, we must look at what those limits are.

Traditionally, the main task of doctors has been to respond to the complaints of individual patients suffering from disease, or fear of disease. The profession has always contained a minority, Public Health Medical Officers, Medical Officers of Health, Community Physicians, who are supposed to conserve health in populations rather than restore it in sick individuals; but they are at the periphery, and have not been encouraged or sometimes even allowed to combine the functions of prevention and treatment. Doctors think of themselves as practical men who pretend no philosophy other than common sense, but their acceptance of this essentially passive social role does in practice amount to a philosophy. By responding to demands but not seeking needs, it has led to failure to apply the effective medical science we already have to a large part of the sick population, to say nothing of those who are well. The nature of medical science is now rapidly evolving in ways which will increase this gap between what could be done, and what actually is done, because it increasingly permits effective action at a presympomatic stage.

We saw in Chapter 1 how from 1922 to 1940 about 3,000 children a year continued to die from diphtheria although it was preventable by immunization, because the main thrust of medical effort was directed at individually presented symptoms; early diagnosis by throat swabs, treatment with antitoxin, admission to diphtheria wards of hospitals, and emergency tracheostomy. By a few heroic cures, the profession distracted its own and the public's attention from failure to prevent by simpler, less costly and far more effective means. At the same time it claimed immunization as an exclusively medical procedure. Not for the last time, doctors claimed territory they were unable or unwilling to occupy.

The Shopkeeping Inheritance

Like it or not, the working tradition from which present general practice stems was a local sick shop where the doctor, unconvincingly disguised as a scientific gentleman, remained a shopkeeper; but a shopkeeper paid increasingly by the state rather than customers. His generally miserable, threadbare surgery, a small shop in working-class districts, his front parlour in the genteel suburbs, far from inviting customers, seemed designed to deter all but the most determined seekers for prescriptions and certificates. Harassed and under-equipped, he alone was responsible for investment in a business which was simpler and more profitable to run if he gave it all of his time but none of his money.

All this was the polar opposite of the hard-selling, extravagantly procedural medicine of Continental Europe and the United States, where each consultation and every medical activity (except learning, teaching and listening) made the till ring. Clinical enterprise in Continental Europe and America generated fees: in the UK it generated costs, above all in time. This, as much as scientific caution, maintained our national tradition of valuable scepticism but complacent passivity, compared with the uncritical enthusiasm of the world medical market.

Origins of Modern Medical Professionalism

Modern British medical professionalism developed during the first half of the 19th Century, culminating in the Medical

Act of 1858. With difficulty, the Act brought together three hitherto almost entirely separate occupations: a few hundred physicians in London and Edinburgh, with gentlemanly status, a knowledge of latin and greek, but virtually no practical training; a few teaching-hospital surgeons; and several thousand provincial surgeons, apothecaries, and surgeon-apothecaries already calling themselves GPs, without gentlemanly status, but with practical training in surgical procedures and the dispensing of medicines.

Though an uncertain majority in all three groups eventually found a common interest in legislation for a single profession of medicine, this view was contested in the parliamentary committee which prepared the Act. It was suggested that a less qualified grade for everyday care of the poor, more or less equivalent to the feldsher grade in tsarist Russia, might be a cheaper and more realistic alternative. The British Medical Association (BMA) successfully resisted this proposal, using an important argument:

> Every attempt to create an inferior grade of medical men of limited education and with aptitude only for the ordinary exigencies of practice should be resisted. Disease affected people wherever they were, and so the same degree of medical skill should be available for everyone.[1]

The British medical profession therefore owed its birth to an egalitarian social argument. This theme has recurred time and again since, despite the obvious fact that it denies the validity of a medical market, with some consuming more and others less medical care than they need. Both ideas, medical care as a human right and medical care as a marketed commodity, have persisted ever since, in uneasy alliance or open conflict, and neither has ever had complete ascendancy. Even the fee-earning private market had to adopt a sliding scale related to supposed income (traditionally based on rent or estimated house value), ostensibly from compassion, more realistically because poor people would not and could not pay large fees, and most people were poor. Medical care was therefore never simply sold as a commodity with a market price, and few British doctors were ever comfortable with the

concept of medical trade. On the other hand, medical care
was not supplied as an equal service by right until 1948,
because to defend its income the profession had to maintain
a difference between the quality of care received as a state-
assisted charity, and what could be bought privately on the
fees market, and no government was willing to meet the cost
of an optimal public service.

Association with Gentry and Science

The currently accepted model of what a good doctor is
became fully developed around the start of the 20th Century,
when medicine began to make serious claims to association
with science. It is most easily dated from 1910, when implementation in the United States of the Flexner Report on
medical education, drawing on British, German and French
experience, elaborated an international professional model
which essentially persists today.

Almost simultaneously, doctors acquired status as gentlemen. Until the close of the 19th Century the social standing
of the medical profession as a whole was precarious. For
example, Queen Victoria could not bring herself to present
personally a Victoria Cross to Surgeon-Major Reynolds after
the battle of Rorke's Drift.[2] Army surgeons were eventually
allowed to win the VC, but were then excluded from a royal
ball for VCs at the palace in 1859, and were not officially
accepted as guests until 1891. Florence Nightingale
campaigned on behalf of the doctors for gentlemanly status,
writing in 1864 that

> . . . we are exacting duties from the medical officer such as sanitary
> recommendations to his commanding officer which especially
> require him to have the standing of a gentleman. . . we are doing
> such things as dismounting him on parade, depriving him of presiding
> at boards, etc, which in military life, to a degree we have no idea of
> in civil life, deprive him of the weight of a gentleman amongst
> gentlemen.

Much of the professionalization of medicine was a search
for higher social status, by identifying the general run of

doctors with the wealthy minority of physicians and surgeons serving the aristocracy and dominating the teaching hospitals. Perhaps because this gentlemanly status was reached so late and with such difficulty, its outward appearance was important for doctors at all levels. A patient in Hackney in the East End of London recalls the appearance of GPs in the slums on the eve of the First World War:[3]

> They all had the same routine: the silk hat, walking cane, white gloves and a Gladstone bag in which they had their stethoscope and other items. The usual formula when my father was ill was that the doctor would be shown into the parlour, the best room of the house, and the first thing he would do would be to take one glove off, then the other glove off, put them both on the table, then put the walking stick on the table, then the top hat and then go upstairs and see the patient.

Flexner added enormous power to this upward movement in social rank. He defined the doctor as a science-based, autonomous professional, relating to society through intimate, individual contacts, whose principal task was the relief of sickness as it came to his door. His unpaid care of the poor gave him access to fees for care of the rich. Either way, doctors derived their authority from associations with science and with gentlemen.

Sir William Osler[4] was the most influential example of, and advocate for, this professional model. His advice to students at Yale in 1913[5] typifies the vigorous, productive, but socially conformist spirit of the times:

> The way of life that I preach is a habit to be acquired gradually by long and steady repetition. It is the practice of living for the day only, and for the day's work, life in day-tight compartments. . . Shut out the yesterdays, which have lighted fools the way to dusty death, and have no concern for you personally, that is, consciously. They are there alright, working daily in us, but so are our livers and our stomachs. And the past in its unconscious action on our lives, should bother us as little as they do. . . Shut off the future as tightly as the past. . . The future is today—there is no tomorrow! The day of a man's salvation is now—the life of the present, of today, lived earnestly, intently, without a forward-looking thought, is the only

insurance for the future. Let the limit of your horizon be a twenty-four-hour circle.

The new doctors needed no understanding of the anatomy or physiology of society, nor of the social history of medicine, for these might divert them from acquisition of the apparently limitless facts of medical science, and were in any case useless, since society was shaped not by man but by God, who manifested Himself, then as now, chiefly by shifts in the market.

This is a travesty of what Osler actually said and wrote; he was a giant figure, of unquestionable greatness, who posed many of the fundamental questions which still face us today, and which undermine the position he himself established.[6] But it is an accurate description of what his contemporaries and subsequent hagiographers actually heard, and Osler, an actor if ever there was one and very sensitive to audience response, knew well enough what he was doing. His aim was to educate doctors to clinical inquisitiveness, a passionate belief in the application of science to the solution of diagnostic puzzles. It is easy for those who already possess this skill to dismiss its importance and effectiveness, but experience of working with doctors who have never acquired it (they do exist) would soon bring such theorists back to earth. Osler's concept of clinical medicine, bringing bedside practice into association with laboratory science, was a huge and necessary advance, but it was obtained at very heavy cost. It was essentially a pursuit of personal excellence, based on the assumption that excellence was not and never could be a universal objective. It must be borne in mind that all Osler's work, and the entire conception of the scientistic medical gentleman, was developed within the walls of voluntary teaching hospitals, the social atmosphere of which are conveyed by the prayer recited by patients at Guy's Hospital:[7]

Bless all the worthy governors of this hospital; excite in our hearts a grateful sense of their charitable care for our welfare, and grant that they may plentifully reap the reward of their labour and love, both in this life, and that which is to come.

Just as it was necessary for doctors to pursue medical knowledge in blinkered isolation from its social context, the good doctor was supposed to fix his gaze only on the patient in hand, in 'patient-tight compartments', forgetting the other 30 in the waiting room or the thousands outside, to reach clinical perfection for a few rather than what was possible and useful for the many. The only way to get on with good clinical medicine was to exclude all demands other than those of the case in hand and give that case total priority. This model of care, impossible in the real circumstances of practice serving unselected whole populations, was and still is taught in teaching hospitals.

The way doctors and their public still like to think of themselves is shown in Luke Fildes' famous picture (Fig. 3.1) exhibited at the Royal Academy in 1891, of which over a million reproductions were sold.

The doctor sits in a labourer's cottage, beside a child with pneumonia, watched by the parents. He stares pensively at the child, willing him to survive. A bottle of medicine stands on the table, but hope centres on the presence of the doctor. He is a man of dignity and education, not too grand to be accessible to the deserving poor, but wise beyond their understanding. In fact, he was unable to influence the course of illness (the painting was prompted by Fildes' experience of the death of his own child) but he had the moral qualities which both doctors and patients wanted and would later need, when medical science had developed effective weapons. The moral authority of Fildes' picture was incorporated into Osler's new scientistic practice, and despite huge technical advances, the whole of current hospital practice could still be fitted into it.

There are two kinds of truth in this sentimental and idealized picture. First, the doctors of the time really did sit through the night with cases of pneumonia, in which fever really did rise to a crisis resolved either by death (in about 20% of cases) or rapid but incomplete recovery, followed by a convalescence prolonged over weeks or months. Doctors worked incredibly hard, at the cost of their own health, to maintain the illusions they were paid to provide, partly

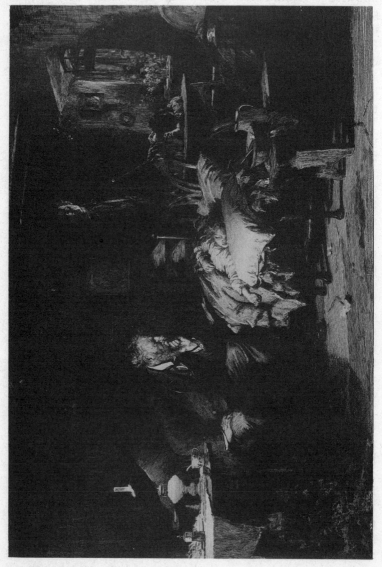

Fig 3.1   Sir Luke Fildes 'The doctor'. Tate Gallery, London.

because there was ruthless competition and most doctors lived close to poverty, but also because their experience taught them that hope was usually the only weapon they had, and compassion expressed as work was the only way to deliver it.

Secondly, it shows management of acute illness rather than conservation of health as the heart of medical practice. Both doctor and parents knew that good food, a dry, warm house and education in the elementary requirements of healthy living, could reduce susceptibility to pneumonia and make survival of an attack more likely. They needed no brilliant insights from academics to perceive this, but both patient and doctor were by circumstances compelled to ignore this knowledge they already possessed, and to put their faith in futile attempts to defy consequences rather than attend to causes. Up to the end of the 19th Century, doctors were as socially necessary, but as biologically ineffective, as parsons or undertakers. They helped people to tolerate an intolerably sad world by sustaining hope and by proving that everything had been done that could be done. When the form and content of our professionalism were defined, medical practice was a world of illusion and the doctor's function was more social than biological. Science was beginning to have some positive impact on diagnosis, but almost none on treatment and the outcome of illness. Though medicine was still almost entirely ineffective, its association with science already made it more credible than religion, both to patients and their families, and to governments requiring legitimation of their rule. GPs were beginning to replace parsons and priests as the most important local representatives of established authority.

The Science of Certainty, and the Science of Doubt

Science was not, and to a large extent still is not, the basis for everyday medical care. For the first time in history, popular experience of science in the 19th Century gave the medical profession a credibility based on more than desperate wishful thinking. It was an experience of railways, dynamite, steam engines and electric light, machines of calculated and predictable performance. In the popular mind, the characteristics of science were exactness, certainty, the elimination of doubt.

That was how science appeared, and for small, everyday science the appearance was true; the most certain of all faiths, and a continuous creator and reinforcer of common sense. But big science, the science of great leaps forward in understanding of nature, was completely opposite to this understanding; it was based on measured doubt, on rejection of all permanence, on acceptance that scientific experiment never leaves anything as it first appeared and that none of its conclusions are ever complete or permanent. Medicine adopted the outward style and authority of science, and used some interesting bits of machinery based on scientific understanding, but this did not make doctors into scientists, any more than driving a car makes a man an engineer. This is the difference between the scientific, and the scientistic.

This misrepresentation of medical science as the solid, simple, Newtonian certainty of engineering, rather than the fluid, complex, Einsteinian doubt of biology, has misled not only the public, but the profession itself. Less in Britain than elsewhere, but still too often, advances in medical technique have been sold as machinery, too complex to be explicable and therefore accepted by most people in the same way that they accept television, as a kind of magic. On the buoyant market of the post-war Welfare consensus, this seemed to suit all interests. Patients were encouraged to believe that given sufficient fees or taxes, every kind of organ damage could sooner or later be salvaged by some feat of medical or surgical engineering. Hospital departments responsible for fulfilling this impossible promise, but desperate for resources, had every incentive to endorse it, at least as a goal for the future. The illusion was bound to crash, not because medicine contained too much hard science and too little compassionate art, but because the engineering model was incomplete, alienating and ultimately unscientific from the start.

Ever since Galileo,[8] science has suffered from the compromise he and all his descendants were forced to make, to secure the patronage on which their work depends. Obliged to guarantee its servility to the men who paid, science isolated itself from common people, treating them as passive, uncomprehending objects rather than participating, intelligent subjects. Medical science was no exception. All the best medical scientists have recognized that effective human biology must accept and use the intelligence of its subjects, but very few of them have felt strong enough to challenge professional and service structures which deny that intelligence. There have been many reasons for this, but not the least of them was that at the time when medical professionalism acquired its modern science-associated form little could be done to change the outcome of any illness, with science or without it. For another 30 years, medical science would remain almost entirely a matter of observation and forecast rather than useful intervention. The entire culture of medicine was built around the need to maximize professional authority (of doctors, but not of anyone else offering help) and lay credulity, as vehicles for hope, faith and the placebo effect.

The Placebo Effect

The effects of suggestion, reinforced by faith and hope, are transiently substantial in virtually all diseases; simply seeing an apparently competent professional and swallowing his pills will have a measurable positive effect in about one-third of all subjects, a remarkably constant proportion in nearly all scientifically controlled trials. Blackwell[9] reported a class experiment on medical students which should be a standard part of the curriculum. The students were given inert blue or pink capsules and told that these would have either a sedative or stimulant effect. The class was asked to divide into pairs to measure pulse rate, breathing rate, and record the subjective feelings of each student over the next 30 minutes. A doctor was available for anyone who felt seriously distressed by any side effects of either the blue or the pink capsules. Of 56 students in the trial, only 3 reported no change in their feelings; 30 felt drowsy, 21 felt more relaxed, 5 felt more cheerful and talkative, with mainly sedative effects on those who had been given blue capsules and elating effects on those who had been given pink capsules, and effects were greater in those who took two capsules than in those who took one. Side effects, mainly headache, were reported by 18, and two felt so ill that they had to consult the doctor. Pulse rates slowed in 37 students and speeded up in 8, and blood pressure fell in 40 and rose in 10.

The placebo effect of surgery is just as great as of medication. Cobb[10] and Dimond[11] showed that about one-third of patients reported substantially less anginal pain after both real and sham operations for internal mammary artery grafts to the heart muscle (a once fashionable but now wholly discredited operation). Apart from a few surgical and obstetric procedures, the placebo effect was almost the only weapon we had in Osler's day. An elderly GP in Port Talbot, Donald Isaac, looking back on his experience as a medical student at University College Hospital in the early 1930s, before sulphonamides, recalled the contrast between the hopeful activity of surgical wards and the informed but hopeless contemplation of medical wards. 'How we loved the surgical wards; most of the patients recovered, at least for long enough to go home and for both them and us to imagine that their disease was cured. And how we hated the medical wards; they all had interesting diseases, and they all died. In those days surgery was everything that really mattered in medicine.' And it was for this reason that when the GP surgeons were finally expelled from the hospitals after 1948, it seemed to them to be the end of good general practice.

The Art and scientistic Pseudoscience of Medicine continued to build on the credulity of both doctors and patients, while Science built on measured doubt, but within the laboratory and the hospital, where it was safe to recognize the experimental nature of all medical treatment. Medical science today has not failed; it has simply never been fully or consistently applied to any whole population, because its attitudes and machinery remained confined to hospitals, which cannot and do not see all of the people.

Doctors and the State

The scientistic content of doctoring was exaggerated, because this reinforced the Osler model of Medical Professionalism. The social content of doctoring was ignored, minimized, or sentimentalized into charity for the sick poor because it could not be fitted comfortably in this model. It excluded the possibility that doctors might at that time have been able to achieve more in the struggle against disease as social workers than as clinicians. Within a year or two of his birth, Osler's scientific gentleman was offered just such an opportunity.

Through the Insurance Act of 1911, Lloyd George enabled doctors for the first time to prescribe money as well as drugs to manual workers during acute illness, thus ensuring that they and their families could eat, would not be evicted for non-payment of rent, and would not be driven into pauperism. Lloyd George understood, and sought to break, the cycle through which poverty caused disease and disease caused poverty. The Act offered GPs power to intervene effectively in the course of acute illness in the labouring poor, and also increased and stabilized their incomes, but the profession bitterly opposed it. The same hostility exploded in 1948, when the National Health Service Act again threatened to give doctors more scope for effective intervention by making all treatment free at the time of use, and again threatened to increase and stabilize GPs' incomes by including the whole population. Both in 1912 and in 1948, GPs soon capitulated and joined the service, but with their tails between their legs, in a mood of defeat where they should have been elated by victory. Neither the Lloyd George Act nor the NHS Act were recognized by most doctors at the time as expansions of their power to treat illness effectively, or as improved security for GPs serving populations previously outside the fees-market. The orthodox contemporary medical view was that both Acts were setbacks for good clinical medicine and ideological defeats for the profession.

Both in 1912 and in 1948, opposition was based on the social assumptions of the Osler model of practice. Writing to *The Times* on the eve of the Insurance Act, Sir Clifford Allbutt[12] accused Lloyd George of having

> an antiquated notion of medicine and of medical service; he took for granted without inquiry a notion built of some vague knowledge of village clubs, and of the old-fashioned *vade mecum* way of doctoring. This is, 'for such and such a disease, such and such a drug; take the mixture, drink it regularly, and get well if nature will let you. . .'
>
> Now younger men who are passing from the universities in these years are entering upon medicine as into a new calling, with new ideas and with changed views of their portion in it. . . they are missionaries, carrying with them these new ideas of medicine, and developing new modes of practice. With these men, if not discouraged, lies the future of medicine in its popular sense; and they have chosen medicine as a calling chiefly because of its new scientific values, and of its enormously increasing power over disease. Thus the hereditary maxims and craft rules of the elder medicine, maxims and rules which made current practice easy and comparatively irresponsible, are dissolving into wider conceptions and a larger scope of work which demand a far more arduous and far more responsible service. . .

Allbutt's summary description of the ordinary GP's work has a contemporary ring. So has his description of the new frontiers opening up to young men eager to use the new technologies of the time:

> The modern physician—for such is the modern practitioner, to whatever side of his profession he be given—perceives that the treatment of disease. . . is first and last a matter of searching diagnosis; and every day diagnosis is opening out as a more and more abstruse and costly affair. . . The man who leaves us for practice is schooled in all these methods; he can examine the blood, counting and comparing its corpuscles; he can perform the ordinary bacterial examinations; he can estimate the chemical values of secretions and excretions; he is skilled in the use of instruments of precision, of blood pressure gauges, endoscopes for the eye, the larynx and other internal parts. . .

Allbutt goes on to discuss in concrete terms the newly-discovered Wasserman test, permitting accurate diagnosis of syphilis (then a common and dangerous disease), and verification of successful treatment by Salvarsan, the first effective antibiotic available to medicine, the 'silver bullet' recently developed by Ehrlich:

> A working man, of about the age of 40, complains of hoarseness: nowadays he is not sent off with marshmallow and tolu, his larynx is examined; one vocal chord is seen to be palsied; and thus an aneurysm in the chest is betrayed. A specific cause for this is suspected; and a so-called Wassermann test is applied; upon the response to this test depends at least six months of continuous and active medication, and at least two years more of occasional vigilance. Now, to perform the Wassermann test takes at least four hours of continuous attention; most general practitioners will no doubt have it done for them by an expert, but will all this be done under a contract at a low rate of pay? The test alone, for skill, time, apparatus, &c, cannot be put at less than 20 shillings. Are we to say that these proceedings are to be denied to the poor country-man who is able to do some work and cannot spend all his time in a hospital?
>
> Now if we are to say that the general practitioner is to be but a stop-gap and that every malady of importance is to be sent to some central institution, is not this to take the heart out of our very efficient students, and to degrade the career of medicine? Gloss it as we may, contract practice will stand lower in public esteem, and will be of lower average efficiency and much less humane; it will damp the aspirations and blot the high-minded ideals with which I, who know, say that the young physicians of today are entering our profession; and it will push them back to old-fashioned routine and to ill-remunerated and therefore undervalued service. . . It must be admitted that, where clubs made the bulk of a practice, it was very perfunctory work, and fell into the hands of perfunctory men; but where a club formed no great bulk of a practice the work has been done better, often admirably, because it has been regarded as hospital work has been regarded by consultants, and been done for love of the profession, for good fellowship and humanity, and, it is fair to add, for some advantage of status and experience; but not for pecuniary profit. But even then such a medical man of a club usually makes his members understand that he does not undertake to give them more than ordinary attention. . . The solution is no contract, but payment for work done on a standard tariff.

The Realities of Working-Class Practice

Allbutt was an exceptionally gifted, publicly responsible, and socially perceptive professional man, who towered above his contemporaries. He was either ignorant of, or considered irrelevant to his argument, the real conditions of practice for GPs serving the mass of the population. Many people simply had no care at all; 5% of non-accidental deaths in England and Wales, 30% in Scotland, were medically unattended.[13]

The conditions of care for the working class had been exposed by Britain's oldest medical journal, the *Lancet*, in a classic of medical journalism, 'The Battle of the Clubs'.[14] The *Lancet* sent a medical correspondent around coal-mining, industrial and maritime communities to investigate the terms and conditions of service of GPs serving the clubs, Medical Aid Societies and Boards of Guardians of the Poor Law, the only sources of primary care for the labouring population. Rates of pay for GPs were generally around 9 pence a month for care of each man earning £1 a week or more, 8 pence a month for men earning over 15 shillings, and 7 pence a month for men earning less than 15 shillings a week. Women were cared for at a cost of 4 pence a month and children for 3 pence a month. These were flat rates, unrelated to the actual number of consultations, and included the cost of medicines. In Southampton a quarter of the population was attended under club schemes at an annual cost of 4 shillings a head, and 2,000 indigent poor were attended on behalf of the Board of Guardians at an annual fee of £5. In 1893 these 2,000 people had 500 visits from the doctor, so the pay averaged 2.5 pence for each visit. The situation in Portsmouth was worse. There the Dockyard Medical Benefit Society obtained primary medical care and medicines for its members at a weekly cost of 0.5 pence a head. One GP went through his books to show he had made 1,958 visits and 4,650 surgery consultations for a total income of £38, 11 shillings and 11 pence; 1.4 pence per consultation.

These earnings covered the ordinary, superficial symptomatic or placebo care of minor injuries, chronic disease and terminal illness in the home. Doctors were not called to an uncomplicated birth. For the difficult births they attended, the Portsmouth doctors had charged £1, 'but some six years ago the Society resolved to reduce them to 15 shillings'. The obstetric fee for miners' wives in Nottingham was 10 shillings and 6 pence. Standard fees of the Bexhill Provident Medical

Association were £5 for amputation of a leg, treatment of a compound fracture of the thigh, or of a strangulated hernia; £3 for a simple fracture of the thigh; and £1 for a fractured clavicle or a dislocated shoulder.

Though doctors did the best they could to get better terms, they were realistic in their expectations; they knew there were not enough rich people to support all the GPs in search of a living and opportunities to practice the kind of medicine they had been taught in hospitals. The *Lancet* correspondent reported the general opinion:

> . . . it is better that the miners should belong to clubs, otherwise their medical attendant will get no pay at all. A penny, twopence, and even sixpence a week can be obtained without difficulty, but shilling fees or 18-penny fees with medicine included are never paid.

The GPs in York believed the formation of clubs had been brought about by the greed of their colleagues, and gave the example of a medical bill of £15 presented to a servant girl

> whose annual wage barely amounted to that sum. Then a bill of perhaps £30 would be presented to the head of a family whose income might not exceed £200.

What Lloyd George did in his Act was to nationalize the only machinery for popular care that actually existed, the same clubs, Medical Aid and Provident Societies whose squalor had been exposed by the *Lancet*. To Allbutt and the other teaching hospital consultants it looked like the end of the world. Threadbare GPs, fearful of losing their only apparent means of escape to financial security and clinical self-respect through fee-earning practice and clinging to the Osler method of practice they had learned in their medical schools, allowed themselves to be led by gentry against a government with more understanding of social realities than they had themselves.

Allbutt saw good clinical standards and effective medical care as inextricably bound with fee-earning autonomy. This was a reality only to the small minority of successful doctors in the carriage trade. They viewed medicine from above, from teaching hospital consultancy, and from GPs who had done well in the best residential areas and wealthiest market towns. They saw that rich doctors with rich patients had the training, staff, equipment and above all the time to work within the Osler model, to take trouble with their patients. Poor doctors with poor patients were by circumstance forced to accept conveyor-belt methods that violated both medical science and the better customs of teaching hospital medicine. Their natural strategy for progress was a downward spread of fee-earning practice throughout the population, gradually displacing the ugly reality of working-class practice, the good doctors of the rich gradually displacing the bad doctors of the poor. How could they be anything but hostile to demagogues who proposed to build a service for the whole nation on the cheap and nasty systems of care endured by the poor?

For the poor doctors of poor people, there never was any question of counting corpuscles, performing bacteriological examinations, estimating chemical values of secretions, or of skill in the use of instruments of precision. In his preface to *The Doctor's Dilemma*, George Bernard Shaw[15] described the effect of the squalid conditions of work endured by the contract GP and his patients in 1911:

> The only way he can preserve his self-respect is by forgetting all he ever learnt of science, and clinging to such help as he can give without cost merely by being less ignorant and more accustomed to sick-beds than his patients. Finally he acquires a certain skill at nursing cases under poverty-stricken domestic conditions, just as women who have been trained as domestic servants in some huge institution with lifts, vacuum cleaners, electric lighting, steam heating, and machinery that turns the kitchen into a laboratory and engine-house combined, manage, when they are sent out into the world to drudge as general servants, to pick up their business in a new way, learning the slatternly habits and wretched makeshifts of homes where even bundles of kindling wood are luxuries to be anxiously economised.

Shaw did not exaggerate. A Glasgow slum GP observed in 1916 dealt with more than 70 patients in three hours; at the end, patients were being seen three at a time.[13] An Essex GP writing to the *British Medical Journal* in 1950 recalled how when working as a locum in a South Wales mining practice he saw about 100 patients in the morning surgery, did 70 home visits, and saw abother 100 patients in the evening surgery.[16] Acting as a locum in Ferndale, Rhondda, in 1960, I saw about 60 patients in the morning session, another 60 in the evening, and visited 25 patients at home. Most doctors qualifying before 1960 who have worked in industrial areas have had similar experiences. GPs sunk to this state had no independent ideology. They valued the Osler model not as a relevant frame for their own work, but as another world to which they, or more likely their sons, might one day escape. Publicly financed care at a civilized standard for the mass of the people was not a credible alternative, and was not on offer from any of the big political parties. Their few private patients appeared to be the only hope of a secure future and of opportunity to practise good clinical medicine. They could be roused to the defence of Harley Street, because though not their own, it seemed more relevant to their preferred image of themselves, and more politically credible than a good service planned for all of the people.

Social Function of Doctors Under the Lloyd George Act

The teaching hospital consultants who led the BMA in 1912 were unrealistic about the clinical functions of GPs serving the common people, and the GPs knew it; never in this life were they going to perform Wassermann tests or count corpuscles. What really ensured their hostility to the Lloyd George proposals was that any future extension of their meagre clinical functions would, as Allbutt's letter showed, be concentrated in hospitals, which would eventually be monopolized by specialists; and their remaining skills would be subordinated to their social function as gatekeepers to insurance benefit, and eventually wither away.

These fears were justified. Lloyd George was shrewd, he understood the limited scope of effective medicine at that time. Access to primary medical care, if it had any importance at all, mattered only as evidence that the State was not completely indifferent to the fate of its citizens, but government was not at that time under much pressure to improve access to the different bottles of mixture which passed for treatment. What both he and the public did understand was the importance of having money to pay the rent, buy some food, and keep off the creditors when the family wage-earner was ill. The principal function of GPs under the Act, and the only reason they were included in it, was to adjudicate fitness for work, and thus prescribe access to cash benefits.

GPs regarded certification and legitimation of the sick role as tasks unfitted to their training, unconnected with the good Oslerian doctor who could diagnose and sometimes predict the course of illness, even if he rarely changed it. But it also put them in a different relationship with the patient. When they were working for the club or local Mutual Aid Society, there was local social pressure on claimants not to abuse the system; the GP could be reasonably sure of support from the local community if he refused benefit, though even then it was an unpleasant thing to do. Once the State took over the small local clubs and societies, much of this support disappeared, and the doctor was left on his own as Lloyd George's policeman.

If medical training had been truly scientific, relating medical care to measurable outcomes in reduced mortality, disability and unhappiness in the population as a whole, what appeared only as a defeat could have been interpreted positively. Creation of a national system of welfare benefits for working men with acute illness was a huge step forward, which by reducing pauperism not only for the worker but also for his dependents, certainly had bigger effects on health than any of the clinical advances of that time. No such conclusion was possible within the Osler model; medical training was not geared towards improvement of health or continuing care of disease in the whole population, but to the creation of a force of men with episodic or crisis-oriented skills for salvage of serious disease, increasingly concentrated in specialist hands in hospitals. Palliation of otherwise untreatable pain and misery, and treatment of minor or self-limiting acute illness, were left to custodial hospitals outside the teaching hospital system, a few wards in workhouses, and above all to care by their own families in their own homes, supported by GPs. GPs with clinical ambition were expected to combine general practice with hospital specialism, or to escape from general practice altogether. The GP with scientific pretensions was recognizable by the degree to which his practice in the community resembled that of a specialist in hospital.

This entire package was flatly contradicted in every aspect by the Lloyd George proposals. Instead of basing state support for general practice on clinically respectable private fee-earning practice for the middle class, it based it on the clubs and Medical Aid Societies of poor working men. Instead of basing it on fees for each item of service, it based it on flat rate capitation, encouraging GPs to take on as many patients as they could get, and then do as little as possible for them. Instead of helping GPs to secure a foothold in hospitals, it thrust them irretrievably into the drudgery of certification, repeat prescribing, and industrialized mass production of token care.

Resistance to the Lloyd George Act

Led by the consultants, the BMA held enthusiastic mass meetings of GPs all over the country, everywhere obtaining almost unanimous support for a boycott of the Lloyd George Act by refusal to register for panel patients (as State Insurance patients came to be known). The situation was vividly described by John Wigg,[17] describing his father's experience as a GP in Camden Town:

> 1911 was a year to remember. My father knew that if he did not accept panel patients he would be ruined. If he did so, he would arouse the violent antagonism of those powerful doctors who cared for the wealthier half of the community. . . The division in the medical profession in those days was almost complete. The hostility between the two parties was intense.

The Act passed its first and second readings in the House of Commons unanimously, and was clearly the will of the country. Better than the doctors, Lloyd George understood the divided nature of the profession. 'A deputation of doctors', he said, 'is always a deputation of swell doctors: it is impossible to get a deputation of poor doctors or of slum doctors.'[18] Having no wish to strengthen local lay control of general practice, which might make much bigger demands on central finance, he had accepted nearly all the demands of the BMA to strengthen the role of GPs and weaken that of the local clubs and societies in administering the Act, and it was already clear that most GPs would financially be much better off than they were before. The BMA secretary, Smith Whitaker, bowed to the inevitable and accepted a seat on the National Insurance Committee to help in administering the Act, supported by a vote of 38 to 3 on BMA Council.

By this time, however, gut-felt hysteria had triumphed over intelligence. Sir James Barr, president of the BMA, announced that health insurance 'would impair the independence, increase the sickness, and hasten the degeneracy of a spoonfed race'. Dr Fred Smith, a consultant at the London Hospital Medical College, wrote a letter to *The Times* denouncing 'the Great Betrayal'. At a mass meeting at Queen's Hall at which Sir Victor Horsley, past chairman of the BMA, was shouted down as a traitor, and with encouragement from Lord Rothermere's *Daily Mail*, GPs reached a new pitch of hysteria. A special representative meeting of the BMA was called which confirmed a policy of total intransigence, and another meeting in December 1912, three weeks before the Act was due to come into operation, voted more than four to one to boycott the panel.

Even as this meeting took place, the BMA secretary had in his possession scores of letters and telegrams from local BMA secretaries showing that a majority of GPs had already joined the panel, though almost all of them had signed pledges that they would never do so. He informed the meeting of this, but led by a Manchester consultant, delegates refused to listen and reaffirmed their stand.[18]

A month later 15,000 GPs had signed contracts with

Insurance Committees and the lists were almost complete. For the BMA, it was a self-inflicted rout. By the early 1920s there was not only overwhelming support by GPs for the Act, but much concern to retain it.

The NHS Act and the Rout of 1948

The leaders of the BMA were not fools, either in 1911–12 or 1946–48. In the run-up to 1948, they knew their own history and feared its repetition. In the 1930s, despite the conservative outlook of the profession, the BMA made difficulties for socially brutal government policies by drawing public attention to the effects on child health of mass unemployment and malnutrition, by proposing extension of free primary care to the dependents of manual workers, and by encouraging discussions on post-war health services in the BMA's wartime Medical Planning Commission, which even included representatives of the Socialist Medical Association. The Commission's interim report (no final report ever appeared) condemned 'the continuance of traditional individualism into an age where division of labour and co-operation are essential factors in social service', admitted that 'the principle of the organisation of general practice on a group or co-operative basis is widely approved', and went on to recommend extension of health insurance cover to 90% of the population, leaving only 10% for traditional fee-earning practice.

From 1940 to the Labour landslide election of 1945, there was a huge swing of public opinion against pre-war Conservative policies of *laissez-faire* economics and appeasement of Fascism. Tasks of social planning and organization which were supposed to be impossible in peacetime suddenly became possible after 1940, when society was mobilized seriously for war; not just any war, but war against Fascism, which was at that time clearly perceived as the creature of big business and the darling of aristocracy. The experience of successful state planning, and the critical role of the USSR in the ground war against Hitler when defeat seemed all too probable, created a durable mass electoral base in favour of collective and egalitarian social policies.

The springboard for this movement in opinion was the Beveridge Report[19-23] on post-war social services, published in December 1942. This had been commissioned by Arthur Greenwood, a veteran Labour minister in Churchill's coalition government. It outlined a grand design for a comprehensive Welfare State which would abolish pauperism, and include medical care at all levels as a human right. A quarter of a million copies of the original version of this dry civil service document were sold within a few weeks, and then another 350,000 of an abridged version. In a public opinion poll two weeks after publication, 19 out of every 20 adults were familiar with its contents;[21] no government publication before or since has ever had such a mass appeal. The BBC broadcast its provisions to Nazi-occupied Europe in 22 languages, and it quickly became the most important positive part of Britain's war aims.

Only a month after its publication, Churchill secretly informed the cabinet that he had no intention of implementing the report until after the war, and even then would make no firm promises; his Labour coalition partners fell in with this. He intended the report to have the same propaganda function in the Second World War as Lloyd George's empty promise of 'homes fit for heroes' in the first. When first debated in parliament in February 1943, the government's obvious reluctance to commit itself resulted in a rebellion by Labour back benchers led by Aneurin Bevan; 97 Labour MPs defied their party whip to vote for a motion of censure. Finally beginning to understand the grip which the Beveridge Report now had on public opinion, Churchill broadcast a speech giving it his general, though still very unspecific, endorsement.

At the height of this shift in opinion in 1944, even the BMA came under its influence. Its leaders were concerned to develop informed liberal opinion in the profession and thus avoid a repetition of the humiliating events of 1912 in future negotiations with government, which they well understood were bound to come after the war. There was evidence that many younger doctors had begun to accept that post-war general practice would and should be organized nationally as a social service.

The BMA sought the views of its members in 1944 on the wartime coalition government's White Paper on post-war health services, which proposed group practice from health centres, a mixture of salaried and private general practice, and measures to ensure a more equal distribution of GPs across the country.[23] Despite the difficulties of balloting doctors in the armed forces, which favoured higher returns from established elderly doctors, 69% of all votes, 79% of service votes, were in favour of a free hospital and consultant service available to the whole population; 60% of all votes, 73% of service votes, were in favour of a free, comprehensive GP service available to the whole population; 57% of all votes, 68% of service votes, were in favour of controlled distribution of GPs; 68% of all votes, 83% of service votes, were in favour of general practice from health centres; and 62% of all votes, 74% of service votes, were in favour of salaried service from health centres.[22] For any post-war government intending to create a National Health Service on radically new lines, there was a clear mandate from the profession.

Only four years later, all this was lost. What in fact occurred was an almost exact repetition of the events of 1911–12. The BMA leaders, Charles Hill and Guy Dain, retreated from the position they took in 1944, and mobilized the membership against the alleged threat of a socialized service to clinical standards. At the BMA annual representative meeting in May 1946, Dr Dain described Aneurin Bevan, the Labour Minister of Health, as a dictator, and Dr Alfred Cox, secretary of the BMA in 1913, claimed the NHS was 'the first step, and a big one, towards National Socialism as practised in Germany'. Delegates voted against nationalization of hospitals by 210 to 29, against controlled distribution of GPs by 214 to 2, and against abolition of buying and selling of practices by 229 to 13. One delegate predicted that the status of GPs under the NHS would be that of West Indian slaves.[24]

Opportunities for Specialists, Drudgery for GPs

There was an important difference from 1911-12; this time, opposition was led by the GPs, not the consultants. Bevan made investment in nationalized hospitals the central feature of his plans for the NHS. He conceded a great deal of power to the consultants, guaranteed their wealth (confessing to Brian Abel-Smith that he 'choked their mouths with gold'), but above all he offered them means to expand and improve their clinical work. Behind the backs of the BMA leaders, President of the Royal College of Physicians Lord Moran ('Corkscrew Charlie') made a deal. He and the Presidents of the other Royal Colleges, the Surgeons and the Obstetricians (the College of General Practitioners was born later, as one consequence of the NHS Act) appealed publicly for reasoned negotiations, and the President of the Society of Medical Officers of Health described the Act as 'the greatest thing that had ever been done in social medicine in any age or country'.

The Spens Report,[24] which showed average net GP income on the eve of the war as £938 a year, proposed a 13% increase in net earnings after adjustment for fall in the value of the pound, and this was fully accepted by the minister: GPs now had a guarantee that, as in 1912, they would be better off after the Act. Finally, parliament had already passed the Act by 261 votes to 113. These concessions and political facts of life had no more effect in 1948 than in 1911-12. To strengthen their hand in negotiation, the BMA leaders had already set the hounds in full cry, and though opportunities for negotiation were obvious, they were unable to call them back without being bitten themselves. Egged on by *The Daily Mail* and *Daily Express*, both of which ran smear campaigns on plans for the NHS, the BMA maintained its stand against any negotiation with the Minister, with furious denunciations of the treachery of the Royal Colleges. The *British Medical Journal* published a lecture by Dr Reginald Payne to the Royal College of Surgeons in which he asserted

> no patient or doctor will ever feel safe from interference by some ministerial edict or regulation, and no independent institution

connected with medicine will feel safe from interference, expropriation, or dissolution. The Minister's spies will be everywhere and suspicion and intrigue will rule.[24]

Though there was no evidence that the government wanted a salaried GP service, which would have been more costly than leaving GPs to pay for their own generally frugal premises, staff and equipment, Charles Hill told a mass meeting of GPs not the truth, but what they wanted to hear:

The events of recent months have made it absolutely clear that these proposals mean and are intended to mean a whole-time salaried service under the State. . . It is now or never for the profession to which we belong.

Calling for a boycott of the service as in 1912, Dr Guy Dain said:

This Act is a paper service and nothing more. The people who have been promised a free-for-all service available to everybody are going to be very disappointed. The service will not and cannot be there on 5th July or any reasonably approximate date. . . The failure of the Service must recoil on the people who produced it well knowing that it was impossible to implement.[24]

Statements like this helped to obtain a 95% vote by GPs, and a 90% vote by all doctors, against service under the Act, on an 84% poll. Most of the press supported the campaign of vilification of the Minister and the Act. The *Observer* called for Bevan's resignation, and the *Daily Sketch* acclaimed the doctors' vote as:

the first effective revolt of the professional classes against Socialist tyranny. . . There is nothing that Bevan or any other Socialist can do about it in the shape of Hitlerian coercion. . . the State medical service is part of the Socialist plot to convert Great Britain into a National Socialist economy.

Two months after the NHS began right on time on 5th July 1948, 93% of the population was registered with GPs, and 90% of GPs were enrolled under the Act. Just as in 1912,

the doctors had done all that was possible to obstruct a major
advance in the social organization of medical care, and had
isolated themselves from public opinion. Speaking in parliament in February 1948, Bevan described this moral suicide:

> I should have thought, and we all hoped, that the possibilities
> contained in this Act would have excited the medical profession,
> that they would have realised that we are setting their feet on a
> new path entirely, that we ought to take pride in the fact that,
> despite our financial and economic anxieties, we are still able to do
> the most civilised thing in the world—put the welfare of the sick in
> front of every other consideration.[24]

The profession had no credible reply. It was fifteen years
before the medical establishment made its apology, and by
then few open opponents of the NHS were to be found anywhere. President of the Royal College of Physicians Lord
Platt summed up what was by then a general guilt, though
characteristically expressed in patrician terms:

> The methods of the BMA were those of trades unionists, not
> appropriate to the leadership of a great profession. . . A generation
> of doctors had been taught to disparage British medicine, to regard
> the Ministry of Health as its enemy, and to speak of the Health
> Service in terms of contempt.[26]

Why Did They Do It?

Since the BMA leaders were not fools, and faced a situation
similar to that before the Lloyd George Act, why did they
repeat the same humiliating follies? Up to the last absurd
moment they were backed by over 90% of the profession.
Though the specialists made their own backstage deal through
the Royal Colleges, this guaranteed only grudging co-
operation. The great majority of consultants, particularly in
teaching hospitals, did not conceal their personal hostility to
the social principles of the service.

We are therefore dealing with a set of fundamental beliefs
shared by nearly all doctors, so deeply rooted that they were
unable to learn from their own historical experience, and
were blind to social reality. They were bound by the limits

of the Osler model, by now an established paradigm:[27] gentlemanly, scientistic, ahistorical and socially isolated medical care. The government's positive programme of investment in hospitals won positive support from a minority and neutrality from the majority of specialists, but GPs had no similar guarantees of a better clinical future, only the prospect of more (though better paid) drudgery. There was therefore no material basis for a settlement with the GPs similar to that with the specialists.

Fee-for-service

To most GPs, the NHS looked as though it would universalize bad practice. A typical view from a 'good' GP was expressed by Geiringer[28] in the *Lancet*, 10 years after the NHS began:

> bad practice. . . originated at the turn of the century, partly from genuine attempts to provide some kind of general practitioner service for the poor, partly as a result of the panel system. . . Under the per capita method of payment this type of pauper medicine is still profitable, and is no longer, as formerly, confined to the poorest section of the community. . . the natural and surest way [to be cleared of these shameful relics] would be a fee-for-service system which would eliminate them in a few years. . .
> The real tragedy of the present situation lies in the relentless process of passive hospitalisation which forces even the best practitioners into doing bad general medicine. . . The attraction of a fee-for-service system is that it would automatically rehabilitate general practice, simply by the working of economic laws. . . [it] would be a hotbed of abuses. But at least it would allow good medicine to survive.

A fee-for-service system, with part-payment by the patient as a brake on overtreatment, is what most British GPs wanted both in 1912 and in 1948, and what their counterparts in Western Europe, North America, Australia and New Zealand actually got when their governments organized partial or complete public primary care services after the Second World War. A fee-for-service system, state-subsidized extension of fee-earning private practice, appeared to GPs to be most likely to preserve or improve their status, earnings and skills, minimize bureaucratic control, and preserve their autonomy. It would be gentlemanly (status, earnings and autonomy), scientistic (clinical skills used and preserved), and though admittedly isolated from social reality and (if anyone bothered to ask) ahistorical, these seemed no great matter to most of the doctors. Better, they thought, to start with good work for a few, later filtering down to the many, than degrade medicine to an egalitarian veterinary service, and destroy the machinery of a future progress which they assumed simply to be more of what they already had.

The word 'gentleman' has many meanings, but it is generally agreed that it should include social responsibility as well as authority, autonomy and affluence. In English culture particularly, though it has been possible and indeed desirable for businessmen to be gentlemen, a certain tension between these roles was always assumed; gentlemen were motivated by the public good as well as by greed, and their necessary search for profit was supposed to be restrained by the bounds of paternalistic social responsibility.

The outcome of Allbutt and Geiringer's Osler paradigm as applied to general practice can be seen in the United States. After 25 years of a state-subsidized fee-for-service system, there is growing affluence but declining social responsibility; though doctors are rich, fees for service have not preserved gentlemanly status. Technical skills have been preserved and developed, but the effect of this has been not to strengthen general practice, but to destroy it; GPs found it more profitable to become specialists. By the 1960s, family practice in the USA was disappearing and there was a large surplus of specialists fighting for trade in prosperous areas, together with shortages of all medical staff in the countryside and areas of industrial decline. Far from reducing bureaucratic overhead costs, the administrative controls necessary to restrain over-diagnosis, over-treatment and fraud resulted in 22% of the US health budget (public and private) going to administrative costs in 1983, compared with only 6% in Great Britain.[29] Far from guaranteeing autonomy, isolation of US doctors as small businessmen in lucrative self-employment left them open to take-over by bigger business-

men, employing doctors at big salaries in competing corporations, in which clinical decisions and even professional
objectives were subordinated to search for profit.[30,31] The
detachment of Oslerean ideology from social responsibility
was fully confirmed; the US care system has never been
accessible to all of the people, and remains least accessible
to those most in need. As for history, it stayed where it
always was, an antiquarian hobby for retired doctors, not the
central thread of all art and all science; people who need
history only to decorate and reinforce their current status
will not develop it as their principal means of understanding
and thereby contributing positively to the social changes
within which they live.

All this has been achieved at ruinous cost. Whereas health
expenditure in Britain has never exceeded 6.2% of Gross
National Product, in the USA by 1986 it was near 11%
despite vigorous government efforts to restrain it. Average
US per capita expenditure on medical care is roughly four
times as large as in Britain, without any evidence of an
overall difference in age-standardized mortality between the
two countries in favour of the fee-for-service system. Unless
US electors rediscover collective solutions for collective
problems and insist on a rationally planned National Health
Service, their doctors will become well-paid cogs in a machine
which neither they nor the public will control.

Cheap Doctors

Experience abroad has proved fees-for-service to be an
illusory alternative, but fears that the clinical skills of the
Osler paradigm would not survive within the general practice
of the Lloyd George Act and later the NHS have been largely
confirmed. Allbutt's predictions that the GP would become
'but a stop-gap', that 'every malady of importance' would
'be sent to some central institution', that most working-class
and much genteel middle-class practice would remain
perfunctory work by perfunctory men, have been sub-
stantiated time and again by objective and responsible
observers.[32,33] Geiringer's warning of 'the relentless process

of passive hospitalisation' which would force even the best
practitioners to give up their technical skills, was largely
correct. In 1938-9, British GPs were estimated to have
performed about two and a half million surgical operations,
an average of three per doctor each week.[34] By the early
1960s, GP surgery had almost vanished.

Already by 1912, more so in 1948, it was clear enough
that specialized technical skills were increasingly important
for effective medical care, and could only be acquired and
maintained in hospitals, which concentrated cases of illness
and experience in dealing with them. The end of amateur
surgery was a terrible blow to the self-respect of many fine
and devoted GPs, but it was an undeniable advance for
patients.

It was less obvious but equally true that systems of second-
ary specialist care in hospitals could only function effectively
and efficiently if their patients were selected through a
referral system based on skilled primary care by generalists.
Despite sentimental rhetoric from both consultants and
politicians that the good GP would always be the keystone
of the service, both groups were almost entirely ignorant of
the skills required for effective primary care, and even of
those required for efficient selection for referral. Writing in
1977, John Horder[35] described accurately the view of
general practice held not only by specialists, but by many
GPs, before he helped to devise an independent ideology of
general practice in the 1960s:

> Specialists thought of the problems which patients present to
> general practitioners as mostly minor ones, of which a high pro-
> portion were psychological or social. A general practitioner was
> therefore nearly the same as a social worker, except that he had
> some medical knowledge, most of which was wasted. His main
> diagnostic task was to sort out what was minor from what was
> major and to refer the latter to specialists. General practice was
> mostly common sense. The practitioner was a very busy man and
> so, much as he would have liked to, he seldom had time to listen
> to patients, examine them, do tests, or talk to them. He could not
> afford to be as precise or scientific as the specialist. All this being
> so, the less intelligent doctors should go into general practice,
> which was most suitable for people good at games. There was no

need for them to have a special training, because common sense cannot be taught. If a general practitioner found himself discontented with this role, he could hear about hospital medicine on a ward round at the local hospital, or do a bit of it as a clinical assistant...

This also was, and probably for the most part still is, the view of politicians, because they get most of their impressions of medicine from specialists. High-born conservatives had little personal experience of GPs, for like other rich men they generally bought care privately from whichever specialist appeared most appropriate or fashionable. Low-born radicals had personal experience of perfunctory care, and what they had seen did not favour general practice as a field for public investment. The costs of general practice consisted almost entirely of payments to GPs, and the cost of prescribed drugs. Everything else, receptionists, nurses, cleaners, office and medical equipment, furniture and buildings, came from the GP's pocket, a public service privately administered. It was, and was intended to be, a formula for cheap service and petty corruption, farming out an important public responsibility to private contractors, whose personal income and leisure time varied inversely with their investment of money in staff and equipment, and time in postgraduate training.

Government ministers, Ministry of Health civil servants, specialist doctors, GPs and the public at large all saw the hospitals as the only significant site for clinical growth and innovation. Though recent development of antibiotics had in effect greatly expanded the potential scope and effectiveness of clinical care within the community, GPs remained divided and isolated, incapable of planning clinical growth and innovation because they had not adapted hospital traditions of teamwork and peer review to community care on their own initiative, and would not tolerate innovation from anyone else. In the eyes of the profession, the government and the public, general practice had an essentially passive role; to go on responding to individual patient demands which were either too trivial for specialists, or still beyond the reach of medical science. The tasks of general practice were residual, to cope with whatever was either beneath the notice of hospitals, or still too difficult for them. Being a public service paid from taxation by governments controlled or influenced by people who did not use the NHS themselves by normal channels, hospitals were permanently underfunded, and therefore able to do less than medical science made possible. The NHS promised to do all that was possible to care for the sick, whoever and wherever they were. Without general practice to fill the gaps, this promise could not even appear to be fulfilled, so it remained necessary, but more as a convenient social illusion than as a clinical reality. Inevitably, on this view, medical progress would eventually relegate the GP to an insignificant clinical role.[19]

General practice was quantitatively extended to cover the whole population, but qualitatively unchanged because it received no significant public investment. Despite much talk in 1944 of health centres and a salaried service, neither of these was on offer by 1948. Six months before the Act was to come into force, without any debate in parliament or constituency Labour Parties, the Ministry of Health circulated Local Authorities with an instruction to discard all future plans for health centre construction, and stop work already in progress. The excuses were alleged higher priority for housing, and medical opposition. In fact 1948 was the peak year for house building, reaching 284,000, and from then on the rate of municipal rehousing declined; the real priority was the futile attempt to retain a world military role which has dragged down the British economy ever since. As for medical opposition, nothing had been done to popularize health centres among GPs, or build on the interest shown in work from health centres in the 1944 BMA plebiscite. Even in 1948, the BMA published a report saying that 'the logical future development will be the provision of specially designed health centres from which both general practitioner and the present Local Authority services can be provided. . . Early experiment is advisable'. Talbot Rogers, a solitary progressive among the fiercely reactionary leaders of the BMA, told how bitter the opposition had already become at the periphery,[36] but no effort was ever made by the Minister to press either for health centres, or any other serious public investment in primary care. Had he done so, a critical mass of support for the Act might have been achieved among GPs, as it was among the consultants. Elder[37] recalled the bitter mood of many doctors returning from the war:

> We returned to the familiar state of isolation with every man for himself in a general atmosphere of cynicism. There was a horrible and demoralising sense of disillusion, and relationships between doctors were worse than they had ever been.

Another correspondent wrote to the *Lancet*:[38]

> the disillusionment and resentment felt especially by the young doctors who had been promised, in section 21 [of the Act] lavish equipment and specially designed premises.

Even in 1952, when interest in health centres was supposed to have died, the BMA found that 48% of randomly-sampled GPs approved of the health centre idea, against 47% who opposed it.[39] If the government had really believed in general practice, and committed substantial resources to it as it did to the hospital service, there would have been a social base for action, even within the profession.

Somerville Hastings, a Labour MP in the 1945 parliament and a consultant at the Middlesex Hospital, summed up the position GPs had got themselves into, isolated from the mainstream of medical advance and hostile to the mainstream of social advance:

> During the negotiations that preceded the National Health Service Act the GPs came together to oppose it. They were also concerned, quite rightly, with their remuneration under the scheme, but gave little thought to their rightful place in it or opportunities for doing good work under it. They only asked to be left alone, and they have got what they asked.[40]

If we are serious about democracy, there can be no public investment without public accountability, a lesson GPs still find hard to accept. We could, of course, forget about democracy, and delegate our social responsibilities to the blind but, so we are assured, ultimately just decisions of the market. We could then stop even pretending to be either gentlemen or scientists; we would be in business, enriching society by enriching ourselves, exactly in tune with the times in which we now live.

The ideology of general practice in 1948 was backward-looking, self-deceptive, sentimental and nostalgic, centred on the already lifeless notions of GP surgery and amateur specialism, indifferent to the many real medical problems people had for which hospital specialists had no answer, and ultimately dependent on the Osler paradigm of professionalism imparted to GPs by their teaching hospitals. The independent ideology they needed to begin making decisions of their own lay in the future, and is the subject of the next chapter.

NOTES

1. Brotherston, J., 'Memorandum of evidence of the BMA'. In, McLachlan, G., McKeown, T. (eds.), *Medical history and medical care*, London: Oxford University Press, 1971.
2. Cantlie, N., *A History of the Army Medical Department*, vol. 1, Edinburgh: Churchill Livingstone, 1974.
3. Hackney Workers' Educational Association, *The threepenny doctor: Dr Jelley of Hackney*, Hackney WEA & Centreprise Publishing, London, 1974.
4. Sir William Osler (1849-1919) has generally been considered the greatest all-round physician in the English-speaking world, as an innovator of clinical method and as a teacher. Born a Canadian, he became Professor of Medicine at Philadelphia, and then joined William Henry Welch at Johns Hopkins Medical School, which pioneered the implementation of the Flexner Report, which first placed US medical teaching on a foundation of laboratory science. He became Regius Professor of Medicine at Oxford in 1905. The first edition of his textbook, *Principles and Practice of Medicine*, appeared in 1905, and continued with posthumous editions until after the Second World War as the most widely used general textbook of internal medicine in the English-speaking world. He probably had a greater influence on the ideas and practice of medicine all over the world than any man since Galen.
5. Osler, W. (1913), in: *A way of Life and Selected Writings of Sir William Osler*, New York: Dover Publications, 1958.
6. Seipp, C., *The ambiguities of greatness: Sir William Osler, 1849-1919*. Unpublished MS 1981. Health Services Research Centre,

University of North Carolina, Chapel Hill.
7. Woodward, J., *To do the sick no harm: a study of the British voluntary hospital system to 1875*, Routledge & Kegan Paul, London, 1974.
8. Brecht, B., *The Life of Galileo*, London: Eyre Methuen, 1963. Brecht began writing his play in 1938-39, after Hitler had imprisoned or expelled all scientists of integrity and imagination in what was then the world's most advanced scientific nation, and conscripted the rest; after Stalin had almost wiped out all objectively formed and imaginative opinion in the USSR; and after Britain and France had turned their backs on the murder of the Spanish Republic and Czechoslovakia. He completed it in 1945-47, following the destruction of Hiroshima and Nagasaki by nuclear weapons, and the first years of the balance of nuclear terror. He shows Galileo's capitulation as a turning point in the development of science.
9. Blackwell, B., Bloomfield, S.S., Buncher, C.R., 'Demonstration to medical students of placebo responses and non-drug factors', *Lancet 1972*; i:1279-82.
10. Cobb, L.A. et al., 'Evaluation of internal-mammary-artery ligation by double-blind technic', *New England Journal of Medicine 1959*; 260:1115-8.
11. Dimond, E.G., Kittle, C.F., Crockett, J.E., 'Comparison of internal mammary artery ligation and sham operation for angina pectoris', *American Journal of Cardiology 1960*; 5:484-6.
12. Allbutt, T.C., 'The Act and the future of medicine'. Letter to *The Times*, 3 January 1912.
13. Gilbert, B.B., *British Social Policy 1914-1939*, London: Batsford, 1966.
14. *The Battle of the Clubs*. A reprint of the reports of the special commissioner of the *Lancet* appointed to enquire into the Medical Aid Societies, London: *Lancet*, 1896.
15. Shaw, G.B., 'Preface to *The Doctor's Dilemma*', London: John Constable, 1911.
16. Levers, A.H., 'The GP at the crossroads' (correspondence), *British Medical Journal 1950*; i:1369-70.
17. Wigg, J.W.E., Horder, J., 'The biography of a general practice', *Journal of the Royal College of General Practitioners 1967*; 14:84-90.
18. Cox, A., *Among the doctors*, London: Christopher Johnson, 1966.
19- I know of five reasonably accessible, reliable and imaginative
23. sources on the Beveridge Report in relation to the birth of the NHS, by Honigsbaum, Foot, Logan and Eckstein.
19. Honigsbaum, F., *The division in British medicine: a history of the separation of general practice from hospital care, 1911-1968*. His interpretation throughout is diametrically opposed to mine, but this is a very useful history. His main theme, the origins of the separation between specialists and GPs in England, and differences between England and other countries in this respect, are dealt with more originally by Rosemary Stevens in her *Medical Practice*

in Modern England, New York: Yale University Press, 1966.

20. Foot, M., *Aneurin Bevan: a biography*, Vol. I, 1897–1945, London: McGibbon & Kee, 1962. This gives a good political account of Beveridge, especially of the in-fighting in Churchill's cabinet and the attitudes of the Labour leadership and Labour Left; nothing seems to have changed since then. The battle for implementation of the Act is dealt with in Vol. II.

21. Forsyth, G., *Doctors and state medicine: a study of the British National Health Service*, 2nd ed., London: Pitman Medical, 1973. This is the best readily available short account of the early politics of the NHS.

22. Murray, D.S., *Why a National Health Service? The part played by the Socialist Medical Association*, London: Pemberton Books, 1971. This is now difficult to find. Though over-optimistic about the role of the SMA in the run-up to the NHS, it is full of useful material not available elsewhere.

23. Eckstein, H., *The English Health Service*, London: Oxford University Press, 1959. This remains the best detailed account of the birth of the NHS.

24. Foot, M., *Aneurin Bevan: a biography*, Vol. 2, 1945–1960, London: Davis-Poynter, 1973.

25. Report of the interdepartmental committee on remuneration of general practitioners (Spens report). Cmnd. 6810, London: HMSO, 1946.

26. Platt, R., *Doctor and patient: ethics, morale, government*, London: Nuffield Provincial Hospital Trust, 1963.

27. The concept of 'paradigm' was introduced by Kuhn in his 'Structure of scientific revolutions', (University of Chicago Press, 1962). A paradigm is a very general, comprehensive theory dominating the assumptions of science over a substantial period, tending to define the questions scientists ask and the answers they find credible. Examples are Newtonian physics, a paradigm which disintegrated with development of particle physics early in the 20th Century, and was ultimately replaced by a new paradigm. The word has been extended to include any generally shared set of assumptions governing teaching and research in any scientific subject, and has been a favourite among medical educationalists.

28. Geiringer, E., 'Murder at the Crossroads, or the Decapitation of General Practice', *Lancet 1959*; i:1039–45.

29. Himmelstein, D., Woolhandler, S., 'Cost without benefit: administrative waste in US health care', *New England Journal of Medicine 1986*; 314:441–5.

30. Freedman, S.A., 'Megacorporate health care: a choice for the future', *New England Journal of Medicine 1985*; 312:579–82.

31. Starr, P., *The social transformation of American medicine*, New York: Basic Books, 1982.

32. Collings, J.S., 'General practice in England today', *Lancet 1950*; i:555–85.

33. Wilkes, E., 'Is good general practice possible?', *British Medical Journal 1984*; 289:85–6.

34. Hill, A.B., 'The doctor's day and pay', *Journal of the Royal*

Statistical Society 1951; series A 114:1-37.
35. Horder, J.P.P., 'Physicians and family doctors: a new relationship', *Journal of the Royal College General Practitioners 1977*; 27:391-7. This was published simultaneously in the *Journal of the Royal College of Physicians of London.*
36. Rogers, A.T., 'Looking forward with hindsight', *Proceedings of the Royal Society of Medicine 1972*; 65:109-18.
37. Elder, H.H.A., 'Forty years in general practice', *Journal of the College of General Practitioners 1964*; 7:328-41.
38. Graham-Little, E., 'Letter to the editor', *Lancet 1950*; i:737.
39. Hadfield, S.J., 'A field survey of general practice', *British Medical Journal 1953*; 2:683-706.
40. Hastings, S., 'Letter to the editor', *Lancet 1950*; i:882.

Chapter 4
NEW IDEAS IN OLD STRUCTURES

The NHS revolutionized the distribution, staffing, equipment, planning and administration of hospitals by nationalizing them all, initiating a centrally planned programme of co-ordinated development. Three quarters of all hospitals in use in 1948 were built before 1914, half dated back to the 19th Century, one-third were former workhouses with a custodial rather than a caring tradition. Half the hospitals had fewer than 50 beds. In 1947 only 8% of all doctors were hospital-based specialists, limited to a few large cities; by 1960 consultants were available in every district general hospital, they comprised 20% of all doctors, and were in charge of two-thirds of all NHS spending and 87% of all health service personnel. Regional planning ensured that compared with other countries, Britain had a rational and relatively equal distribution of specialist units throughout the country. In the first 25 years of the NHS, there was a 12% rise in population, an 80% rise in hospital admissions, and a 10% fall in the number of hospital beds. This huge rise in productivity was achieved by rational deployment of resources and a large rise in medical and above all in nursing manpower. Between 1949 and 1971, the number of hospital medical, nursing, administrative and clerical staff each more than doubled. Over the same period the number of GPs increased by only 16%, though they were gradually redistributed to reduce over-doctoring in wealthy areas, and increase the number of GPs in poor areas.

The members of Regional Hospital Boards, who controlled

the hospital service, were not locally elected, but appointed by the Minister from lists of the local great and good traditionally associated with hospital charities. An analysis of the social composition of four Regional Boards in 1964[1] showed that of 108 members, 46% had a medical background (including 2 GPs), and one was an industrial worker. Of 360 chairmen of Hospital Management Committees, 24 were Lord Lieutenants or Deputy Lieutenants, 17 were Lords or their wives, widows and offspring, 8 were retired admirals or generals, and one was a retired ambassador. Of a sample of 92 Hospital Management Committees, a quarter of the chairmen were company directors and not one was a wage earner. Planning and control were oligarchic, leaving the power of the consultants virtually undisturbed by local criticism, and much augmented by the new resources they controlled. Private practice diminished at first, never disappeared, and now prospers among part-time consultants. The main features of the Osler paradigm were enhanced as medical science gave specialists more effective weapons. Though government funding was always insufficient, it grew as national wealth expanded. In general, the form of the hospital service seemed suited both to its functions as seen by local oligarchs, and to the requirements of Osler professionalism as seen by the consultants.

In hospitals, doctors felt no need for a new ideology. As patients slowly became less willing to be pushed around, the traditional arrogance of specialists became more civilized, but though reform in this respect appears substantial to people of my age who remember the truly feudal relationships of the 1950s, it remains obvious to each new generation that meets it.

General Practice 1948–66

The situation in general practice was a stark contrast. Private practice was virtually wiped out, with little regret from GPs. Even in 1953 Hadfield, the BMA's observer of a random sample of GPs, noted general relief that billing patients was a thing of the past.[2] By 1964, Ann Cartwright[3] found that only 3% of patients ever consulted a GP privately, and about half of her random sample of GPs actively discouraged private patients, finding them snobbish, inconsiderate and unable to accept what they (the GPs) saw as a reasonable doctor-patient relationship. If Geiringer was right in considering fee-earning private practice the head of general practice, it certainly was decapitated.

An Australian doctor, J.S. Collings, visited 55 practices all over England, sitting in on surgeries and giving a vivid account of what he found one year after the start of the new service:

> . . . the buildings which serve as the doctor's workshops. . . are usually located in what was once a shop, or a residence above a shop, or in the downstairs rooms of a house tenanted by some person who takes care of the surgery, or occasionally by the doctor himself. . . As a rule two adjacent rooms serve as waiting and consulting rooms. . . I did not see a single industrial surgery which was built for its purpose. In most cases the waiting rooms are too small, cold and generally inhospitable. In peak hours in big practices it is usual to see patients standing, waiting their turn. . . and it is not uncommon to see them standing in the garden. . . or queuing in the street. . . In several of the surgeries I visited there were no examination couches; in many there were no filing cabinets, and such records as were kept lay around the room either loose or in boxes; in one there was a chair for the doctor only (the patient remained standing throughout consultation and examination). . . Few skilled craftsmen, be they plumbers, butchers or motor mechanics, would be prepared to work under conditions or with equipment as bad. . . as that tolerated by many doctors working in industrial practices.[4]

In middle-class practice, Collings found a more genteel appearance, but clinical function was little different.

These poor conditions and low expectations were common in general practice in most countries at that time. The quality of care found in similar surveys in USA in 1953[5] and Canada in 1958[6] was little better, but the structure of NHS general practice seemed designed to inhibit progress and discourage investment and innovation. More than 20 years after the NHS began, study of a random sample of general practices in 1969[7] showed that 16% had no room for a secretary, 31% had no typewriter, 62% no dictating machine, 29% no toilet available for patients, 15% no equipment for urine analysis,

22% no equipment for skin suture, 32% no vaginal speculum, 65% no haemoglobinometer, and 90% no electrocardiograph. While entrepreneurial practice abroad invested in modern premises, office equipment and supporting staff (and slid away from general practice to more lucrative specialism and pseudo-specialism), general practice in Britain remained stagnant.

This was the material evidence of professional demoralization, expressed even more dramatically in the way GPs now thought of their patients, their work and themselves. More than at any time before or since, GPs were defined not by what they were, but by what they were not. Taught entirely by specialists in hospitals, GPs were men who had failed to become specialists and were unable to work in a hospital.

Lord Moran's Ladder

This view was candidly expressed by Lord Moran in his evidence to the Review Body on. Doctors' Remuneration in 1966:[8]

> *Chairman:* 'It has been put to us by a good many people that the two branches of the profession, general practice and consultancy, are not senior or junior to one another but they are level. Do you agree with that?'
> *Lord Moran:* 'I say emphatically no. Could anything be more absurd? I was dean of St. Mary's Hospital [medical school] for 25 years. . . all the people of outstanding merit, with few exceptions, aimed to get on the staff. There was no other aim, and it was a ladder off which some of them fell. How can you say that the people who get to the top of the ladder are the same as the people who fall off it? It seems to me so ludicrous.'
> *Chairman:* 'But might not general practice be a vocation especially suited to those wishing to serve the community?'
> *Lord Moran:* 'If a man's vocation was obviously trying to help the community, would he not have more opportunities as a consultant?'

Lord Moran's ladder quickly became notorious. His condescension infuriated leading GPs, but it was a correct description not only of the attitude of the overwhelming majority of consultants, particularly in teaching hospitals

('What a waste: brilliant young fellow, but he only wants to be a GP!'), but of most GPs as well. Curwen[9] studied a random sample of GPs in 1963 and found that over half had wanted to become specialists; only one third claimed to have had any positive reasons for choosing a career in general practice.

A GP interviewed for Ann Cartwright's classic study of general practice in 1964[3] spoke for many if not most of his generation:

> We're swamped with trivialities. This isn't the sort of work one spent years at university preparing oneself for. There's the utter futility and humiliation of a professional man who feels his training is wasted. The GP has no status because he doesn't do medicine.

Trained by specialists in hospital for specialism in hospital, blinkered by the customs and assumptions of the Osler paradigm, he was not scientist enough to see what stared him in the face: a huge, largely unmapped field for effective medical care requiring skills unknown to hospital specialism, but badly needed by his patients.

The College of General Practitioners

British medical professionalism developed in the first half of the 19th Century around the waxing Royal Colleges of Surgeons and Physicians and the waning Society of Apothecaries. Efforts were made in 1845 to set up an independent Royal College of General Practitioners, resulting in over 100 references to this issue in the medical literature around that time. The movement was opposed by the two senior Colleges, mainly to protect their power to control undergraduate teaching, and thus to define the clinical and social content of medical professionalism. When the GPs gave up their attempt to form an independent College, they effectively conceded social and professional leadership to the physicians and surgeons and accepted a subordinate role. By the end of the century, centralization of technical care in hospitals finalized this arrangement, apparently for all time.

When the NHS finally expelled GPs from all but subordinate roles at the fringes of hospital work, they had nowhere to go but a College of their own. The BMA was not a feasible alternative. It represented all doctors, specialists as well as GPs, and its essentially trade-union function accorded badly with the claim of all the Royal Colleges to be concerned only with the quality of practice, rather than its terms and conditions. The BMA was in any case at that time an unconvincing vehicle for any attempt to revive confidence in NHS general practice, being still heavily influenced by GPs who hankered for a return to private practice, and could not accept the finality of the NHS. After two years of negotiation in corridors of medical power, and against the opposition of the three existing Royal Colleges of Physicians, Surgeons, and Obstetricians, the College of General Practitioners (not yet Royal; its viability was still uncertain) was born in 1953.

Initially the College was chiefly concerned to survive and establish its respectability in traditional terms. The first President, Will Pickles, was internationally recognized for his research on infectious diseases in his own practice in Wensleydale, much less known for his quiet but lonely local support for the NHS when all around him lost their heads. The first secretary, John Hunt, was still in entirely private practice in Sloane Street, where Harrods was the local grocer. The image of the College was comfortably non-industrial, but a principal spur to its creation was undoubtedly a generally recognized need to rectify the clinical squalor described in the Collings Report. A member of the Provisional Foundation Council of the College, Geoffrey Barber, had contributed to discussion of that Report in the *Lancet*:

> We all know too well that twenty years of general practice brings far too many of us down to the level described by Dr Collings. . . the root of the matter lies in the width of the gulf between the conditions under which the medical student is prepared for general practice, and the actual conditions he finds there. . . to teach general practice with real understanding, clinical teachers must at some point have been in general practice themselves for a sufficient time to understand the conditions under which the ordinary doctor

works. The student must be so prepared for general practice and for the difference between what he is taught to expect and what he actually finds, that he will adopt a fighting attitude against poor medicine—that is to say, against hopeless conditions for the practice of good medicine. The young man must be taught to be sufficiently courageous, so that when he arrives at the converted shop with the drab battered furniture, the couch littered with dusty bottles, and the few rusty antiquated instruments, he will make a firm stand and say 'I will not practise under these conditions; I will have more room, more light, more ancillary help, and better equipment.' . . . It ought to be possible for domiciliary medicine to compete favourably with treatment in hospital for many conditions which nowadays are thought of as the sole prerogative of the specialists; but this will be possible only if the general practitioner is well trained, and equally well equipped, and if—most important of all— he is able to devote adequate time to his patients.[10]

Better training was on the way, eventually including at least token teaching from general practitioners. The implications of more room, more light, more ancillary help, better equipment and more time devoted to the patient, though central to the College's task, were the most difficult to tackle. Under the independent contractor system, all must one way or another be subtracted from the GP's income. The structure of the NHS protected and encouraged squalid practice, while exposing individual GPs rather than government to complaint. In opposing intolerable conditions of practice, the College was bound to collide with the immediate economic interests of many of the GPs it sought to influence and recruit. In its early days, the dilemma was postponed by selective recruitment of GPs with large consciences, small lists, or in market town groups uncontaminated by the worst features of club practice; but it has never gone away.

Balint and the New Ideology

Locked out of the hospitals, forced to accept Lloyd George practice where imitation of their specialist teachers had to be attempted at their own cost, GPs in search of self-respect were forced to look for alternatives. Progress with body-care was difficult, but care of the soul looked more promising.

Material for this was provided by Balint in 1957, with his book *The doctor, his Patient and the Illness.*[11]

Balint was a refugee from Hungary, a Freudian psycho-analyst of unusually practical bent, who found British psychiatrists generally hostile to all forms of psychotherapy as time-consuming and therefore impractical in an almost exclusively public service (private couch-psychiatry and psycho-analysis on the US and Paris model scarcely exists in the UK except for a little private practice in London). He turned to GPs as a possible alternative source of psychotherapy for the many unhappy people treated either by pills or Electro-Convulsive Therapy, who really needed a skilled listener. He defined a wide area of need that was currently ignored or rejected by specialists, and was not recognized as a medical task in the Osler paradigm. Of all patients referred for hospital outpatient investigation by specialist physicians, about one-third had no evidence of organic disease.[12] Instead of repeating futile investigations of increasing complexity and cost, and then telling these people there was nothing wrong with them, Balint taught active search for causes of anxiety and unhappiness, and treatment by remedial education aiming at insight, rather than tablets aiming at suppression of symptoms. He showed GPs that far from being inferior to hospital specialists in this role, for this large group of patients they might be more effective and less dangerous. He also taught that in order to be effective in this work GPs must learn to look as objectively as possible at their own personalities, and accept that they might have to change.

The Balintists met in small groups analysing themselves, each other, and their most difficult patients. Theirs was always a minority movement, and probably never involved more than about 5% of GPs. Even today, a much larger minority of GPs in actively hostile to it, but they are die-hards who tend to be hostile to all innovation; the Balintists held the ideological initiative. For the next 25 years Balintry was the principal innovating ideological force in British general practice, and was particularly influential among the younger GPs forming the second generation of leaders for the College of General Practitioners, now becoming Grand

Old Men.

Psychosomatic medicine, which once appeared to be its central feature, proved to be a shallow concept amounting to little more than recognition that all patients have thoughts and emotions, and both health and all forms of disease are modified by them (though to many doctors these seem still to be novel ideas). However, three features of Balint's ideas became permanent achievements, foundations for an ideology of general practice independent of hospital specialism. First, he gave GPs confidence in their own potential worth, without resorting to sentimentality and nostalgia. Second, he showed how inappropriate their undergraduate training was to common problems confronting them, and therefore posed the questions how GPs were to organize their own remedial education, and how they should change their practice. Finally, he showed them that to be effective they must do more than passively respond to the immediate demands of patients; active search for the hidden needs behind overt demands was essential to effective care.

These three assumptions may now be taken for granted by most GPs, at least for their model of ideal practice, but initially they had to be fought for against powerful and pervasive inertia, and even now can never be taken for granted. Abdication of professional leadership to hospital-based medicine was and still is easier than the hard road of collective self-improvement championed by the College. Most GPs still wanted to be left alone. Six months after its foundation, membership reached over 2,000, about 10% of all GPs. By 1986 this had risen to over 13,000, over one-third of all GPs, but only a small minority were active members.

Rediscovery of General Practice

During the first 13 years of its existence, the ends preached by the College were virtually unsupported by means other than what GPs spent from their own pockets. The self-critical, reforming approach enjoined by the College on its members was unrewarded, and incurred costs because its

implementation required more time for the patient and more
supporting staff. It was voluntary, and most GPs were not
volunteering. Earnings depended almost entirely on capitation,
so that the most successful doctors were those with the
biggest lists (the legal maximum in those days was 4,000),
and therefore the least time available for their patients.
Though GPs still insisted on independent contractor status,
they wanted the government to pay for any improvements
in the service. The general practice share of the NHS budget
fell from 12% in 1950 to 8% by the early 1960s.

There were no hospital postgraduate centres or libraries
open to GPs, postgraduate education was limited to lectures
by consultants and a few residential courses at teaching
hospitals, 27% of GPs had no office staff of any kind, not
even a receptionist,[7] and 85% had no appointment system.
In 1964, 11% of randomly-sampled GPs said they got little
or no enjoyment from their work, and 56% estimated that at
least half their consultations were trivial, inappropriate or
unnecessary.[3] The most able young doctors were conscripted
to general practice by shortage of consultant posts rather
than recruited positively by ambition to work at community
level. The Royal Commission on Medical Education[13] found
that only 23% of final-year students wanted a career in
general practice, though about 50% ended up there.
Mechanic[14] studied the opinions of another random sample
of GPs at the height of dissatisfaction on the eve of the
Package Deal settlement of 1966. Asked to list problems
they found fairly serious or very serious, 68% quoted the
time available for each patient, 64% the level of their own
income, 49% the number of patients they had to look after,
and 48% the high proportion of consultations for trivial or
inappropriate problems. Few GPs seemed concerned with
better working conditions, buildings, staff, professional
isolation or access to diagnostic services. He noted that GPs
perceived their problems subjectively, and looked for personal
rather than organizational solutions. This is interesting in the
light of the solutions finally negotiated through the Package
Deal, which, apart from better pay, generally addressed
problems which individual GPs (though not their

organizations) ignored.

Low morale in general practice in the mid-1960s coincided with a transient shortage of medical graduates because of cuts in medical school intake after the war. By itself this probably would not have worried the NHS authorities, but the quality of GP care was at last beginning to be recognized internationally as both a cause and a potential means of containing escalating hospital costs.

News about this came from the most influential possible source, the USA. The proportion of GPs in the US profession had fallen from 76% in 1940 to 36% by 1965, and most of these were old men. In the wealthiest country in the world, 40% of the people had no personal doctor. Between 1965 and 1970, people going to hospital emergency rooms increased by 49%, more than half of them people who had no other source of medical advice.[15] The big money was in specialism, not friendly and efficient local first-contact and continuing care; but without GPs, specialists could only pseudospecialize, and costly hospital equipment could not be used rationally or economically. There were eight times as many specialists per million population as there were in Britain, but large parts of the USA still had inadequate specialist cover. In New York, 196 neurologists served 6.5 million people, while 2 neurologists served 2 million people in West Virginia;[16] plenty of doctors, not enough medical care. The lesson from North America was clear: GPs were a dwindling national asset; nations lucky enough to still have them should take care, or they might disappear.

The 1966 Package Deal

The obvious and effective way to help general practice was the way the NHS had already helped hospital-based specialism; public investment in appropriate education, better buildings and equipment, and more office and nursing staff.

None of the medical schools then gave any significant teaching in or about general practice or by general practitioners, little postgraduate education was available and virtually all of it was by specialists. A Royal Commission on Medical

Education was appointed in 1965 and published its conclusions in the Todd Report of 1968[13], which proposed:

1) a sustained increase in medical manpower to double output by 1990.
2) recognition that no newly qualified doctor can ever be competent in all fields and that the aim of undergraduate training should be to produce educated health workers able to continue specialist education throughout their working lives.
3) that general practice was itself an important speciality requiring substantial time in the undergraduate curriculum and a planned programme of postgraduate vocational training, partly in hospital and partly in the community.

The Report was a landmark in thought about medical education, and gathered important data about the social composition, attitudes and experience of medical students. It naturally encountered fierce resistance from the medical schools Establishment, and its aims are still incompletely realized, but all except Bristol medical school now have a department of general practice of some kind, though so eminent a school as Oxford is still unwilling to fund its own department. This book is not about medical education, and this important subject must be left there.

Other than these minor changes in undergraduate training, channels for public investment in general practice were contentious. Public investment in buildings and staff had often been advocated, but were always opposed by the BMA because public investment implied public accountability, and would therefore threaten independent contractor status. GPs who accepted buildings, staff and equipment from the state would be in no position to withdraw from the NHS and revert to private practice, the only sanction the BMA could conceive in any dispute with government.

There was a growing consensus among leading GPs of all persuasions that the future lay with group practice from purpose-built premises, and full supporting office and nursing staff; the BMA was prepared to support this if full autonomy was guaranteed. Already in the late 1950s, GPs had agreed through their BMA negotiators to encourage group practice

by introducing a substantial extra payment for groups of
three or more GPs working from a single centre, but the BMA
had no plans of its own for further public investment, even
with a government now eager to help. The Labour Minister of
Health, Kenneth Robinson, was the son of a GP and both
sympathetic to and well informed about general practice; the
Chief Medical Officer at the DHSS, Sir George Godber, was
the best friend progressive general practice ever had there;
Hugh Faulkner in the Medical Practitioners' Union (MPU)
had prepared a workable policy for teamwork in general
practice, and the BMA had a newly imaginative and intelligent
leader in Jim Cameron who was prepared to modify this
policy, sweetening it with some fees-for-service, and present
it for the BMA; the opening for a new advance into public
funding was obvious.

Recruitment to general practice began to fall in 1960, and
fell at an accelerating pace through 1965, with mounting
dissatisfaction among GPs, finally leading to a new round of
resignation threats, with the BMA collecting promises of
withdrawal to strengthen its arm in negotiation for better
pay and improved conditions of service. This time, however,
the BMA leaders knew when to compromise;[17] they dropped
their objections to public investment in general practice, and
acquired a fully costed policy (the Family Doctors' Charter)
by lifting it virtually unchanged from its minuscule rival,
the MPU. The MPU had always supported the principle of the
NHS, and had developed a detailed set of proposals based
largely on the experience of a few progressive GPs who had
developed their own fully staffed group practices in better
buildings, in a spirit of co-operation rather than rivalry with
Local Authority nurses, midwives and public health medical
officers.

The agreement which emerged, agreed in 1966 and implemented in 1967, has been known ever since as the Package
Deal or the GP Charter.[18] There is general agreement on all
sides that this was a turning point for British general practice.
It had seven main features:

1. GPs' pay was substantially increased, to make the average GP's
   NHS earnings roughly equal to the basic NHS earnings of

specialists. Specialists with Merit Awards or in part-time private practice could still earn more, often very much more, than GPs, but newly-appointed consultants were often worse off than established GPs in large practices. The basic salary component of income was increased, and the proportion from capitation was reduced.

2. The full rent of suitable premises became reimbursable by government, together with the first large programme for health centre building. Cheap loans were made available to GPs to encourage them to buy and develop their own purpose-built buildings, which then became their property. Capital appreciation on many of these buildings, often on commercially attractive sites, went to the GPs, not the NHS.

3. Each GP could claim reimbursement of 70% of the wage costs of employed office and nursing staff, up to a total of two Whole-Time-Equivalent (WTE) staff for each GP.

4. Seniority payments were introduced to help older GPs to maintain earnings while reducing workload, initially contingent on attendance at a small number of postgraduate lectures each year; this was later abandoned on the insistence of the BMA that this condition was insulting, whereupon attendance at postgraduate meetings fell by 80%. Vocational training payments were introduced to encourage young GPs to undertake postgraduate vocational training before going into practice (this was not yet compulsory).

5. There had been a trainee scheme of sorts ever since 1948, but it had fallen into disuse because trainees were virtually bound apprentices, and in the new conditions of doctor-shortage none were to be had. To implement the recommendations of the Todd Report, substantial extra payments were introduced to selected GPs to act as trainers in the vocational training scheme, with similar payments to District Course Organisers who began organizing day-release courses.

6. Local Health Authorities were encouraged to redeploy community nurses, health visitors and midwives from compact populations defined geographically ('patches') to relatively dispersed populations defined by registration with a practice ('GP attachments').

7. Limited fees-for-service were introduced to encourage GPs to take responsibility for contraceptive care and advice, and to do cervical smears.

The Package Deal had three main effects. It was the first evidence that any government was really concerned about the quality of general practice or its future, by committing new material resources which were not all routed via GPs' pockets.

This had a profound effect on morale, and created an atmosphere of goodwill which helped to break down earlier hostility between GPs and NHS administration. Secondly, it encouraged GPs to adopt elementary office organization and delegate some of the work they should have been doing (but were often unable to do) to office workers and nurses. This expanded unit of employed and attached staff has, with varying credibility, been referred to ever since as a 'Primary Care Team'. Thirdly, it introduced a subset of practices selected for vocational training which were generally innovative, better equipped and staffed, accepted some degree at least of audit and peer review, with some commitment to change, for if they had none of these they could and increasingly did, lose their privileged status. Roughly 15% of GPs are now trainers and 25% of practices are training practices.

Renewed Growth

The Package Deal underwrote the College by giving its independent ideology of general practice a material base. Most of the disincentives to investment in staff, premises and equipment were removed, and the College acquired a practical task supported by public funding, the development of vocational training. General practice became a more attractive career. By 1980, it was the first career choice of 37% of pre-registration doctors, twice the proportion favouring the runner-up, hospital internal medicine.[19] For the first time, many of the most successful students opted for general practice rather than consultancy.

There was a rapid expansion of vocational training schemes led by the College, which provided ideology and structure for postgraduate training superior to any other speciality, as well as 74% of the GP trainers. Two books, *The future general practitioner*[20] and *Teaching general practice*[21] became landmarks in medical education.

Sample surveys of training practices in 1970[22] and 1981[23] showed that the average training practice was indeed better staffed, organized and equipped than the average non-teaching practice: the results are shown in Table 4.1.

Table 4.1 Percentages of randomly-sampled training practices and all practices showing certain features in 1969, 1970, and 1981.

	all practices 1969[7]	training 1970[22]	training 1981[23]
Working from purpose-built premises	17%	40%	61%
Attached or employed staff:			
Manager or administrative secretary	—	38%	93%
Attached district nurse	—	80%	99%
Treatment room nurse	—	—	53%
Equipment possessed:			
Typewriter	69%	94%	—
Dictation machinery	38%	66%	—
Age-sex register	15%	65%	88%
Vaginal speculum	68%	97%	100%
Refrigerator	69%	87%	99%
Suture equipment	78%	83%	89%
Peak flow meter	5%	28%	87%
ECG	10%	37%	69%
Hold special clinics:			
Ante-natal	—	82%	90%
Immunizations	—	79%	83%
Cervical smears	—	55%	60%
Child care	—	50%	69%
High blood pressure	—	—	12%
Diabetes	—	—	3%
Patients seen at a rate of 12 per hour or more	—	31%	25%

The College provided organization, authority, and above all some evidence about what actually went on in general practice. It became a powerful medicopolitical body whose opinion had to be sought by government, or any other group with an interest in primary care. It acquired a Royal Charter in 1972, impressive premises in the most expensive part of London, and most of the costly and time-consuming pomposity apparently inevitable in such organizations. To the BMA nationally, and to the Local Medical Committees which guarded the BMA's policy at grassroots level, the

College became too big to be ignored; an occasionally necessary, useful and sometimes more attractive public face for general practice, but for that very reason a potential danger. The role of the Royal College of Physicians in 1948 as alternative negotiator with government was an obvious possibility for the Royal College of General Practitioners.

Limits of the Balint Paradigm

The first attempt by the College to define a credible new and independent territory for general practice lay in willingness to accept areas of psychosocial concern wider than those accepted by hospital specialists and more congruent with the actual concerns of patients. Starting from Balint, a generation of innovating GPs devoted most of their work to deepening and extending the individual doctor–patient encounter, linking this with development of local programmes for postgraduate vocational training.

This strategy was limited by three factors. First, later work[24] showed that, in practice if not in theory, the Balint style was still almost completely doctor-centred; doctors influenced by its philosophy gave patients little more opportunity to define medical problems in their own way than their more traditional colleagues. This weakness is of fundamental importance and will be discussed fully in Chapter 7.

The second limiting factor was more immediately obvious, and seriously reduced its appeal; the new territory claimed for GPs by the Balint style lay outside organic physical disease, the traditional core of clinical practice. The Balint style sought to modify medical behaviour on the psychosocial border territory around the management of organic disease, but left clinical management more or less untouched. The Balint style did imply more listening to the patient, but a general belief still persisted that specialists could remain as tunnel-visioned as before, delivering sound if unimaginative care for organic disease, aided by more sympathetic though technically less competent family doctors who would attend to the soul while specialists dealt with the body. In this scenario, the function of general practice could increasingly become the provision of a well-mannered and sympathetic explanation of clinical work done, more aloofly but also more effectively, by specialists. A philosophy of general practice which covered the periphery but not the centre of clinical medicine was unconvincing and unattractive to most doctors.

The third and final limiting factor was that in practice the Balint style, like the Osler paradigm, ignored social context. It did not ignore society in the ordinary way of complacent philistine technologists, by forgetting the effects of social class, occupation, or interactions with family, friends and personal enemies. On the contrary, like its holistic successors, its adherents took pride in their sensitivity to all the complex environmental factors influencing every case, each patient's problems being regarded as unique for this very reason, requiring personal evaluation and solution; but it continued to ignore the unique asset of British general practice, its defined population base.

An early achievement of independent GP philosophy, developed by James Mackenzie in the first years of the Osler paradigm, was to look at each encounter not as a self-contained episode, but as an event related to previous and subsequent events in the history of the same patient. The best GPs could do this better than most specialists, because they could more easily keep in touch with the patient before and after an illness. As Rosemary Stevens[25] first pointed out, the division of labour between GPs and specialists, uniquely early and uniquely complete in Britain compared with other nations, gave the patient to the GP and the illness to the specialist. Because of the clubs and then the Lloyd George capitation system, requiring registered lists which limited shopping around between doctors, GPs could, unlike the specialists, relate their work to identified populations at risk. Exceptional hospital physicians who understood this, for example John Ryle,[26] were unable to develop the idea fully precisely because they did not have such a listed population at risk. Registered patient lists made possible a scientific approach to management of illness in society, rather than in individual sick people. Specialists could only count the cases they saw, derived from a more or less unknowable and un-measurable source population; GPs could (but rarely did) relate the cases they saw to the local populations from which they came. This made it possible for them, and almost impossible for hospital-based specialists, to look at the most important uncharted territory in medical science; the inter-face between health and disease. A philosophy which perceived and built upon this hitherto neglected opportunity could challenge the Osler paradigm not at its periphery, as Balint had done, but at its centre. And not only challenge it, but defeat it, because the main front for progress in medical science now lies on that interface, rather than further refine-ments in terminal salvage.

Fusion of Epidemiology with Primary Care

The opposite of the one-person clinical medicine which has hitherto dominated GP philosophy is epidemiology, usually described as the study of disease in populations. But popula-tions are not simply collections of individuals, but parts of local communities; communities are parts of a society; societies are organized into states; and states act primarily in the interests of the dominant classes they represent to preserve and increase their wealth and power. The language of epidemiology is statistics, a word derived from the same root as the word 'state'. Epidemiology is inescapably a political subject, incapable of social neutrality. The assumptions of epidemiologists about society and its history necessarily and inevitably affect their choice of questions for study, the way they are asked, and the solutions they find credible, however much they conceal this from themselves and their readers by 'value-free' terminology.

Immediately before, during, and for a short time after World War II, epidemiology grew rapidly as a vigorous, innovative, and optimistic discipline, but the first generation of post-war GP philosophers did not connect with this; the Balint approach rarely looked beyond the family for its context.

Large-scale surveys of non-infective disease, such as the Framingham study of coronary heart disease in the USA, demonstrated the possibility of early diagnosis by active screening of populations, rather than later diagnosis by waiting for symptoms to be presented. In the USA this led to a profitable new frontier for fee-earning practice, the health-check industry, which now takes more time in US primary care than the management of disease. The effectiveness of such health-checks was never validated, but as they were sold to the public as a commodity, it never had to be. In Britain, presymptomatic screening threatened to extend primary care from a reactive to a proactive role, which would have incurred costs to the State. This was headed off by the full weight of established epidemiological authority.[27,28] The idea of presymptomatic screening was subjected to tests so severe, designed by people so lacking in street-wisdom, so innocent of the real problems and opportunities of primary care that adaptation of screening to general practice, and of general practice to screening, were confused, discouraged and delayed for a generation.

The socially crude techniques of screening used by epidemiological research were indeed generally ineffective for early diagnosis. In the Netherlands, Van den Dool,[29] assisted by a university team, screened his rural practice population of 4,000 three times, with successive response rates of 80%, 85% and 90%. Despite this high contact rate, he found this technique of repeated invitation or command call-up inappropriate to general practice and wasteful. Instead, he proposed what he called 'anticipatory care', but Establishment epidemiologists preferred to call 'case-finding'; systematic use of normal consultations initiated by patients, to create and maintain an updated, continuous record of variables important for health care and early recognition of reversible disease, whether or not they cause symptoms. Slowly at first, now at gathering speed, this is becoming the central feature of progressive general practice and its philosophy. Because in the NHS every person has their own GP, and GPs are gatekeepers to the whole medical care system, it is a potential basis for supercession of the entire Osler paradigm.

Anticipatory Care and Prevention

On the initiative of John Horder, President of the College, a working party was set up in 1980 to look at the GP's role in preventive medicine. The group decided to look at four very different fields of work in some detail, in order to make sure that its conclusions were so far as possible concrete, practical and usable by primary care teams in their ordinary conditions of work. These fields were family planning, child rearing and child health, psychiatry, and arterial disease; alcohol problems were added later, but handled in the same spirit. The reports of this Working Party and its subgroups[30-36] could, and probably will, become a turning point in development of the College and of British general practice.

In order to look systematically at what GPs were already doing about prevention, they had to match achievement against registered populations at risk. It was not long before they realized that this was necessary not only to study prevention, but also to look objectively at any other aspect of their work, including what had always been their central function, the management of disease; and also to realize that they were in this respect far in advance of hospital specialists, who were unable to evaluate their work in this way because they could not identify their populations at risk with precision. The practical tasks of prevention fused with systematic management of disease in the registered population in a single task of anticipatory care, verifiable by the simple but powerful technique of clinical audit, simply reviewing randomly-sampled patient-records in various groups. Combined with rapid advances in information technology, it began to seem possible that primary care teams serving registered populations could become largely self-regulating basic units in a fully rational health service, serving the health needs of the people with optimal effectiveness and economy.

The End of the Beginning, or the Beginning of the End?

Population-based primary care, planned and verified by local health workers, began to seem feasible by the early 1980s, but it faced four formidable difficulties: the threatening nature of the truths revealed by audit, the new resources and structure needed to deliver proactive care, the new social orientation required for effective accountability, and the rising political pressure to replace a unified health service serving all of the people by a two-tier service, with over-sold clinical extravagance for the rich, and perfunctory evasion supplemented by crisis-management for the poor.

The first of these difficulties is the theme of the next chapter. The last is the easy option for the substantial number of doctors who hope to be employed by rich people in a divided society, the privateers. The Osler paradigm helps them to retain credibility and self-respect. Though in a two-tiered service they would evade the real difficulties of the service and therefore the most socially relevant realities of medical science, they would control enough of the latest technology to give them a convincingly scientistic appearance. A majority of doctors, however, would still have to serve the losers in such a society, who would increasingly present the most serious medical problems. To them, the Osler paradigm will appear exhausted and unhelpful in solving the central clinical problem they will have to face, which the privateers evade; how to deliver medical science effectively, humanely and economically to the whole population, and continue to do so as science advances.

NOTES

1. Stewart, M., 'Unpaid public service', Fabian Pamphlets no. 3. London: Fabian Society, 1964.
2. Hadfield, S.J., 'A field survey of general practice 1951–2', *British Medical Journal 1953*; ii:683–706.
3. Cartwright, A., *Patients and their doctors: a study of general practice*, London: Routledge & Kegan Paul, 1967.
4. Collings, J.S., 'General practice in England today', *Lancet 1950*; i:555–85.
5. Peterson, O.L., Andrews, L.P., Spain, R.S., Greenberg, G.B., 'An analytical study of North Carolina general practice', *Journal of Medical Education 1956*; 31:1.
6. Clute, K.F., *The general practitioner*, Toronto: University of Toronto Press, 1963.

7. Irvine, D., Jeffreys, M., 'BMA Planning Unit survey of general practice 1969', *British Medical Journal 1971*; 4:535–43.
8. Review Body on Doctors' and Dentists' Remuneration (Danckwerts Committee), Seventh Report, HMSO, 1966.
9. Curwen, M., 'Lord Moran's ladder: a study of motivation in the choice of general practice as a career', *Journal of the College of General Practitioners 1964*; 7:38–65.
10. Barber, G., 'General practice today', *Lancet 1950*; i:781.
11. Balint, M., *The Doctor, his Patient and the Illness*, London: Pitman, 1957.
12. Forsyth, G., Logan, W.P.D., *Gateway or dividing line? A study of hospital outpatients in the 1960s*, Oxford: Oxford University Press, 1968.
13. Royal Commission on Medical Education 1965–68. (Todd) Report. Cmnd. 3569. London: HMSO, 1968.
14. Mechanic, D., 'General practice in England and Wales: results from a survey of a national sample of general practitioners', *Medical Care 1968*; 6:245–60.
15. Fulton, W.W., 'General practice in the USA', *British Medical Journal 1961*; i:275–82.
16. Batistella, R.M., Southby, R.M., 'Crisis in American medicine', *Lancet 1968*; i:581–6.
17. Klein, R., *The politics of the National Health Service*, London: Longman, 1983. This gives a good short account of the conflict before the Package Deal on pp. 87–9.
18. British Medical Association. Charter for the family doctor service, London: BMA, 1965.
19. Parkhouse, J., Campbell, M.G., Parkhouse, H.F., 'Career preferences of doctors qualifying in 1974–1980: a comparison of pre-registration findings', *Health Trends 1983*; 15:29–39.
20. Working Party of the Royal College of General Practitioners, *The future general practitioner: learning and teaching*, London: British Medical Association, 1972.
21. Cormack, J., Marinker, M., Morrell, D., *Teaching general practice*, London: Kluwer Medical, 1981.
22. Irvine, D., 'Teaching practices'. Report from general practice 15. London: Royal College of General Practitioners, 1972.
23. Freeling, P., Fitton, P., 'Teaching practices revisited', *British Medical Journal 1983*; 287:535–7.
24. Tuckett, D., Boulton, M., Olson, C., Williams, A., *Meetings between experts: an approach to sharing ideas in medical consultations*, London: Tavistock Publications, 1985.
25. Stevens, R., *Medical practice in modern England*, New York: Yale University Press, 1966.
26. Ryle, J., *Changing disciplines: lectures on the history, method and motives of social pathology*, Oxford: Oxford University Press, 1948.
27. Wilson, J.M.G., Jungner, G., 'Principles and practice of screening for disease', *Public Health Papers no. 34*, Geneva: WHO, 1968.
28. Hart, J.T., 'A theory of screening in primary care'. Chapter 2 in, Hart, C.R. (ed.), *Screening in general practice*, London: Churchill

Livingstone, 1975.
29. Van den Dool, C.W.A., 'Opsporing van chronische ziekten', in 'de huisartspraktijk mogelijkheden tot secundaire presentie', *Huisarts en Wetenschap 1970*; 13 pt 1:3–9. 'Surveillance van risicogroepen; anticiperende geneeskunde', *Huisarts en Wetenschap 1970*; 13:59–64.
30. 'Health and prevention in primary care: report of a Working Party appointed by the Council of the Royal College of General Practitioners', *Report from general practice 18*. London: RCGP, 1981.
31. 'Prevention of arterial disease in general practice: report of a Working Party appointed by the Council of the Royal College of General Practitioners'. *Report from general practice 19*. London: RCGP, 1981.
32. 'Prevention of psychiatric disorders in general practice: report of a Working Party appointed by the Council of the Royal College of General Practitioners'. *Report from general practice 20*. London: RCGP, 1981.
33. 'Family planning—an exercise in preventive medicine: report of a Working Party appointed by the Council of the Royal College of General Practitioners'. *Report from general practice 21*. London: RCGP, 1981.
34. 'Healthier children—thinking prevention: report of a Working Party appointed by the Council of the Royal College of General Practitioners'. *Report from general practice 22*. London: RCGP, 1981.
35. 'Promoting prevention: a discussion document prepared by a Working Party of the Royal College of General Practitioners'. *Occasional paper 22*. London: RCGP, 1983.
36. 'Alcohol—a balanced view'. *Report from general practice 24*. London: RCGP, 1986.

Chapter 5
MEASUREMENT OF OMISSION

When doctors began to measure their work, they measured what they saw and did, not what they didn't see and therefore couldn't do. Cobblers don't assess their work by counting barefoot children; like other entrepreneurs, doctors perceived their customers, not the population as a whole.

In 1966, before immunization against rubella (german measles) was available and abortion was legal only if a mother's life was in danger, I was consulted by a 42-year-old woman with an unplanned and unwanted sixth pregnancy. There were no reasonable grounds for abortion, though that is what I would have recommended, and what she would have wanted (we have discussed the matter since), had the 1967 Abortion Act then been in force. She had no apparent ill-health during the pregnancy, but her daughter was undersized at birth and had cataracts in both eyes, not large enough to impair vision, but sufficient to indicate the possibility of rubella damage during the first twelve weeks of pregnancy. This was later confirmed by impaired hearing and severe brain damage. She became autistic; withdrawn, self-mutilating and destructive. As she grew she became more difficult. She smashed all the windows in the house, which became like a cave. In the insensitive jargon of health economists, she became a high consumer of services, first on a largely futile journey around rival experts, later for special educational support, finally, as her exhausted relatives died or capitulated, for full-time residential care. All her older brothers and sisters were damaged in various ways by the demands made on them and their parents. Her father coped by heavy smoking and drinking and died of coronary thrombosis and diabetes in his early fifties.

Rubella vaccine became available in 1969, making it possible and ethically mandatory to prevent tragedies of this kind. DHSS policy was to immunize girls aged 11–13 at school. Knowing that school absence was normally about 20% on any one day, I wrote to the Medical Officer of Health for the District, asking for a list of Glyncorrwg girls who had not been immunized so that I could contact them and make sure they were all done. 'I can give you a list of the ones we did,' he replied, 'but how am I to know the ones we didn't?' What we needed then, and need now for all work not prompted by patient demand, was exactly that; not a list of acts, but a list of omissions.

Measuring What We Do

DHSS policy since 1970 has been to immunize all girls aged 11–13 through the schools medical service, screen all women of childbearing age for rubella antibody at ante-natal clinics, and immunize those still susceptible to infection; the programme has therefore relied on a variable and relatively uncoordinated mixture of initiatives from salaried school doctors, salaried hospital specialists and staff in training, and self-employed GPs in loosely-defined contract to provide primary care, with responsibility for the demands of individual patients, but not for their needs as a local population. Had this programme been fully implemented, rubella-damaged babies would be born only to mothers with a conscientious objection to abortion under any circumstances; in fact, malformations associated with rubella in pregnancy have not fallen significantly, nor have terminations of pregnancy for rubella exposure.[1]

David Andrewes,[2] a GP in Telford new town, set up an age-sex register for his practice as his starting-point for a locally-organized campaign to implement DHSS policy in his own population. Figs. 5.1 and 5.2 show the planned change he brought about.

Fig. 5.1 Analysis of Telford practice age-sex register on 1 July 1980 to show percentages of 'rubella-protected' and 'rubella-risk' patients by age.

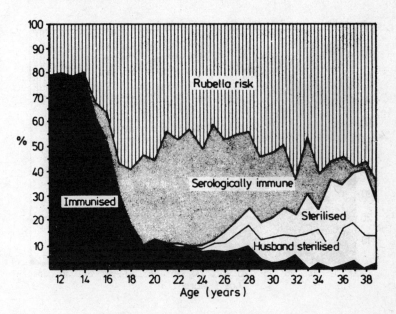

Source: Fig. 1. Andrewes, D.A., 'Rubella immunization: whose baby?' *British Medical Journal 1983*; 287:1769–71.

In 1978, before his reorganization, half the 3,143 female patients aged 10–40 were still at risk for rubella. After reorganization, verified by three cycles of audit and action over five years, only 15% were at risk. He concluded that the GP team is better placed than any other agency to implement prevention policies of this kind, because it can set up an accurate register of the target population, is in frequent contact with it and has its confidence, and already has access to personal, often highly confidential data (in this case, vasectomies and hysterectomies) necessary for accurate decisions.

He also analyzed costs: it cost the practice £30 to identify and immunize each non-immune patient aged 14–40. The DHSS fee paid to the doctor was £2.80. The relation between

Fig. 5.2 Analysis of Telford practice age-sex register on 1 July 1983 to show percentages of 'rubella-protected' and 'rubella-risk' patients by age.

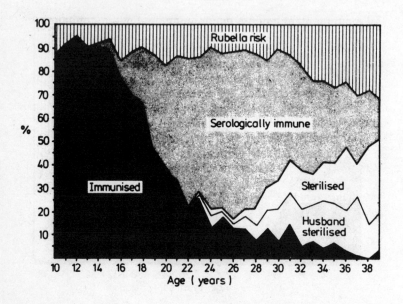

Source: Fig. 2. Andrewes, D.A., 'Rubella immunization: whose baby?' *British Medical Journal 1983*; 287:1769–71.

costs and practice earnings has not changed since.

This example shows that in the particular case of foetal rubella damage, an important new scientific advance has been generally delivered to only about half the people who could benefit from it, despite the existence of a National Health Service freely accessible to the whole population. Failures may be occurring at four points. First, the strategy was devised centrally, probably with little attention to the views and experience of the various health workers who would actually have to implement it. Secondly, insufficient thought may have been given to co-ordination of national health education campaigns with work by local GPs, primary care teams, and school medical services.[3] Thirdly, specific local targets were not set, local audit procedures were not planned, and divisions of labour and responsibility between the three possible sources of care were not agreed, probably not even discussed. Finally, the balance of income and expenditure for independently contracted GPs was not considered; economic disincentives were ignored, and little was done to motivate staff by focusing attention on local evidence of the social costs of failure, the scale on which failure persisted, or on their eventual achievement.

The Rule of Halves

Not only rubella immunization, but a wide range of other clinical work, is delivered to 50% or less of the people who need it.

The 'Rule of Halves' was first described by Wilber and Barrow[4] in the USA, for detection and management of high blood pressure; half the people with high blood pressure were not detected, half those detected were not treated, half those treated were not controlled. Numerous studies have confirmed similar or worse figures in Britain,[5-8] with damning evidence of consequent premature and preventable deaths from stroke, heart failure and accelerated kidney failure.[9] The Rule can be broken and made obsolete, using precisely the repeated cycles of audit and action used so successfully by Andrewes to improve his local population's protection from rubella; but it does not change spontaneously, without organized effort. Without permanently sustained work, passivity and inertia reassert themselves. The examples I quote are from practices willing to allow their work to be evaluated objectively, and therefore represent above-average practice. The rule is obsolete only where vigorous pioneering work has been done and then maintained for at least one generation of staff. No one seriously suggests that this has yet occurred in more than a small minority of practices, certainly not more than 10%.

Depending on definitions and social class, high blood pressure affects from 7% to 25% of the adult population. It is one of four principal underlying causes of arterial brain damage (stroke) and coronary heart disease, the others being smoking, high blood fat (cholesterol) and diabetes. Smoking is also the commonest and most important cause of most chronic lung disease, closely followed by asthma (reversible airways obstruction). Atmospheric pollution, which was a major cause of chronic lung disease until the Clean Air Acts of 1956 and 1968 transformed Britain's urban environment with a success we have too quickly forgotten, is now a subordinate cause. Chronic lung disease can also be a cause of heart failure, and in practice disability and early death are more often than not attributable to multiple causes. Knowledge of variables related to stroke, coronary disease, diabetes and chronic lung disease, such as blood pressure, blood cholesterol, blood sugar, Peak Expiratory Flow Rate (PEFR), body weight in relation to height, evidence of early eye damage in diabetes and average daily cigarette and alcohol consumption, are essential to effective limitation of damage to health by these diseases, which together account for nearly two-thirds of all deaths under 65.

The only evidence we have on how much GPs attend to these underlying causes and mechanisms is what they write in their patients' records. For practical purposes, work not recorded is either work not done, or information wasted. Wherever we look at these records, the Rule of Halves (or worse) applies unless and until the cycle of audit and action begins. Four studies including data from 21,296 records relating to patients aged 25-64 held by 103 GPs showed that smoking habits had ever been recorded in only 22-50% of records;[5-8,10] here the Rule of Halves is not even average, but the best quality attained.

Cigarette smoking is now generally accepted as the most important single avoidable cause of ill-health and premature death in Britain, mainly through its effects on coronary heart disease, leg artery disease (particularly in diabetics), lung cancer and chronic obstructive airways diseases (asthma, emphysema and chronic bronchitis). How can doctors manage such diseases or help to prevent them, if they don't even know whether their patients smoke? Respiratory disease accounts for 22% of all GP consultations, by far the biggest single category, but these still tend to be wasted on largely futile reactive treatment for symptoms, and by antibiotics which have at most a brief palliative effect. The most powerful measure of function, predictor of mortality,[11] and educational tool for management of nearly all chronic lung damage is the degree of airflow obstruction, easily measured by GPs with a Peak Expiratory Flow meter. By 1977, 77% of GPs possessed these meters,[12] but of 90 asthma deaths in the West Midland and Mersey regions in 1979 studied by a committee of the British Thoracic Association,[13] serial measurements of airway obstruction had only been made for three out of 26 patients under regular hospital out-patient supervision, and one out of 42 who had regular supervision from their GP. Despite the enormous number of consultations for respiratory symptoms, few are used proactively to build up useful information for prevention of chronic disease.

Evidence on care of diabetics is particularly instructive, because they are a relatively large, well-defined group at high risk, particularly of coronary heart disease, for whom regular monitoring is essential. A minority of diabetics depend on insulin injections requiring frequent monitoring of blood sugar levels and adjustment of treatment. Doctors looking after insulin-dependent diabetics need not only sufficient training (which most of them have), but also sufficient numbers of patients to maintain expertise; these numbers do not exist in single-handed practice, and can only be created in group practice by concentrating patients in one clinic and responsibility for their care in one doctor, still an unusual arrangement in British group practice. We are in a period of rapid technical innovation for insulin-dependent diabetes, which requires more rather than less specialist commitment. At least for the next decade, it is unlikely that GPs generally will be able to undertake independent care of insulin-dependent diabetics routinely, and it will for the most part remain a task for specialized hospital clinics or diabetic day-centres of the type pioneered in Ipswich.

The position is entirely different for the much larger number of non-insulin dependent diabetics (maturity-onset or Type II diabetics) who now strain the resources of hospital diabetic clinics, though their care is generally simple, chiefly requiring sustained teaching in the nature of diabetes, the requirements of dietary control and risk factors for arterial disease, and simple monitoring for blood sugar control and arterial, eye and kidney damage once or twice a year. All this is well within the competence of any GP, but it needs protected time which few are organized to provide. Epidemiological screening studies[14] have shown that 2% of the adult population have diabetes, but only 1% are known before screening or intensive case-finding; the Rule of Halves again. Doney[15] looked at all the known diabetics in a practice population of 20,000; roughly a quarter of them were attending a hospital out-patient clinic, another quarter were seeing the GP from time to time, but half were not having any medical supervision for their diabetes, just repeat prescriptions from a receptionist. Worst of all, when he sorted them out into those with and without complications (diseased leg nerves and arteries, damage to the kidney or retina), diabetics with complications were just as likely to be without supervision as the uncomplicated cases. Diabetes is now the commonest cause of blindness, but although diabetic damage to the retina is preventable by laser treatment if it is recognized quickly, only one third of diabetics with retinal damage are recognized early enough to benefit from treatment.[16] Figures from a recent study[17] of seven practices in Southampton with a total population of 50,500 were better than in Doney's study, with 56% of all known diabetics seeing their GP, 46% attending a hospital clinic, and 22% having care from both sources; but 20% of all known cases were still having no regular care from anyone, and the overall prevalence of 0.85% suggests that half their diabetics were not detected. Over half the non-insulin-dependent diabetics without symptoms were originally diagnosed by routine urine tests on admission to hospital for other reasons, suggesting that their GPs were not searching for diabetes routinely in high-risk groups.

A Rule of Halves again, this time for non-insulin-dependent diabetes: half are not known, and roughly half of those known are not getting adequate treatment. This estimate is derived from evidence of audits of the quality of care when patients with uncomplicated non-insulin-dependent diabetes are taken out of a hospital clinic and returned to the care of their GPs. Two large studies of this kind have been published. One in Sheffield in 1980[18] was an audit of the performance of 75% of GPs in the city who had agreed to take responsibility for follow-up of non-insulin-dependent diabetics. It showed that 41% of patients were being seen by their GPs only on the patients' initiative or not at all; only 23% were being seen at regular intervals. About half had high levels of blood sugar, and one-third had evidence of arterial disease in their legs. The second, published in 1987, was in Ipswich,[19] in an area of low morbidity generally considered to provide a high quality of GP care. All but one practice in the town participated in a shared-care scheme in which GPs agreed to follow up their own patients, with review in a hospital clinic two years later. When this was done, 44% had no entries at all in their co-operation records, and 31% had never had any check on their diabetes by their GPs in the whole 2-year period. Even of the 69% who had had some kind of review, 27% had never been weighed, 42% never had blood pressure checked, 44% never had any examination of the eye and 60% had no tests for blood glucose.

Authors of the Sheffield study concluded:

Large clinics are short of staff and must shed some workload: but busy general practitioners attuned to contractual obligations and. . . five-minute appointments may not eagerly seek out extra work. Even if they do, they will probably have to pay themselves for the detection and pursuit of non-attenders. . . we must acknowledge that general practice must not be separated from modern hospital technology. Any excessive use [of technology] in hospital does not excuse its absence in the community, and having demonstrated that 'straightforward' cases may not be so straightforward after all, the practitioner must be enabled to take a detailed interest in patients at special risk.

Does accurate management of diabetes make any difference to outcome? There is now a large, generally consistent body of evidence that strict control of blood sugar is effective in delaying damage to the retina, kidneys and leg nerves,[20,21] that control of smoking delays damage to coronary and leg arteries and to the kidneys,[22] control of blood fats delays damage to coronary and leg arteries, and control of high blood pressure in diabetics prevents strokes and delays kidney failure.[23]

Hospital out-patient clinics, overworked and understaffed, are far from perfect even in providing the simple monitoring and patient education required by most patients, and are expensive, inconvenient, and time-wasting for patients compared with what can be done by a properly organized GP team; but they do as a rule guarantee a minimum level of organization essential to safe care, which is simply not available from most GPs. Hayes and Harries[24] in Cardiff did the critical experiment. After agreement with local GPs on a follow-up protocol, they randomly allocated 200 non-insulin-dependent diabetics attending the hospital out-patient clinic to either continued hospital care, or follow-up by their own GP. The fate of both groups was reviewed five years later. Only 14% of patients in the GP group had their diabetes reviewed at least once a year, compared with 100% in the hospital group, and 18 died in the GP group compared with 6 in the hospital group.

This classic study attracted little attention when it was published, because it seemed only to confirm what specialists already believed: that GPs can't be trusted with even the simplest long-term management of chronic disease, and if specialists want the job done properly they must do it themselves. Reviewing 27 consecutive emergency admissions for diabetic ketoacidotic coma (an immediately life-threatening condition usually caused by neglected gross diabetes), Pyke[25] found that 15 of these were in previously undiagnosed diabetics. In 12 of the 15 urine had never been tested for sugar, although they had visited their GPs a total of 41 times. This picture of frequent incompetence or neglect was confirmed by a larger study of deaths in diabetics under 50 years of age.[26]

Who actually does most of the routine medical work in hospital diabetic clinics? Not consultants, but junior doctors in training, backed by a team of nurses, dieticians, chiropodists and office workers; and most of these junior medical staff will within a year or two become GPs themselves. How do the young princes from the out-patient clinic become frogs in general practice? At British standards of undergraduate medical education, clinical expertise is rarely a problem until lost through disuse, and GPs are better placed than most hospital doctors to adapt advice to patients' individual needs and maintain personal continuity of care, both key factors in obtaining good compliance. The critical differences between specialized hospital clinics and customary general practice are in staffing and organization. In hospital clinics, medical staff have protected time devoted entirely to diabetic care, undisturbed by competing demands; routine tasks are performed according to a more or less standardized protocol, with a division of labour between doctors, nurses, technicians and administrative staff; and patients are followed up actively, given further appointments at planned intervals, with reminders sent to defaulters. Except for a small minority of GPs who have set up their own diabetic mini-clinics, GP care of diabetics is prompted not by the predictable needs of patients for regular follow-up, but by their demands for relief of symptoms, often either irrelevant to their diabetes, or resulting from organ damage which could and should have been prevented.

Management of Chronic Disease

It has often been said that modern medicine has exchanged early mortality for chronic morbidity. Having almost wiped out dangerous acute diseases like pneumonia and other serious infections in relatively young people, it has left the problems of chronic degenerative disease as the greater part of clinical medicine. There certainly is less acute disease today, mainly because most people live better, and what's left is mostly easier to treat effectively; but the burden of serious chronic disease in middle age is also less, not least because premature ageing of organs and body-systems is caused in part by the cumulative effects of successive acute illnesses. The Osler Paradigm concentrated attention on crisis-intervention, and on initial diagnosis rather than long-term management, because it was based on the generally episodic view of disease available to specialists working in hospitals. The management of chronic disease was despised and neglected, and its long-overdue recognition today is itself an important conceptual advance.

The central problem of medical care now is the effective and economic management of chronic disease throughout the whole population, in such a way as to limit damage and conserve health. In Glyncorrwg, starting in 1968 with screening of our whole population aged 20-64 for arterial blood pressure and smoking,[27,28] we have searched through the population for other early indicators of common conditions which shorten or substantially impair life. Supplemented by occasional call-up screening, we have obtained our data by extending ordinary consultations, averaging 4.5 per patient per year, to include measurements of blood pressure (BP), cigarette and alcohol consumption, Peak Expiratory Flow Rate (PEFR), weight and height in the whole population, and biochemical indicators of alcohol damage and diabetes where suspicion of these conditions is high. We have aimed at updating all this information at least once every five years in everyone aged 20-64. Out of a total registered population of 1,656 in 1987, there were 1,185 men and women aged 20 or more. Table 5.1 shows the prevalence in our population of high blood pressure, symptomatic arterial disease, obesity, chronic lung disease, diabetes and alcohol problems of sufficient severity to require active medical management (diagnostic criteria are given below the Table).

Even to cope with diabetes, the least common of these conditions, is too big a task for hospital out-patient clinics, and they are seeing only those patients identified and referred under the Rule of Halves. If all cases of diabetes in the general population were found, and all were referred, the hospital out-patient load would be about three times as great as it is. There is no way that more than a small minority of patients with these and other common and important conditions such as epilepsy, rheumatoid arthritis, atopic dermatitis, psoriasis or schizophrenia, can all be followed up regularly in hospital

Table 5.1 Prevalence of six common chronic conditions in Glyncorrwg adults aged 20+ in 1987.

Condition	Number	Per cent
All adults 20+	1,185	100%
Chronic lung disease	275	23%
Obesity	208	18%
High blood pressure	129	11%
Alcohol problems	94	8%
Arterial disease	81	7%
Diabetes	35	3%

Criteria for diagnosis: Chronic lung disease = PEFR 50% or less of expected value for age and height; obesity = Body Mass Index 30+; high blood pressure = mean diastolic BP 105 mmHg or more age 40+, 100 mmHg or more under 40, mean of 3 separate readings; arterial disease = typical symptoms of angina pectoris, claudication, or cerebro-vascular disease; diabetes = blood glucose >12 mmol or glycosylated haemoglobin >8%.

out-patient clinics. The minority who really need consultant care are those presenting special difficulties in management, and are unsuitable for routine care by inexperienced junior medical staff.

Doctors who have not worked outside big university centres may imagine that this intelligently divided and shared responsibility between specialists and GPs is what we have now. In industrial areas at least, it remains exceptional; for the most part, GPs and hospital consultants seem to run two entirely independent services, operating at different social and technical levels, with different sets of expectations from both doctors and patients. Patients get referred by GPs not because they need specialist skills, but because, for whatever reason (not enough time, not enough organization, not enough reading or clinical discussion, not enough confidence), the GP cannot cope with them; and specialists finally return patients to their GPs not because they think the primary care team will do a better job than the hospital team, but because they consider patients' problems to be solved, insoluble, trivial or imaginary. Doctors in charge of both systems seem to be so hurried that few have the energy, optimism, imagination or time to attempt any rationally planned division of labour between the two, and the structure of the NHS is such that if neither GPs nor consultants are prepared to organize the interface between them, nobody else will.

Hospital Outreach

Like all good doctors, specialists trying to advance their subject also want to move beyond salvage to anticipatory care. Having little confidence that GPs will undertake regular supervision of important chronic disease, they usurp their functions by expanding out-patient facilities, sending out teams for home care, encouraging direct self-referral by patients in emergencies, and even by organizing their own community screening clinics. In the least deprived areas where progress is possible, hospital clinics or day centres are set up not only for long-term care of diabetes, but for high blood pressure, epilepsy, asthma, migraine, premenstrual tension, phobic neuroses, rheumatoid arthritis, multiple sclerosis, psoriasis, and virtually every other complaint that is neither self-limiting nor curable, but requires some kind of continued medical supervision. In cities, and particularly within easy reach of teaching hospitals, general practice can become a clinical desert where GPs abdicate responsibility not only for major episodic disease, but also for conservation of health and continuing care of chronic illness.

Passive transfer of elementary care to hospitals is reinforced by the expectations of patients. Ann Cartwright[29] found that 42% of people randomly sampled in 1964 would expect to refer themselves directly to the nearest hospital casualty department (emergency room) for a cut leg which seemed to need stitching. Other similar questions were repeated in her 1977 study,[12] permitting an estimate of trends: 37% in 1964, rising to 51% in 1977, would expect their GP to refer them to hospital for cutting out a small cyst, 30% (32%) for a blood test, 18% (14%) for a vaginal examination, and 12% (23%) for a sprained ankle. 24% of adults in the 1964 sample (36% in 1977) had been to hospital as an out-patient some time during the previous 12 months. Two thirds of these were referrals by GPs, the rest were referrals from dentists, works medical departments, self-referrals to Accident and Emergency, and recalls by the hospital itself for continued follow-up, with little change between 1964 and 1977. Nearly a quarter of those who had been to hospital out-patients had been attending for the same condition for a year or more, and 5% had been attending for 5 years or more. The data suggest a slowly increasing tendency for clinical responsibility to slide toward hospital outpatient care.

DHSS data generally confirm this, but the increase in outpatient referrals is not uniform and may be tapering off, possibly indicating improvement in the quality of GP care. Fig. 5.3 shows the trend for numbers of new out-patients referred from 1971 to 1985. It also shows the trend for new patients seen in Accident and Emergency departments; this is rising more rapidly, with no indication that the rate of increase is diminishing.

In 1981-2, hospital out-patient costs represented 12% of all hospital expenditure, at an average cost to the NHS of about £50 for each new referred out-patient, compared with £5 for each patient who consults a GP, and nothing at all for patients who discuss their ailments with their local chemist, as a Conservative Health Minister, Dr Gerard Vaughan, pointed out in a speech to the Pharmaceutical Association in 1984. 'We have a climate for change,' he said, 'and the government is willing to contemplate it. . . we could see some quite rapid changes.' We could indeed, and regardless of evidence on the quality of GP care of chronic disease compared with hospital out-patient clinics, further extensions of hospital outreach are unlikely to be encouraged by the DHSS. Nor is it likely to encourage screening campaigns to identify more cases of early and more treatable disease; if hospital diabetic and high blood pressure clinics are overworked now, why double their burden by finding all the people who would benefit from skilled management of their health problems?

Fig. 5.3 New patients attending NHS hospital Out-patient and Accident & Emergency departments in the United Kingdom, 1971–85.

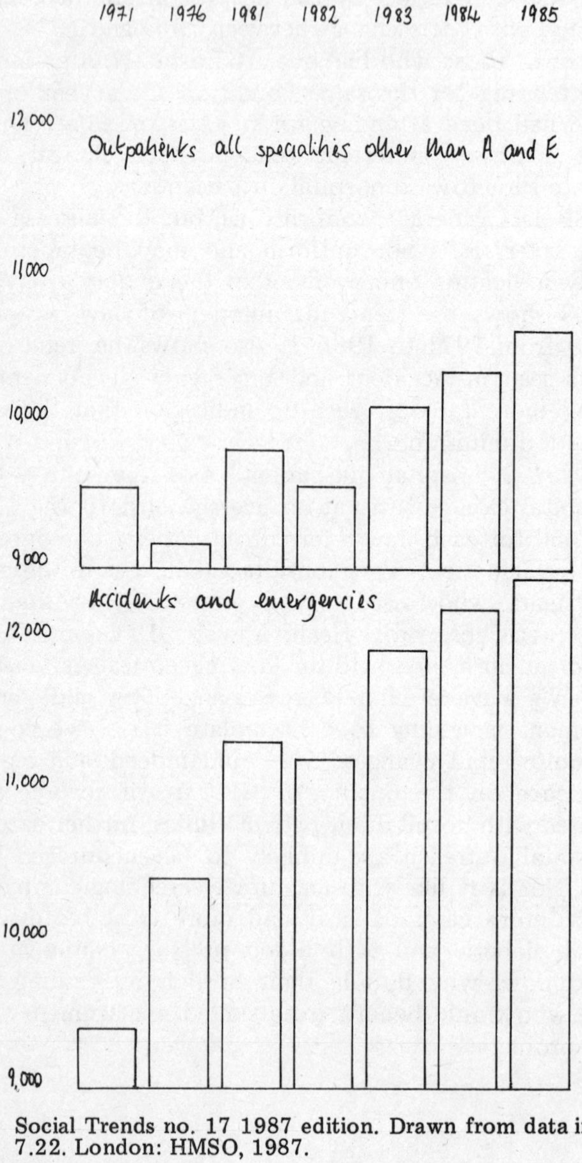

1971   1976   1981   1982   1983   1984   1985

12,000

Outpatients all specialities other than A and E

11,000

10,000

9,000

Accidents and emergencies

12,000

11,000

10,000

9,000

Source: Social Trends no. 17 1987 edition. Drawn from data in Table 7.22. London: HMSO, 1987.

Reactive and Proactive Care

This chapter has given evidence that medical care as now organized for the general population is failing to deliver simple and effective scientific advances, which require little technical skill to implement (though considerable social skills), and lie at the heart of traditional clinical medicine.

In the Osler Paradigm, patients initiate episodes of medical care, prompted by symptoms of disease which they can perceive and are eventually unable to ignore. Patients initiate medical transactions as customers, and doctors respond passively to their demands, however active their treatment may later become. If patients are well off, they pay; if they are poor, a civilized society sees to it that care of some kind will be provided. Either way, medical care is reactive to patient initiative.

In the new paradigm, doctors must still respond to demand, for this is the only ultimate guarantee that patients' wants will be included in the medical definition of needs. The right of patients to direct access to their own personal doctor and to present their own demands, so that their definitions of what is important have ultimate priority over the opinions of doctors or any other health workers, is a necessary and important element of democratic control which to some extent at least people already have, and should never give up. The new paradigm should, in this as in most other respects, include and surpass rather than eliminate the old.

Even so, however, patients are not customers, but joint producers (with professionals) of solutions to their problems, and as care concentrates less on salvage and more on prevention, as it adopts a more anticipatory style, its initiation must depend less upon symptomatic demand, and more upon perceptions of need, which initially at least must be medical perceptions. As better living, better care, and more effective medical science make gross end-stage disease less common and crises exceptional, GPs will have actively to search for needs, and take the initiative in organizing health maintenance in the small local populations for which they are responsible. People with chronic lung disease should not have to be blue in the face, coughing up a cupful of sputum a day, barely able to climb the stairs in their own home, and then have to face the fact that their lungs are irreversibly damaged and untreatable. Overweight people should not already have irreversible arthritis in their knees and hips or diabetes, and only then be told that they must change the eating habits of a lifetime and join a long waiting list for new joints. People with high blood pressure should not have to wait for a stroke before their exceptional risk is recognized and controlled. People with alcohol problems should be helped before their lives have been wrecked, and diabetics should be helped to get their blood glucose controlled before they go blind, their kidneys fail and their toes drop off. All these conditions start with few or no symptoms, and all of them are more simply, easily and effectively treated early rather than late in their otherwise inevitable progression.

Wherever we look in medicine, we find the same pattern; early recognition and management of disease is simpler, cheaper and more effective than salvage. There is good evidence, for example, that epilepsy becomes more difficult to control the longer it continues without effective treatment,[30] and that delay in initial management of schizophrenia is associated with poor control of the disease later on.[31] Experience shows that optimal control of epilepsy in the community urgently requires both organized anticipatory care by GPs, and locally agreed divisions of labour between GPs and specialists.[32] The entry point seems immaterial; whatever disease we choose, the answers seem to be the same; we need earlier, more active diagnosis, a more open attitude to patients and to our colleagues, and an anticipatory style that begins to take some of the panic out of medical care.

People do not, in general, demand treatment for causes of diseases they don't yet have. A customer-provider relationship even in a free service supported by the State, must always mean delayed and less effective treatment of people who, at least initially, cope with risks by denying them; and that means most people, most of the time. This cannot be corrected by encouraging doctors with fees, for over-diagnosis and hasty treatment may then easily become more dangerous than the marginal risks they claim to control. If medical science is to be delivered effectively to the people, anticipatory care must stop being regarded as an optional extra, to be encouraged by this or that special incentive; it must become the heart of good practice. If the terms and conditions of GP service discourage this, they must be changed.

The Authority of Hospital Specialism

The much greater authority of hospital specialists makes them appear to the public and to government as the only conceivable innovators in applied medical science. Patients may conform with advice from a hospital specialist which they would ignore from their own GP, because the specialist is associated with big, dangerous, but effective medical care which they ignore at their peril. They see GPs, on the other hand, as generally perfunctory men, who need not be taken more seriously by their patients than they appear to take themselves; the only defence offered for the GPs in the Sheffield and Ipswich studies of diabetics was that when patients were returned to the care of their own GPs they generally interpreted this as evidence that they were 'cured', despite explicit advice that they were still diabetic and needed follow-up as much as before. If, they may have reasoned, they really had an important problem, surely they would not have been returned to the care of a mere GP?

The authority of hospital specialists has been built up by nearly a century of social custom and experience, reinforced by deference, fear and the popular belief that scientific attitudes can be expressed only through incomprehensible jargon and intimidating technology used by men in white coats. The future authority of GPs and primary care teams will have to be earned by public experience of work done more efficiently, more humanely, more effectively and in fact more scientifically (though less scientistically) in community care than in hospital clinics, limited as they are by excessive size, discontinuity of staff, and isolation from the other problems patients face in managing changed behaviour or chronic illness. Hospital outreach clinics close to the community, like the diabetic day-centres pioneered in Ipswich after the failure of the initial trial discussed earlier in this book, which are being taken up with enthusiasm by the British Diabetic Association as a model for future care, may prove a useful half-way house, transmitting the organizational traditions of specialists to general practice. However, there are potential difficulties, particularly for older non-insulin dependent diabetics, who nearly always have multiple problems. At some point there will either be wasteful duplication and re-creation of the skills of general practice at a new site, or the care of diabetes and its complications will become isolated from anticipatory care of other causes of ill-health. Creation of a wide range of specialized day-centres, for example for asthma, epilepsy, obesity, schizophrenia or rheumatoid arthritis, would only be workable either if cases were carefully selected, as they are supposed to be now for outpatient referral, or if the entire strategy of general-practice-based primary care were abandoned in favour of primary specialism on the Soviet polyclinic model, leaving whatever would be left of clinical general practice to wither on the branch. In general, it seems to me they will work well if they are used as a bridge aiming at expansion of the range and quality of primary care rather than its replacement, but GPs cannot defend territory they have failed to occupy.

Anticipatory care should also be based on realistic estimates of risk, which are often small in absolute if not in relative terms; even a man who is two or three times as likely to die from a heart attack as his average neighbour usually has only a small risk of dying within the next year or two, and fear of death is ultimately a less effective educational weapon than love of life.

In the eyes of government, the advantage of GPs and primary care teams over hospital specialists is that they are relatively cheap. Once we accept that clinical and organizational standards in community care could and should be as high as in hospitals much of the price advantage of general practice disappears; it is a fundamentally weak argument, which GPs and their professional organizations use at their peril.

The real advantage of GPs is that they are closer to the population. Fig. 5.4 illustrates the point. On the left hand side is the familiar medical career pyramid of the Osler paradigm, with a few clever people at the top doing expensive things to a few highly selected patients, and a lot of less successful doctors at the bottom, who have fallen off Lord Moran's ladder to do unexciting, undemanding work in the general population. On the right we see the pyramid pushed over, perhaps by some such cataclysmic social event as the 1945 election. Having been trained almost entirely by specialists in hospitals, young doctors still tend to roll down to the bottom, where as many as possible become consultants. Those who cannot become specialists still try so far as possible to mimic them, and therefore feel more comfortable with sick patients than people at risk, apart from the fact that they are generally far too busy dealing with illness to think much about health. In search of the sort of substantial organ damage they were trained on in hospitals, they get as far away as they can from the source population, and therefore also pile up on the right, their faces still turned to the hospital and their backs to their communities.

Now let us suppose that a disease becomes newly recognizable and reversible at a pre-symptomatic stage, so that late presentation with symptoms represents clinical failure rather than success: then the GPs halfway down the inclined plane are in a better position to reach the population at risk than the specialists, though even so, their orientation must change if they are to get there.

The number of diseases detectable at a presymptomatic stage is now increasing, and will do so faster as molecular biology begins to influence medical practice. A *Lancet* editorial[33] bravely entitled 'Cancer of the cervix: death by incompetence' provides a simple example of the practical implications of this trend. In England and Wales cervical cancer kills about 2,000 women each year. Since cytological (cervical smear) screening began on a large scale in 1964,

Fig. 5.4

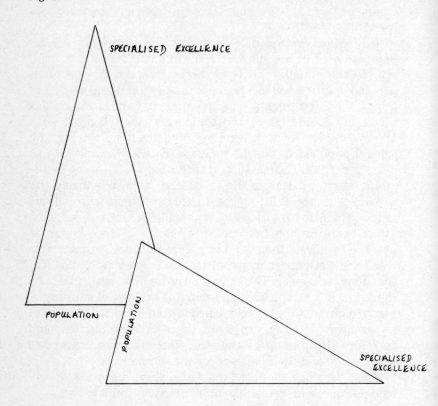

Left: the professional pyramid of the Osler paradigm.
Right: the inclined plane of population-based anticipatory care.

mortality from cancer of the cervix has fallen at a rate of about 1% a year, about the same as the rate at which it had been falling for several decades before screening began, though there are many more hysterectomies for other reasons (and therefore fewer women at risk). We are now doing about 3 million smear tests a year, about 40,000 smears per life saved; hardly an efficient performance. The position is the same in Norway, which like Britain adopted a policy of leaving the initiative with GPs, hospital specialists, and clinic doctors to use the laboratory service in whatever way they wished, without any organized plan.

By contrast, in Aberdeen (where Dugald Baird fought for and achieved a unique gynaecologically liberated area), and in Finland, Denmark, Iceland and Sweden, with resources and costs similar to our own, mortality has fallen and continues to fall, and prevention programmes are cost-effective. These successful programmes have three features in common:

1. They are organized as public-health cancer-control programmes, specifically directed towards a reduction in mortality; that is their explicit objective. They are not simply laboratory services for providing clinical investigation facilities to be used at doctors' discretion.
2. They call up the age-groups at greatest and most immediate risk (30+) and they keep on trying. They concentrate first on women who have never had a smear at all. They use population registers.
3. Real people are in charge: they have names and telephone numbers and can be held to account.

The failed programmes in Britain and Norway, the *Lancet* went on to say, have none of these. Their objectives are stated only in terms of process (to provide a cytology service) rather than outcome (to reduce mortality). No one is in charge, and no one is either praised for success or rebuked for failure. Instead we have a clumsy all-carrots and no-sticks policy, offering a fee to GPs for one smear every 5 years in women over 35, but no other pressure on GPs to provide a service. Despite the fee-for-service incentive, most GP smears are performed in young women, and in the same women again and again, proving once more that most GPs still do not plan their work even to maximize profit, but respond passively to patient demand. Young women are better informed and have higher expectations than older women at higher risk, their expectations have rightly been raised by women's magazines and discussions on TV and radio, and by experience at Family Planning clinics which work to protocol. The result is that a minority of better-informed, generally younger women of higher social class and at relatively low risk return regularly for tests every two or three years, while many in the highest risk-groups remain untested.

Fig. 5.5 shows how the percentage of women in Glyncorrwg aged 35–64 who had cervical smears within the previous 5 years rose from 20% in 1982 to 83% in 1986.

We were able to make these measurements because we knew the names and addresses of our whole population, we knew who had a uterus and who hadn't, and we knew who only answered the back door because she owed money to a debt-collector. All this knowledge, though accessible to us more easily than any other agency, required work to obtain, and our point of departure (20% of women with smears done in the past 5 years) was the same as that estimated for all practices in the National Morbidity survey of 1971.[34] As the *Lancet*'s editorial suggested, our objective was to wipe out cervical cancer as a cause of death in Glyncorrwg, and so far we have succeeded (the last two deaths from the disease both occurred here in 1963), but until 1986 this was more by luck than good judgement. What happened in 1986? We employed a nurse to call up the age-groups at greatest risk and keep on trying; she has a name, a telephone number, and gives account of her work to the practice team. We meet the *Lancet* criteria, and can do so more easily, more sensitively, more effectively, and more cheaply than any other local agency.

This example is too simple to serve as a complete model for the whole of anticipatory care, because few other diseases are so simple to recognize and treat at this very early stage, but the basic principles are the same. Cervical cancer is not the only area in which Britain is losing its post-war position as one of the world's healthiest nations; Britain now has

Fig. 5.5 Percentages of women in Glyncorrwg aged 35-64 who had cervical smears within the previous 5 years in 1982, and in 1986.

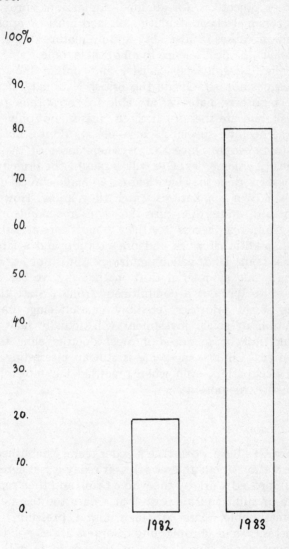

Western Europe's highest all-causes death rate in middle age.[35] These three principles, specified outcome rather than process objectives for defined populations, proactive care and personal accountability, can and must be applied to all common causes of disability and premature death, if we are to deliver medical science to all of the people.

Unlike hospital specialists, and unlike most of their colleagues abroad, GPs in the British National Health Service have registered patients, are able to know their population at risk, and are therefore able to measure not only what they do (as hospital specialists have always done), but what has yet to be done. Since that is where most of the future of clinical medicine lies, GPs will in fact be the principal natural innovators, once they have learned to make clinical discoveries in their own populations which they know. However, they need to do more than turn their eyes and minds in this new direction; real access to their population at risk requires much additional work and organization and a larger, more diverse team, all of which incurs costs. It is not just a spiritual change, but a material shift in the way we use our social resources. Without a commitment from a State that shares these social priorities, credibly guaranteeing that this re-direction of social investment will actually take place, we should not be surprised if most doctors cling to the old paradigm. Clinical medicine is still an interesting and well-paid occupation, even when practised incompletely and far below its true potential.

Conclusion

Where GPs have worked in a wider team, established baseline information about their work as it really is, set agreed targets for improved work by the whole team, and then repeated the cycle of audit and innovation at a pace the team can accept as reasonable, care of high blood pressure,[36] type II diabetes,[37] and chronic lung disorders are as good as in any hospital clinic, and better in that patients with multiple problems (that is, most patients) can be dealt with by people they know, close to their own homes. The same is, or soon could be, true of most of the major chronic disorders which shorten and impair life.

Such practices are exceptional, and within the present contract (even with the tinkering modifications of the 1987 White Paper) will remain so, because general practices are still small independent businesses, and large, imaginative extensions of workload and operating costs cannot be accurately compensated by fees for service. Fee-for-service systems of any kind will always lag behind the best practice, and must create new burdens of accounting and verification to avoid systematic fraud. However, progress can be made if the GP contract is well defined and tightly administered, if the salary element already present is increased and capitation reduced, and if allowances are made for the widely different workload in different neighbourhoods, differences which must increase if health indices in the worst areas are to approach those in the best.

There is good evidence that a high proportion of GPs, probably a majority, are .willing to measure their work, set objectives, and verify their attainment. The Northumberland Local Medical Committee, an elected group representing all 51 practices in the area, sent questionnaires to all of them, with a response rate of 95%.[38] Replies included data on qualifications and postgraduate training, professional commitments outside patient care, and the range of clinical services offered by each practice. For example, the data showed that 88% of practices had special sessions for ante-natal care, 84% for immunization, 71% for child health surveillance, and 35% for family planning. To get beyond this initial stage requires practical assistance rather than exhortation. Already about half the 85 practices in the Oxford Family Practitioner Committee area, covering a population of 300,000, have carried out clinical audits during the past three years, with substantial practical assistance from Community Physician Dr Muir Gray and lecturer in general practice Dr Godfrey Fowler (Oxford colleges can afford rare wines but not a Professor of General Practice) and their departments, and nurse-facilitators Elaine Fullard and Aislinn O'Dwyer.[39] The scheme was funded by a special grant from the Chest, Heart and Stroke Association, not the DHSS, and even though it is now getting some government support, there is no indication so far that this will become general; the funding of FPCs and practice nurses envisaged in the 1987 White Paper fall far short of what would be required for any general expansion of this kind.

Moreover, such audits are only the first step. Practices which have initially accepted a commitment to raise the quality and coverage of care in one area of special interest, say high blood pressure or asthma, soon find it is not possible to limit their integrity to a single clinical problem. Once the process begins it must extend, year by year and one step at a time, to a comprehensive anticipatory approach which includes everything from family planning at the beginning of life to terminal care and bereavement counselling at its end. GPs are and must remain clinical generalists, whose special interests and loyalties are devoted to a locality and its population, not to a disease, organ or system of the body.

British general practice as it is now has the potential for such a revolutionary shift to anticipatory care, but there is no way this can be more than begun within the traditional contract, in which quality and extent of care depend on what GPs are prepared personally to afford. This chapter has had to document the consequences of leaving a major public responsibility in private hands, without effective accountability. Effective anticipatory care of chronic disease in the whole population is a huge new function for a system of general practice hitherto geared only to passive response to symptoms, transferring the crises that result from this policy to hospital specialists. It is absurd and unreasonable to imagine that this system can, without radical changes in staffing, organization, and equipment, take on new tasks of this size.

Attempts by both government and the profession to preserve the material limits of the Osler paradigm, but somehow transcend them by a magical birth of selflessness in a society which embraces Mammon as a new state religion, are leading to a fundamental crisis in medical thought and practice, and to a collision between a large part of the

profession and its erstwhile sponsors. Recent indications of
that still developing crisis are the subject of the next chapter.

NOTES

1. Weatherall, J.A.C., 'A review of some effects of recent medical
   practices in reducing the numbers of children born with congenital
   abnormalities', *Health Trends 1982*; 14:85-8.
2. Andrewes, D.A., 'Rubella immunization: whose baby?' *British
   Medical Journal 1983*; 287:1769-71.
3. Hutchinson, A., Thompson, J., 'Rubella prevention: two methods
   compared', *British Medical Journal 1982*; 284:1087-9.
4. Wilber, J.A., Barrow J.G., 'Hypertension—a community problem',
   American Journal of Medicine 1972; 52:653-63.
5. Ritchie, L.D., Currie, A.M., 'Blood pressure recording by general
   practitioners in north east Scotland', *British Medical Journal 1983*;
   286:107-9.
6. Heller, R.F., Rose, G.A., 'Current management of hypertension in
   general practice', *British Medical Journal 1977*; i:1442-4.
7. Kurji, K.H., Haines, A.P., 'Detection and management of hypertension in general practices in north west London', *British Medical
   Journal 1984*; 288: 903-6.
8. Michael, G., 'Quality of care in managing hypertension by case-
   finding in north west London', *British Medical Journal 1984*;
   288:906-8.
9. Whitfield, A.G.W., 'Young medical deaths: their cause and prevention', *Update*, February 1981:1249-54.
10. Fleming, D.M., Lawrence, M.S., 'Impact of audit on preventive
    measures', *British Medical Journal 1983*; 287:1852-4.
11. Peto, R., Speizer, F.E., Cochrane, A.L., Moore, F., Fletcher, C.M.,
    Tinker, C.M., Higgins, I.T.T., Gray, R.G., Richards, S.M., Gilliland,
    J., Norman-Smith, B., 'The relevance in adults of air-flow obstruct-
    ion, but not of mucus hypersecretion, to mortality from chronic
    lung disease', *American Review of Respiratory Diseases 1983*;
    128:491-500.
12. Cartwright, A., Anderson, R., *General practice revisited: a second
    study of patients and their doctors*, London: Tavistick Publications,
    1981.
13. Research Committee of the British Thoracic Association, 'Death
    from asthma in two regions of England', *British Medical Journal
    1982*; 285:1251-5.
14. Sharp, C.L., Butterfield, W.J.H., Keen, H., 'The Bedford survey',
    Proceedings of the Royal Society of Medicine 1964; 57:193-204.
15. Doney, B.J., 'An audit of the care of diabetics in a group practice',
    Journal of the Royal College of General Practitioners 1976; 26:
    734-42.
16. Gloag, D., 'Avoidable disability', *British Medical Journal 1986*;
    292:507-8.
17. Burrows, P.J., Gray, P.J., Kinmonth, A-L., Payton, D.J., Walpole,
    G.A., Walton, R.J., Wilson, D., Woodbine, G., 'Who cares for the

patient with diabetes? Presentation and follow-up in seven Southampton practices', *Journal of the Royal College of General Practitioners 1987*; 37:65-9.

18. Wilkes, E., Lawton, E., 'The diabetic, the hospital and primary care', *Journal of the Royal College of General Practitioners 1980*; 30:199-206.

19. Day, J.L., Humphreys, H., Alban-Davies, H., 'Problems of comprehensive shared diabetes care', *British Medical Journal 1987*; 294: 1590-2.

20. Pirart, J., 'Diabetes mellitus and its degenerative complications. A prospective study of 4,400 patients observed between 1947 and 1973', *Diabetes Care 1978*; 1:168-88.

21. Dornan, T., Mann, J.I., Turner, R., 'Factors protective against retinopathy in insulin-dependent diabetics free of retinopathy for 30 years', *British Medical Journal 1982*; 285:1073-7.

22. Christiansen, J.S., 'Cigarette smoking and prevalence of microangiopathy in juvenile-onset insulin-dependent diabetes mellitus', *Diabetes Care 1978*; 1:146-9.

23. 'Long-term antihypertensive treatment inhibiting progression of diabetic nephropathy', *British Medical Journal 1982*; 285: 685-8.

24. Hayes, T.M., Harries, J., 'Randomized controlled trial of routine hospital clinic care versus routine general practice care for type II diabetes', *British Medical Journal 1984*; 289:728-30.

25. Pyke, D.A., 'Diabetic ketoacidosis', *Journal of the Royal Society of Medicine 1980*; 73:131-4.

26. Tunbridge, W.M.G., 'Factors contributing to deaths of diabetics under fifty years of age', *Lancet 1981*; ii:569-72.

27. Hart, J.T., 'Semicontinuous screening of a whole community for hypertension', *Lancet 1970*; ii:223-6.

28. Hart, J.T., 'The marriage of primary care and epidemiology: continuous anticipatory care of whole populations in a state medical service', *Journal of the Royal College of Physicians of London 1974*; 8:299-314.

29. Cartwright, A., Tables 36 and 37, pp. 128-9, in *Patients and their doctors: a study of general practice*, London: Routledge & Kegan Paul. 1967.

30. Reynolds, E.H., Elwes, R.D.C., Shorvon, S.D., 'Why does epilepsy become intractable? Prevention of chronic epilepsy', *Lancet 1983*; ii:952-4.

31. Johnstone, E.C., Crow, T.J., Johnson, A.L., MacMillan, J.F., 'The Northwick Park study of first episodes of schizophrenia. I. Presentation of the illness and problems relating to admission', *British Journal of Psychiatry 1986*; 148:115-20.

32. Taylor, M.P., 'Epilepsy in a Doncaster practice: audit and change over eight years', *Journal of the Royal College of General Practitioners 1987*; 37:116-9.

33. Editorial, 'Cancer of the cervix death by incompetence', *Lancet 1985*; ii:363-4.

34. RCGP, OPCS, DHSS, 'Morbidity statistics from general practice 1971-2: second national study'. *Studies on medical and population subjects no. 36*, London: HMSO.

35. Catford, J.C., Ford, S., 'On the state of the public ill-health: premature mortality in the United Kingdom and Europe', *British Medical Journal 1984*; 289:1668-70.
36. Hart, J.T., *Hypertension*, 2nd Ed., Churchill Livingstone, 1987.
37. Singh, B.M., Holland, M.R., Thorn, P.A., 'Metabolic control of diabetes in general practice clinics: comparison with a hospital clinic', *British Medical Journal 1984*; 289:726-8.
38. Hutchinson, A., Mitford, P., Aylett, M., 'Creating a general practice data set: a new role for Northumberland Local Medical Committee', *British Medical Journal 1987*; 295:1029-32.
39. Muir Gray, J.A., O'Dwyer, A., Fullard, E., Fowler, G., 'Rent-an-audit', *Journal of the Royal College of General Practitioners 1987*; 37:177.

Chapter 6
A CRISIS OF ACCOUNTABILITY

Though most thoughtful and well-informed GPs now accept the need for more staff, equipment and postgraduate training, they are uncertain about what new investment is needed, and even more so about how it should be made.

The only answer fully consistent with autonomy in the Osler paradigm would be that GPs should invest their own money as entrepreneurs, selling their services as commodities in an open market. In Britain, though not in many other developed countries, this had lost majority professional support by the 1920s and after 1948 its few remaining adherents became isolated. So long as the State was prepared to underwrite the cost of providing a service to the whole population free at point of use, return to the private market was bound to narrow medical employment and clinical opportunity. However attractive ideologically, it made no sense at all in terms of income, employment and security for doctors.

Marketed medical care remains the 'natural' solution to Margaret Thatcher and the politicians of New Conservatism. As the public hospital service lags further behind advancing medical science, their remedy is to encourage high quality growth in the private sector, leaving the public sector to cope as best it may. The eventual goal is to achieve high-quality marketed care at both hospital and GP level for a core population in stable employment at high rates of pay, with a salvage service for peripheral populations in casual employment, or unemployed, the nature and quality of which will depend on political pressures.

Most doctors have until recently seemed to accept decline of the NHS as inevitable, just as they formerly accepted its permanence. Like any other occupational group, their first concern was to find a safe haven for themselves. If most of them were prepared to look for security in a transitional economy, moving away from a comprehensive NHS toward a frankly two-tiered service even at GP level, the New Conservative strategy would succeed. Judging from the unusual caution so far shown by Conservative Ministers of Health, the government is far from sure it can get away with it. The attitude of GPs to privatization of the health service has not been tested by a frontal attack, and probably never will be. An approach by stealth is already going on which will soften the impact, but an eventual collision is inevitable between public and professional expectations and a government withdrawing sponsorship for growth in the public service.

On the best-informed and most responsible independent projections of medical school output, NHS career posts, and demographic trends, about half the students now entering British medical schools will be unable to work in the NHS by 1997, even if the rising proportion of medical women and lower GP lists are taken into account.[1] Most medical students and junior hospital doctors now appear to be adapting to this prospect, but seem unaware of the real nature of the alternative private medical market. If effective medical care now requires a transformation of the GP service into locally-controlled, population-based, need-orientated anticipatory care, the genteel medical shopkeeping to which these doctors think they might return would conflict far more with good clinical medicine than it did before the NHS. The real nature of a new medical market can already be seen in the USA, though in a much wealthier society which can better afford its extravagance; primary medical generalists as well-paid but strictly controlled cogs in impersonal, for-profit corporations selling medical care to those who can afford high-premium insurance, or have good jobs in growth industries.

We are entering an era of struggle in medical ideology, a

battle of ideas arising from fundamental conflicts of interest, pitched not in some hypothetical future when medical care has been restored to its 'natural' place as a commodity sold to individual consumers by competing suppliers, but in the present, when all but a handful of GPs earn their living from the Welfare State. Even today, the only realistic point of departure must still be the relation between GPs and the State established by the Lloyd George Act of 1911.

Public Service Privately Administered

For the Osler paradigm, the best alternative to a private market in fees was public funding without public accountability, public service privately administered. Without noticing this paradox, let alone asking themselves how it was achieved, this is what GPs finally got; so strongly had they resisted public service on any terms, that they hardly noticed how easily government conceded their continued independence to run their practices pretty much as they liked, providing it didn't cost more money. In fact, Lloyd George favoured the doctors in order to rid himself of the local power exerted by the thousands of small local Friendly Societies which had run the club practices he nationalized. The medical profession and its obsession with autonomy was the weapon he used to break the power of the locally-based insurance societies, and ensure that all lay control would lie with central government. The Insurance Committees which administered the Act were soon dominated by the local doctors and by central government appointees, and the Friendly Societies, which had represented some degree of local democratic control, were steadily squeezed out.

Despite paranoid BMA forecasts of clinical decision by committee and the end of clinical freedom in 1912 and again in 1948, both contracts were administered with a disinterest difficult to distinguish from indifference. In theory, first the Insurance Committees, then the Executive Councils, now the Family Practitioner Committees[2] (always the same organization, only names changed) had responsibility for ensuring that GPs provided a good clinical service from adequate premises and that they maintained proper records. In practice, the administration of general practice, even more under the NHS than under the Lloyd George Act, was, and for most areas still is, entirely passive and negative, limited to the organization and supervision of GPs' earnings and prescribing costs. Though generations of newly appointed chief FPC administrators have wanted to do something more positive, they have never been given the staff or office organization required for an imaginative approach to planned primary care; after a year or two enthusiasm has given way to cynicism, and eventually to entrenched bureaucracy. Providing GPs did not cheat on a big enough scale to guarantee successful prosecution for fraud, did not absent themselves from their practices completely, did not certify unfitness for work without even seeing their patients, and did not prescribe more than 50% more per head than their local colleagues, neither excellence nor incompetence, indifference, ignorance or exhaustion attracted administrative action, either supportive or punitive. Administration of general practice had, and for the most part still has, no defined objectives other than containment of costs and minimizing of complaints.

Until the 1987 White Paper, the legal definition of GPs' work in the NHS was contained in the Regulations of the NHS Act of 1977.[3] For the 39 years since 1948 the duties of GPs were:

> to render to their patients all necessary and appropriate medical services of the type usually provided by general practitioners.

In other words, if GPs did the same as most other GPs, they'd stay out of trouble. George Bernard Shaw would have been amused to see this definition of medical conscience, confirming his own in his preface to *The Doctor's Dilemma:*[4]

> Doctors are just like other Englishmen: most of them have no honor and no conscience: what they commonly mistake for these is sentimentality and an intense dread of doing anything that everybody else does not do, or omitting to do anything that everyone else does. This of course does amount to a sort of working or rule-

of-thumb conscience; but it means that you will do anything, good or bad, provided you get enough people to keep you in countenance by doing it also.

Shaw's cynicism was more justified when he wrote than it is now; since the NHS took Shaw's advice and virtually abolished fee-earning in general practice, many individual GPs have pioneered work which everybody else does not do, and have had the courage to discard much that everyone else still does. Yet up to the 1987 White Paper there was little evidence that either district or central administration was as interested in the outcome of care as Lloyd George[5] threatened they would be in 1912, when speaking in parliament on his plan to increase from 6 to 9 shillings per head the proposed annual payment to panel GPs:

If the remuneration is increased, the service must be improved. Up to the present the doctor has not been adequately paid, and therefore we have had no right or title to expect him to give full service. In a vast number of cases he has given his services for nothing or for payment which was utterly inadequate. There is no man here who does not know doctors who have been attending poor people without any fee or reward at all.

I have got three conditions which I am going to lay down as the result of this increased provision. One is that the doctor who acts on the panel shall agree to give, without further charge, those medical certificates which an insured person will require to enable him to get sickness or disablement benefit. . . Secondly, we shall also ask that those practitioners who act on the panels shall keep simple records of the patients whom they treat, the illnesses from which they suffer, and the attendances given. This is new in respect to the industrial practice of this country. Though we are providing increased remuneration, I frankly admit we are also asking for increased service. We know that doctors dislike book-keeping above all things but we also know that they desire the advancement of medical knowledge, and we feel that they will co-operate with us in this matter. We on our part undertake that the records required shall be of the simplest character that will give the necessary information.

Thirdly, and chiefly, the service must be improved in certain definite respects, as compared with what it has been possible to give in the past. It will be the duty of the Commissioners. . . to see that a proper standard is reached and maintained, not merely in the number of visits paid or the number of times a patient is seen at the doctor's surgery, but also in respect of the amount of time and attention given, and also that where necessary the practitioner should resort to those modern means of exact diagnosis the importance of which I am advised is increasingly recognised in the profession.

This promised administrative interest in the more easily measured aspects of clinical work was never implemented by Lloyd George or any other Minister, either under the Insurance Act or the NHS. The initial hostility of GPs was not enough to explain this; by the 1920s, the greatest fear of most GPs was that Conservative governments might repeal the Liberal legislation they had once opposed, and had the government wished to press for improvement in the quality of GP service, it had the power to do so. The most obvious explanation for this indifference was that governments were more concerned with economy than with the quality of the service. Concern displayed for clinical effectiveness has as a rule been rhetorical, unless some charitable foundation or commercial interest could be found to pay for material change in some token project. Relatively well-paid doctors running a cheap service remained an attractive formula for all politicians from all parties. If it meant that many practices were nasty as well as cheap, this was seen as a moral problem for GPs, not an administrative problem for government, which concerned itself not with the low standards and expectations of average general practice, but with individual complaints against individual GPs for exceptional acts and omissions.

Better work requires not more exhortation, but more time, more space, more staff, better equipment, time-consuming development of self-criticism and peer-criticism and continued postgraduate education, all of which depend on greater investment in primary care. Investment of public money through the GP's pocket has proved as erratic and uncertain as would be the standards of schools, if they were funded through the pockets of head teachers. If public work is put out to private contract, the usual way to ensure good standards are maintained is strict accountability to the public body responsible, with process and outcome targets set and regular reports on how far they are achieved. No Family Practitioner Committee (FPC) has ever worked in this way, though there have been a few recent imaginative attempts to break out of the straitjacket by some progressive FPCs.[2] Such an approach to primary care is essentially neither easier nor more difficult than it is for education, whose administration is concerned with standards and resources as well as teachers' pay. Definition of objectives and measurement of their attainment would not of itself solve the problem of increasing public investment in primary care, any more than the existence of state education guarantees that a government will consider that educating our children is more important than tax relief for millionaires or organizing the means to destroy life on earth, but it would at least create the machinery essential for future governments with more humane and intelligent priorities.

Hospital consultants are salaried professionals, not independent contractors. Health Authorities are responsible for providing their resources and ultimately for maintaining standards. Weak though they usually are, national and District Health Authority policies and planning do exist in the hospital service, but are almost entirely absent in the GP service. Administrative controls on specialists have generally been used with discretion, and alleged threats to clinical independence have not materialized; nearly all difficulties in this area have arisen from government attempts to reduce costs, and occasionally from attempts by consultants to do private work at the expense of their NHS contract, not from positive proposals with which specialists disagree.

Three Foundations for Independent Contractor Status

There must be few employed people in any occupation who, given the choice, would not prefer to be self-employed, handling substantial funds without a clear division between personal income and service expenditure and with minimal accountability. GPs are the only professionals in public service permitted to retain this curious 18th Century privilege.

The anomaly of independent contractor status has survived because of the persistence of three hitherto dominant ideas, all of which must keep their hold on both government and profession for it to continue. Two of these ideas have already been dealt with; GP autonomy and government parsimony. The third is the belief that the real work of medical science must always and only go on in hospitals, that general practice is more a social arrangement than a clinical discipline, an almost indestructible, infinitely elastic, generally cheap and largely illusory service whose main function is to fill the widening gap between what medical science makes possible, and what is actually done.

As never before, all three foundations are now in doubt. Of course, like all other creative workers, GPs need autonomy of some kind; but thoughtful GPs, even if few can yet conceive of autonomy without independent contractor status, are beginning to consider what their independence is for, and to recognize that it may limit at least some aspects of their work however much it may appear to facilitate others.[6] For clinical initiative and decision autonomy is essential, but even then only within limits set by their ability to explain their actions and omissions to their colleagues, their patients and an interested administration, and either persuade them they are responsible, or think again. GPs have created their own body of independent research and literature, and medical knowledge in general is becoming as accessible to them as to hospital specialists; these, not Ministry directives, should remain the main sources of innovation in general practice. Practice and community nurses are beginning to follow this autonomous but socially responsible path, which needs to be encouraged if appropriate community care is to surpass inappropriate hospital care in effectiveness and efficiency. But autonomy for delegating more work to underpaid assistants, for taking on more better-paid part-time jobs outside NHS general practice, or even in order to remain on a less rigorous scale of income tax, is publicly indefensible, though these are precisely the arguments principally deployed when the question is debated within the profession. The assumption that all GP autonomy is altruistic is no longer credible even to GPs themselves, who know very well that it is at present more often used to justify search for a quiet life than to accelerate clinical innovation. Many GPs are now groping towards accountability, but can't make up their minds who they can or should be accountable to.

Belief in the cost advantages of general practice is also less sure than it was. General practice is still cheap compared with hospital work, and this accounts for most if not all recent political interest in the subject. For the first time in history, all the major British political parties issued policy documents on primary care in the run-up to the 1987 general election, but at their 1986 annual conference the subject was never debated, it never surfaced during the election campaign itself, and none of the press conferences or detailed political comment in the serious medical press referred to any new ideas about general practice. Though proposals for annual reports by GPs, annual meetings open to patients to discuss them, and elected patients' committees to assist and advise GPs were all contained in a Labour Party policy document published in the run-up to the election,[7] these were completely ignored by Labour Party spokesmen and shadow ministers, as well as by their opponents and by the medical press. Party political argument was almost confined to rival claims about global support for NHS spending, not about how money should be spent or new directions for health service investment.[8] Though we must always live in hope, neither ministers nor shadow ministers have as yet appeared to see primary care as a field for expansion rather than cost containment. They face a dilemma; the GPs and nurses most actively pressing the case for primary care also want it to be upgraded in quality and comprehensiveness, better staffed and equipped, aiming at qualitative parity with hospitals. In theory, a better GP service would take over much of the work now done at higher cost by hospitals, but in reality the immediate effect is to duplicate it. Few leading politicians now have the time for imagination, or the stomach for long-term solutions which are bound to present initial difficulties.

Finally, the clinical scope of general practice is growing too fast to be ignored much longer, even by politicians still ignorant of its potential. No GPs working within the NHS contract can do more than begin systematically to do all the simple and effective things that need to be done for all of their patients, but enough have begun to do some of them to show, very impressively, what is possible. Public expectations are rising, and though some who can afford it will be diverted into health-care acquisitiveness in a growing private sector on the North American and West European model, most cannot and will not. Perhaps for the first time, there is beginning to be serious pressure on government for a better primary care service, reflected in the 1987 Report of the Parliamentary Select Committee on Primary Health Care.[9] The natural tendency of government will be to concede this without cost; at the top by encouraging privatization, at the bottom by stricter enforcement of a contract which may be modified here and there, but will remain orientated to process rather than outcome. Independent contractor status has endured because government and profession jointly agreed on a stagnation comfortable for both. For many different reasons, that collusion is now breaking down.

Limits of Cash-Limits

In seeking a return to the leaner, fitter, more competitive society in which they believe, Margaret Thatcher and her New Conservatives have generally met less resistance than either they or their enemies expected in dismantling the civilizing reforms of a crude market economy achieved by 75 years of struggle and concession, but the GP service has so far been an exception.

When they first won power in 1979, the solution to all social and economic problems appeared the same; privatize the problem, expose it to market competition, let the fit survive and the weak perish. To New Conservative theorists, general practice seemed a particularly suitable subject for this simple treatment. It was still an under-capitalized cottage industry, and many relatively inefficient GPs were there to be shaken out. There were also many energetic GPs impatient to apply new technology to primary care which was already in general use in Western Europe and North America, which was uneconomic under their existing contract. There was a new generation of better paid, better informed, more demanding consumers willing to pay more for better personal care for themselves and their families and eager to pay less in taxes for care of other people. General practice seemed ripe for entrepreneurial expansion into new responsibilities GPs had been unwilling to undertake in a public service funded only for obsolete care, but might willingly provide for fees.

Exactly what happened to this theory we shall never know. At considerable cost, the government commissioned a major independent study on the possibilities for applying cash limits to general practitioner services, so that FPCs would operate within plannable annual budgets. The results of this study, the Binder–Hamlyn Report, have never been published, so the public which paid for it has never been able to see the evidence it unearthed. It seems reasonable to assume that Binder–Hamlyn confirmed that general practice had to remain a demand-led service if its essential buffer function was to be maintained, and that no simple solution was yet feasible for rationing GP access to hospital referral. However that may be, the still secret Binder–Hamlyn Report put an end to proposals for either cash limits or large-scale privatization of primary care, which were publicly buried in the government's Green Paper on the future of primary care in April 1986,[10] though probably in a shallow grave designed for easy resurrection now that a decisive 44% of the British electorate has voted for five more years of conspicuous personal consumption side by side with impoverished public services and an army of unemployed.

Solution of the problems of primary care by straight privatization evidently failed to survive even the briefest exposure to the reality well known to every medical civil servant: that Britain already had the cheapest and most cost-effective health service in the developed world, consuming the smallest proportion of a dwindling Gross National Product, with the lowest administrative overheads, the cheapest medical profession, and for the most part a still very undemanding public with low expectations by West European and North American standards. Every other country which relied on market forces for distribution of medical care had higher costs, lower efficiency, less comprehensive coverage of the population and higher expectations for technical salvage. Privatization of the more potentially profitable parts of hospital care was a different matter, but privatization of general practice threatened only to disrupt a cheap but still popular and credible service, which it would be politically and economically suicidal to disturb for doctrinal reasons.

The Thatcher government therefore had to accept that it could not afford any general privatization of general practice, but it also could not afford to ignore the anomalous position of GPs as the only health service workers with a demand-led and therefore unplannable budget, which was largely responsible for initiating costs in the hospital service. GPs alone appeared to be in a position to control the demands on specialist care in hospitals, but they remained outside the NHS management system. In an ageing and therefore sicker population, hospital throughput, staff workload, in-patient and out-patient waiting lists, and pressure on community nursing, social services and GPs inevitably increased, given an upward twist by each advance in medical science, always widening the gap between what could and what actually was done faster than it could be narrowed by greater staff effort. In any such permanently overloaded system there must be flexibility somewhere; the traditional and most economic point for this was always in general practice, the interface between undemanding apparent health and demanding symptomatic disease, where response was cheapest and could most easily control entry to hospital services.

The Green Paper

Before the government got the bad news from the Binder–Hamlyn Report, it embarked on preparation of a major discussion document on the future of primary care, known as the Green Paper (confusingly but aptly, it eventually turned out to have blue covers, but discussion papers are traditionally known as Green, final proposals as White). This was promised as the first comprehensive review of general practice since the NHS began in 1948, and was generally expected to contain radical proposals for privatization and market incentives. As two, then three years rolled by without publication, it became an open secret that these ideas had been discarded as impractical; the New Conservative radicals were too ignorant of the realities of general practice, and the DHSS experts too entangled with the welfare tradition, to be able to agree on any fresh practical proposals. The BMA was still much clearer about what it didn't want than about positive proposals for reform, and found it difficult to admit publicly that there was any serious or widespread problem about the quality of GP care.

For the first time since its birth, there seemed to be an opportunity for the RCGP to use its *de facto* political muscle, by putting forward positive proposals for better general practice, against minimal professional opposition, with a government which might be grateful for anything that looked like a policy. The General Purposes Committee (GPC) of Council of the RCGP, its main collective policy-making body, began preparing the College's proposals in 1983. All members of GPC (of whom I was one) and probably all members of Council, shared a common point of departure; that the quality of GP care was generally uneven and often grossly deficient, that reform required material investment in time, staff and equipment, and that the new investment available from the 1966 Package Deal was almost exhausted. Though only 15% of GPs chose to employ the full complement of staff permitted under the wages reimbursement scheme, this proportion had not changed significantly for about ten years. As in 1966, the most innovative practices offering the best public service were generally doing so at high personal cost to the GPs in charge of them.

The task given to GPC seems in retrospect poorly defined: to produce a discussion document. Should a discussion document provide a range of options together with relevant evidence which could then be discussed by a wider member-

ship? Or should it present a more or less finished consensus
policy? This choice was never explicitly made. Almost to the
last moment, those who believed in multiple options (myself
among them) deceived themselves that full public discussion
would be encouraged. In fact what emerged was a single
prescriptive view, though no viable consensus existed on
anything but the Status Quo.

Before either the Green Paper or the RCGP's reply were
published, two members of GPC published their own independent proposals. Marinker[11] put forward a complex plan
'based on entrepreneurial competition within the NHS', in
which groups of GPs would be budget-holders exerting
consumer pressure on hospital specialists competing for
referred trade. This was included, and implicitly endorsed,
in a review[12] subsequent to the Green Paper but before its
explosive rejection, jointly authored by Pereira Gray (now
Chairman of the RCGP), health economist Alan Maynard,
and Marinker himself. It was an unconvincing attempt at a
market solution, in tune with the times but wholly impractical, and would have permanently antagonized the
hospital specialists if anyone had taken it seriously. As a
'Left' alternative, I[13] proposed the creation of a new career
option for GPs to act as both personal doctors and community physicians for their own registered populations,
giving account of their work through annual reports both to
District Health Authorities, and to general meetings and
elected committees of their local populations. This gained a
little published professional support,[14] but none within
GPC. Similar proposals were discussed in the intelligent
report on primary care of the House of Commons Social
Service Committee, which had members from all parties in
parliament on the US pattern.[9] It was probably unrealistic
to expect the novel idea of locally democratized, public-
health oriented general practice to be rapidly accepted or
even understood in an election year; the Labour Party is a
conservative organization, in which any imaginative proposal
is quickly dubbed lunacy by what Aneurin Bevan called 'the
most prostituted press in the world' and thus transformed
into an electoral handicap. In fact there was at that time

little real interest in any proposals on primary care from any of the political parties.

The Quality Initiative

While discussions in depth continued on GPC (which seemed to have no effect at all on its final document), the fifty or so members of RCGP Council took back to their own practices proposals for personal audit, the first move in the College's 'Quality Initiative' programme.[15] This aimed to improve standards in individual 'opinion-forming' practices by encouraging quantified review of what GPs actually did, comparing this with what they thought they ought to be doing, particularly in areas of prevention and anticipatory care, such as population management of high blood pressure, diabetes, cervical cancer and immunization. It was (and still is; the movement continues, though rather uncertainly) essentially an exercise in self-help and voluntary peer review in the tradition of professionalism, pre-empting public accountability by offering self-criticism and peer-criticism instead; 'If we don't do it, somebody else will—outside the profession.'

From the College's point of view, the response was encouraging. An impressive range of often imaginative work was begun, on a wider scale than most had dared to hope. But from the point of view of any administrator concerned with progress in NHS general practice as a whole, the exercise must have seemed almost irrelevant; as usual, most of the initiatives were from areas where relatively good standards already prevailed.

However, even this self-help voluntarism was a brave policy for the College, always in danger of isolating itself from the majority of GPs, in or out of the College membership, who considered themselves already at full stretch meeting individually presented demands, without the added burdens of active follow-up for chronic disease, search for needs, or organized practice intelligence on prescribing and referral which provided nearly all the subjects pursued in the Quality Initiative. Whenever the players thought they were getting somewhere, the College seemed to move the goal posts; right for a body concerned with the advance of art and science, but very wrong for many GPs who still saw themselves as practical men in a small way of business. The possibility of an explosion was always there, and early in 1986, when the Green Paper[10] was finally published after three postponements, the roof fell in.

The Good Practice Allowance

Despite claims to be the first thoroughgoing review of primary care since 1948, the Green Paper was no such thing. In general, it made no attempt to define either the objectives of primary care or to assess how far they were being attained, and proposed few fundamental changes. It assumed that general practice was effectively co-terminous with primary care, and there was no serious discussion of how the work of GPs was to be co-ordinated with the work of other primary care health workers or Public Health bodies. Its only substantially new proposals were for an increased capitation element in GPs' pay to encourage competition for patients, vaguely formulated suggestions for 'health shops' in which GPs would join other more overtly commercial entrepreneurs (pharmacists, opticians, private physiotherapists, health food shops and the like) to woo the health-care-acquisitive consumer, and the Good Practice Allowance.

The first two of these fell at the first fence. No GP who remembered the pre-1966 Package Deal years wanted to return to the unprincipled competition for patients and bitter intraprofessional rivalry of those days, and none believed that a return to capitation would encourage better quality of care; all historical experience proved the reverse. The 'Health shops' idea was plainly ludicrous, typical of other absurd attempts to transplant US commercial culture to a society which didn't want it and couldn't afford it. The BMA and the RCGP were opposed to both these proposals, and neither got any significant support or attention from the profession.

The only really novel feature of the Green Paper was the Good Practice Allowance (GPA), but this had clearly emerged not from the Minister, but from the RCGP discussion document. The GPA boldly faced up to the long obvious fact that the service offered by GPs was extremely variable in quality. Like teachers, milkmen, and all other trades and professions, problems existed because there were both good and bad practitioners; pay the good ones more and the bad ones less, and market forces would eventually eliminate bad practice; problem solved. This was not only a matter of quality of service, but had huge economic consequences. According to Donald Crombie at the RCGP Research Unit in Birmingham, data on practice activity from about 1,000 GPs in 1982-3 showed that annual per capita hospital costs initiated by GP referrals varied nearly fivefold between the top and bottom fifths of the distribution (overall mean £257, £106 below the 20th centile, £509 above the 80th centile).[16]

The flaw undermining this simple logic, which few of its original supporters seem to have recognized, is that GPs not only create their practices, but are created by them. The problems faced by GPs seriously concerned to provide an effective service differ from one place to another as much as the mortality and morbidity levels they should be aiming to reduce. Points of departure are hugely different, and innovations that are relatively easy in one area may be extremely difficult in another, above all where needs are greatest but pressure of demand seems to preclude planned development of anticipatory care. As originally proposed in the RCGP discussion document,[17] and elaborated by Pereira Gray, Marinker and Maynard[18] in the *British Medical Journal*, the GPA was to be a reward for achieving certain minimum standards of practice, measured in terms of premises, equipment, information available and accessibility to patients, delays between requests for consultations and their achievement, flexibility of consulting hours, special clinics, group activities, annual reports, and evidence of innovation; a consensus description of the practice nearly all of us want to be in, whether as doctors or patients. The GPA was obviously an additional reward for attaining such a practice or being in one already, but it was not at all clear how it would help the GPs in greatest difficulties to get there.

The gap in quality between 'good' and 'bad' practices would at least in the short term be increased rather than reduced by rewarding better practice with higher income. Whether or not 'bad' practices would or could change their ways in search of higher earnings remains doubtful. Bosanquet and Leese[19] have presented evidence that many GPs do respond to economic incentives for personal investment in group practices serving relatively young communities with good prospects for economic and population growth and practice expansion, but do not invest in areas with ageing populations, and without prospects for economic or social growth; in other words, precisely the areas in which bad practice is endemic and in most urgent need of reform.

British GPs have a long and robust tradition of hostility to all proposals for stratification of primary doctors into superior and inferior grades, either by income or authority. It cannot be described as egalitarianism, because grossly unequal partnership agreements whereby established senior partners exploit their juniors are still common, though much less so than before the NHS. GPs have always opposed grading by quality of either training or performance. They rejected several million pounds of additional income offered as part of the 1966 Package, rather than accept Merit Awards for better practice.

Much of this hostility is based on GPs' view of consultants who can double their incomes with Merit Awards (Distinction Awards), devised when the NHS began to compensate consultants for expected loss of private practice. Every year £50 million is paid to consultants in awards ranging from £4,890 for a grade C to £24,930 for an A+. Once given they are never taken away whatever the quality of the consultant's work, and they go on after retirement as higher pensions.[20] Beneficiaries are chosen in secret by anonymous committees of current Merit Award holders, using secret criteria. It has always appeared to outsiders that the principal quality sought must be resemblance to themselves. Sir Russell Brain, President of the Royal College of Physicians, said secrecy was desired only by those of insufficient merit or distinction to obtain an award, in order to protect their own reputations, but a survey in 1973 showed that secrecy was favoured by 67% of award-holders, compared with 29% of those without awards.[21] Consultants in unglamorous but socially necessary specialties like geriatrics, psychiatry and the non-clinical diagnostic specialties, are consistently under-represented among the chosen, and cardiologists, neurologists and other prestigious specialties are consistently over-represented. For example, in England and Wales in 1984 less than a quarter of all geriatricians got them, compared with over half of all general surgeons. Merit Awards were originally introduced to compensate consultants for their expected loss of private practice, but abstinence from private practice is not a criterion for selection. It is a corrupt system which, whatever its original intentions, discourages imagination and criticism of established practice in young consultants and fails to ensure industry in old ones. GPs wanted none of it, nor anything like it.

The College in Crisis

The Government Green Paper, and its central feature, the Good Practice Allowance, were endorsed with uncritical enthusiasm by the Secretary and Chairman of the College within hours of publication. In an editorial in the RCGP Journal, Chairman John Hasler[22] made belief in the GPA a test of loyalty to the College and commitment to good practice:

> Modern general practice of a high standard provides care which is second to none. The arguments for providing increased resources for those practices which are innovating and striving for improvement are unanswerable. Nevertheless, we must recognise that a significant increase in resources for general practice (as in the mid-sixties) is highly unlikely to be provided without some demonstration of improved patient care and greater accountability. To reject a quality incentive equation is to reject the new resources that modern general practice now needs and our patients deserve. . . The important decision now facing the profession is whether or not to accept and endorse the principle of encouraging quality and rewarding personal investment. The government's proposals for a Good Practice Allowance go some way to achieving that objective. Whatever the profession

decides ultimately about the allowance, it must not lose sight of this underlying principle.

Though over a third of all GPs are now members of the College, a large majority are passive and rarely attend meetings or take part in College activities. The same is true of the other mass organization for GPs, the BMA, and there is a large overlap in membership. The BMA, centrally and in the elected Local Medical Committees which are its real voice and local organization, was furious, both because of opposition to the GPA itself, and because the College appeared to be usurping the General Medical Service Committee (GMSC) of the BMA's function as principal professional body for all negotiations on terms of service in the NHS.[23]

Within three months the Chairman's view was thrown out and the College was in greater disarray than at any time since its foundation. Simultaneously, war broke out between College Council and its large panel of examiners for the College Membership examination (MRCGP), prompted by the sacking of chief examiner Dr Andrew Belton, a bellicose character more in tune with many peripheral GPs than were the College officers. The two issues, independence of examiners and the GPA, not only coincided in time, but reflected the same grievance; the College was seen as 'too political', in other words more political than the membership was willing to be at the time. After a few weeks of bewildered defence, the leadership's position was clearly untenable; Chairman John Hasler resigned, and a new Chairman, Dennis Pereira Gray, took on the difficult task of backtracking on a policy he had fully supported and apparently still believed in.

Practice Allowance or Bad Practice Allowance?

GP entrepreneurs who had most successfully used the terms of the 1966 Package Deal to improve the quality of care, it appeared self-evident that if more practices were to join the pursuit of quality, good work should be rewarded and bad work penalized by a new contract, in which GP incomes would be related to performance; hence their faith in the Good Practice Allowance. To the concerned public it was even more obvious that the first priority for investment should be the practices which had failed to use the 1966 Package, and continued to maximize GP incomes by extending their practice lists and their commitments outside the care of their registered populations; in other words, some kind of Bad Practice Allowance.

The source of this paradox is simple, and clear enough to anyone willing to see it. Bad practice needs investment in more staff, more time, better equipment and better buildings, and more thought about effective service to patients. Since at present few even of the best practices seldom deliver more than about 50% of any reasonably defined target for the services people need (as measured by monitoring the care of common chronic disorders such as diabetes, high blood pressure, asthma, epilepsy or schizophrenia), virtually all practices are in need of a 'Bad Practice Allowance', but the best practices need it least. The barrier to such a policy is independent contractor status, which tends to channel all investment through the GP-entrepreneur's pocket, where some of it naturally tends to remain; if more investment goes to bad practice than to good, independent contractor status ensures that the doctor in charge earns more from bad work than from good.

It is on the whole a sensible idea that GPs who work harder, more imaginatively, and more effectively should be better rewarded than those who do not, but this cannot be done within independent contractor status without further widening the gap between the best and the worst practices, with a steady slide back to a two-tier service. A quality-related contract which retains and develops social equity is possible only in some kind of salaried service, in which the GP's pay is entirely separated from the costs of practice, and all staff, equipment, premises and further training are paid for directly by the employer, the State. It is certainly very stupid to continue as we are now, when the most conscientious GPs have to innovate at their own expense, and further innovation is no longer possible within the

1966 framework.

Tactical Retreat

Still unable to face this obvious conclusion, the College sought more tolerable reasons for its crisis by turning its back on reality. The official diagnosis was poor communication between the centre of the College and its periphery, and improved communication with and dispersion of power to the Faculties was proposed as its remedy. This treatment could do little harm, because peripheral initiative is always more important if there is any; but was there then any real peripheral initiative to prefer? Wherever there is disagreement between centre and periphery failure of communication can be blamed, but what evidence is there that the Faculties had positive policies for NHS reform to communicate in the two or three years preceding the crisis? From 1983 to 1986, I can't recall a single example of any positive proposal for reform of NHS general practice from the periphery which was opposed or ignored at the centre. The truth is that most GPs were reasonably satisfied with things as they were. For most GPs, investments in buildings were extremely profitable and were therefore being made, but only a minority were investing heavily in ancillary staff, computer systems and diagnostic equipment, and felt any urgent need for more money to pay for them. If the price of more government investment in general practice was more accountability, most GPs, in or out of the College, preferred to do without the investment and carry on as they were. The predominant mood was and still is conformist complacency; doing most things that other doctors do, and little that they do not do. There never was a mandate from the mass of the membership for a serious policy of reform in any direction, and once any proposals got beyond the talking stage, and involved the whole membership rather than the small active minority, they would have aroused the same grassroots opposition.

It is said that the College antagonized its membership by venturing into negotiations on the structure of the service, which are supposed to be the province of the BMA, but in practice it is impossible wholly to separate structure from function. Any group genuinely interested in the quality of care must concern itself with terms and conditions of service, and where the line is drawn between medicopolitical and academic functions must be a matter of judgement according to circumstances.

The year before this crisis of confidence the government launched its plans for a limited list of drugs prescribable on the NHS. The idea had been floated many times before, and had always been rejected out of hand by the BMA as an attack on clinical freedom, with apparently vigorous support from the BMA membership. The BMA and, to its shame, the leadership of the Labour Party, rushed to the defence of medical independence, without bothering to find out what GPs actually thought. In fact, GPs had become steadily more sceptical of the claims of the pharmaceutical industry, and more hostile to the way it enriched itself at the expense of the NHS; they were ready to agree to common-sense proposals which might limit the burgeoning power of the multi-nationals, though they knew very well that this was only a cost-cutting exercise, without any larger purpose. In those circumstances, and backed up by a postal ballot of the whole membership, it was possible for the College leadership to take the membership undivided in a socially responsible direction, and to prove itself a more sensitive and adaptable vehicle for professional change than the BMA. This success seems to have led to intoxication; though the GPA proposal had far less support than the limited prescribing list, it was driven through without a membership ballot, and only abandoned when the position was clearly hopeless.

As for the examiners, the MRCGP was drifting irresistibly away from its original function as a ticket of entry to active membership of the College, towards its present *de facto* status as an elegant ticket of exit from vocational training. An exit test is necessary and will continue as one relatively unimportant part of training for general practice, just as the MRCP examination is a necessary but relatively unimportant part of the training of consultant physicians, and I think there is a strong case for making it mandatory, though this is

still a minority view. The examiners were addressing themselves successfully to this task, but it had little to do with the
general direction being taken by College Council, increasingly
(and rightly) concerned with structural reform of general
practice as a whole, rather than with verifying what young
GPs knew at the end of their training. The potential for a
dangerous split is still there.

The 1987 White Paper

Although the specific proposal for a GPA has collapsed, the
search for some means of improving 'bad' doctors by rewarding 'good' ones has not been abandoned, either by the
government and the DHSS, or by the College. The final reply
by the College to the Green Paper[17] still claimed that 'The
key issue now is the way of achieving a link between the
general practitioner's NHS contract and the quality of services
that a practice offers.' How this could be done without
raising the same issues as the GPA was not explained. It
looked very much as though some leaders of the College
(and probably some leaders of the BMA) regarded a two-tier
service as inevitable in a two-tier society, and were simply
waiting for the troops to catch up with the realism of the
general staff.

As I completed the final draft of this book the new health
minister, John Moore, launched the government's White
Paper on primary care,[24] with some proposals to be incorporated in a Bill to come before parliament as this book
goes to press. Most of its proposals, however, will have to be
negotiated with the General Medical Services Committee of
the BMA, and this is likely to be a very prolonged battle,
probably setting the main agenda for the next two or three
years. The White Paper claims to be the biggest shake-up of
primary care services since 1948, but though it certainly is a
turning point in government and perhaps in professional
attitudes to GP autonomy, it is not at all clear what strategy
will replace the present incoherent jumble of unaccounted
resource and unresourced accountability.

The White Paper is a profoundly contradictory document.

It drops the Good Practice Allowance, but states that it has not abandoned the idea of performance-related pay for GPs. As the terms of the White Paper come to be negotiated with the BMA, with the RCGP still a potent force on the sidelines, all the issues raised by the GPA and the Green Paper will resurface. The White Paper does attempt for the first time to define some fragments of a boundary to a verifiable GP contract for proactive care in specific terms of health maintenance, though the bits it has chosen (cervical smears, immunization, developmental assessment in childhood, 'health checks' for the elderly, blood pressure screening and so on) are a ragbag of what is measurable rather than what is important, hastily prepared by people without personal experience of anticipatory care in the community and unaware of the real constraints and difficulties faced by all primary health workers who take this work seriously.

Targets are to be set for immunization rates and various sorts of screening, verified by Family Practitioner Committees which are to be encouraged to take on positive functions in health care planning. There are to be inducement-payments for success in achieving these targets. Though obviously this will be more difficult in high-workload, high-morbidity areas such as inner cities and areas of high unemployment and industrial decay, other incentive payments are proposed to improve recruitment of young GPs to these areas, which are presumably intended to offset higher earnings in areas where high rates for preventive care will be more easily attained.

The limit of two Whole-Time-Equivalent staff to each GP is to be removed, and a wider range of staff can be employed, including physiotherapists, interpreters and other social link workers and counsellors. However, reimbursement of wages for these additional staff are to be cash-limited, presumably implying that the most progressive practices which already employ their full quota and want more staff will get them, but the most backward practices most in need of more staff are likely to find the cupboard bare when they get there; 'buy now while stocks last'.

FPCs will be responsible for setting targets for preventive

work and verifying their achievement. It is not at all clear how this will be done; FPC budgets have just been cut and further cuts have been officially forecast for next year, though at the same time more money is promised to assist these new functions. The White Paper mentions the possibility of annual reports by GPs as part of their contract, but does not seem to see this as a major area for innovation, and naturally ignores the possibility that these could be a pathway for direct accountability to patients, the development of democratic control, and the means of creating a counterbalance to the risks of central bureaucracy in any future salaried service.

In apparent conflict with all these proposals, the minimum list size to qualify for the Basic Practice Allowance (the salary element in GP pay) is to be raised from its present level of 1,000, and the proportion of earnings from capitation is to be increased. The policy makers seem inclined towards the pattern of care long advocated by Geoffrey Marsh,[25] an extended team of nursing and other supporting staff, with a smaller number of GPs with large lists, concentrating on their traditional task of dealing with established symptomatic disease and diagnostic and therapeutic puzzles. These larger lists would be attained by more vigorous competition, assisted by simpler procedures for patients who want to choose a different GP, and by moves towards advertising the range of services offered by different practices.

The White Paper proposes an immediate reduction of the salary element in GPs' pay with a corresponding increase in capitation, to encourage competition and larger lists, and warns that further increases in capitation and reductions in salary are planned for the future. It is interesting that despite the entrenched hostility of GPs to a fully salaried service, both the College and the BMA are fiercely opposed to increases in the capitation element, rightly believing that this will encourage competition for patients in terms which will certainly address consumer satisfaction, but will equally certainly fail to address population needs. The most probable scenario for any shift of British general practice to salaried service is that this will occur not in one single dramatic leap, but by incremental shifts away from capitation and fees-for-item-of-service and towards a proportionally larger salary (basic salary plus salary increments for further training, seniority and difficult areas of practice), together with a more positively planned and verified local contract with proactive rather than reactive FPCs. It is difficult today to conceive of BMA negotiators openly embracing the form of a salaried service, but it is entirely conceivable that they could, faced with uglier alternatives, accept its substance.

A Menu Without a Meal

Though it implies a substantial extension of the scope and responsibilities of general practice, the White Paper proposes an increase in expenditure of only 5% in 1988-9, 2.5% in 1989-90 and 3.5% in 1990-91, all in real terms. The only immediate new money available for this is to be £170 million from charges to patients (for the first time) for examinations by dentists and opticians, a step which obviously contradicts the government's claim to be promoting prevention. FPC budgets are for the first time to be cash-limited in respect of all this proactive care, as opposed to reactive demand-led care, which remains open-ended because even this government has not yet thought of any way of closing it. The White Paper's menu does contain many interesting items, particularly to progressive GPs accustomed to baked beans every day for the last 39 years, but when we come to who pays, it turns out that this meal is to be more a literary than a gastronomic experience.

In strategic terms, the White Paper is a dog's dinner, an incoherent jumble of measures promising something for everybody, but which on the day it was presented to Parliament apparently pleased nobody. It is interesting that the Right was probably more angry than the Left. The White Paper gave a ritual curtsey to The Market ('The Government sees no reason why private primary health care should not be developed in ways that provide both an alternative source of care and means of comparison with NHS services'), but the Director of the Social Affairs Unit (a New Conservative think-tank) writing in *The Times*[26] the next day on 'The great health collision' saw 'no substantial differences' between the policies of the Labour and Conservative Parties, and was clearly disappointed at the failure even of the third Thatcher administration to break with the tradition of welfarism in the NHS:

> The ingredients are all there: scientific and medical progress making available a host of new treatments, rising public expectations that the treatments are a 'right', and cost of treatment rising faster than the general rate of inflation. It is a collision course. . . We are now seeing the acknowledged *rationing* of health care. Unless something is done soon, there will be much more. . .
>
> It is certainly true, as the [White Paper] suggests, that the quality and effort of GPs varies enormously. But, again, this is to be corrected by the politicians and bureaucrats deciding what constitutes a good doctor and giving slightly increased incentive payments for him to do the things they want. . . the overall question of what suits the varied needs of the 750,000 who visit the GP each day is not reflected in these broad objectives. True, the customer is to be given a little more information about the rival merits of GPs but not to the extent that it might inconvenience the GPs, or that trade union, the British Medical Association, that Thatcherism has yet to put in its place. . .
>
> True radicalism would involve facing up to the central problems that health services need a lot more money and it cannot all come from raised taxation, that we need an innovating health system with true competition, and that 'inefficiency' cannot improve unless true costs and preferences are revealed by a market.
>
> True radicalism would not restrict its use of charging to outside the GP service—as [the White Paper] does. It would consider whether innovation, efficiency and consumer satisfaction might not be better served by returning to each family of four who wishes it, the £560 it has contributed in taxation to the nationalised system. . . and letting them spend it on private care. All the evidence shows that many families are willing to add such a sum and spend more, provided they know it is going to the family's health care, not to the general tax coffers.

The contrast between rationing and the market is instructive. Wartime rationing gave us a better-fed nation in war than we had in the peacetime of the 1930s, when markets ruled. The Radical Right never seems to notice that if people have money to spend on private medical care or to contribute to charities, this money could equally, and more efficiently, have been spent on higher taxes for better services which would not have to depend either on the poorly-informed demands of consumers or on humiliating appeals for charity. The fact that many people love themselves more than their neighbours and want to spend their money accordingly seems a poor base for what claims to be a moral argument.

The same issue of *The Times* contains the reports of the White Paper's reception in parliament under the headline 'FURIOUS PROTESTS GREET HEALTH WHITE PAPER'. The fury came not only from the opposition, but from the Conservative back benches, including such Thatcher stalwarts as Dame Jill Knight, Mr Robin Maxwell-Hyslop, and former Conservative Health Minister Sir Barney Hayhoe, who protested at the continued under-funding of the NHS and told his own front benches that if in the next budget possible tax cuts were foregone in order to provide more money for the NHS, the Chancellor of the Exchequer 'would be cheered equally in all parts of the House'. Between its raucous un-elected advisers and its more cautious MPs, the Government has little room for manoeuvre.

As I write, there has not been time for either the College or the BMA to respond to the White Paper. The minister is probably confident that no real alternative, a planned service accountable for health outputs as well as measures of process, has yet been developed or even contemplated either by professional bodies, or by the opposition parties, and in the absence of positive proposals he can negotiate the details with the BMA with an effectively bipartisan policy behind him in parliament for his positive measures. The Labour Party might well prefer the Conservatives to take the blame for any incursions on GP autonomy, while congratulating themselves on the useful precedents set for a future administration.

The White Paper probably defers a clear decision in any direction. GP accountability is to be increased, though how this will be done is not at all clear. In general steps forward towards a more continuous, anticipatory and socially responsive service are roughly balanced (and for the most part contradicted) by concessions to consumerism and competition (inevitably impairing continuity), fees-for-service (which may be inflationary and will certainly increase bureaucracy), and direct patient charges (though not yet within the GP service). Though nothing has been actively done to promote private general practice, pressure from the Radical Right will continue, restrained chiefly by the wish of Dame Jill Knight and other Conservative MPs to be re-elected next time they face the voters.

Doctor-centred or Patient-centred Service?

I have dealt at length with the Green and White Papers story because it is the most recent and dramatic example of the unresolved conflict at the foundation of the health service in Britain, and in sometimes more, sometimes less obvious forms in all other market economies; hospital services cannot work effectively without a primary care base of GPs, the primary care base cannot work effectively without more public investment in medical, nursing and office staff time, and public investment will not be made without public accountability; but GPs are reluctant to accept public accountability and as yet unable to imagine it in terms of local participative democracy rather than central bureaucracy. None of these developments can therefore occur on a mass scale, and governments anxious to hasten as slowly as possible will be satisfied to keep this situation going as long as they can, unless and until escalating hospital costs force them to look again at fundamental changes in primary care.

The GPA, and the quality-related pay proposals in the White Paper, attempted to solve problems of clinical squalor concentrated above all in industrial and inner-city practice, by rewarding already-innovating practices almost none of which are to be found where these problems are at their worst. 'The arguments for providing increased resources for those practices which are innovating and striving for improvement are unanswerable', said RCGP Chairman John Hasler. No doubt they were; but even more unanswerable were the arguments for providing increased resources for practices which were not innovating and not striving for improvement, because these resources were needed for patients, not doctors.

There is only one means of escape from this dilemma; GPs' practices belong not to them personally, but to the communities they serve. Left to themselves, GPs will never accept this in reality, though they may occasionally be willing to talk about it. But in the real world, they are no longer being left to themselves; they are entering a stormy sea, in which secure and well-rewarded mediocrity will no longer be on offer from any political party. At the time of the Green Paper in 1986, the most the College could realistically have hoped to do was to make the various options for reform clear to the membership, together with such evidence as we had, and leave them to make their own choice through their own traditional negotiating bodies, the Local Medical Committees and the BMA. There was, and as yet there is, no consensus support for any major move in any direction; it was folly to believe it could be otherwise, until it becomes obvious to a critical mass of the membership that the status quo is no longer an option. The historic push had to come from the outside, and with a little patience would soon have done so; it is probably doing so now. It was wrong to risk the unity of a socially valuable organization in a vain attempt to lead GPs where they did not want to go, at a time when they were not yet convinced that they had to move at all.

After the election of 1987, Mrs Thatcher and her New Conservatives believe they have a popular mandate to impose radical change throughout society, and general practice will ultimately be no exception. Under the slogan of Parent Choice, 'good' schools are to be encouraged to expand at the expense of 'bad' ones, ignoring the obvious question; why will any parents choose 'bad' schools? The government is gambling on its belief that a vocal minority of parents will believe that their own children will gain from a two-tier system, and that most parents will continue passively to accept whatever schooling is locally available, thereby returning to an educational system which even in childhood deliberately reinforces the division of society into winners and losers. All the arguments for widening the gap by rewarding good schools and pauperizing bad ones, rather than making effective investment where difficulties are greatest to improve standards for all neighbourhoods (because it is tidy or rough neighbourhoods we are really talking about), can be applied to arguments for a two-tier GP service. Individual GPs are likely to be scapegoated for bad general practice in the most damaged parts of our society, just as individual teachers have been pilloried for bad schools, and individual social workers have been sacrificial victims of their permanently overworked and undermanned service. Invited to act as jurors, exasperated patients may serve as willingly as disappointed or frightened parents. Mrs Thatcher knows how to economize in already impoverished educational and social services which have to cope with the results of divisive economic and social policies and drastic cuts in central funding, while blaming the consequences on those who have to operate them. GPs are likely eventually to find themselves in the same line of fire. The easy options will be gone, and GPs, in the College and in the BMA, will have to look for new allies and consider active policies for change.

From Investment without Accountability to Accountability without Investment

The prospect now facing (but not, as yet, faced by) GPs is that having so long refused to pay the price of public accountability for increased public investment, they may get the accountability without the investment. It is not too painful to rationalize distribution of effort within an expanding service, but in a cash-limited service squeezed between the growing needs of an ageing population and the rising expectations of continued scientific advance, it is going to be very painful indeed, not only to patients, nurses and other health workers, but even to doctors. A minority of doctors and patients will solve some of their own problems by moving backward in history to the private sector, but a frankly two-tiered service for patients will also mean two-tiered quality of care and two-tiered careers for doctors.

Increasingly, doctors will question the value of the social components of the Osler paradigm. Gentlemanly status is a waning asset, and the possibility of a different social alignment may become more attractive. Once compelled to accept that we must be accountable to someone, we shall begin to understand that we have a choice, if we have the courage and imagination to make it. Apart from accountability to the individual patient, the only forms of accountability ever considered within the Osler paradigm have either been accountability of the profession to itself (which is what we are supposed to have now, and has generally meant no accountability at all) or accountability to some higher administration, without recent personal experience of the everyday realities of practice, with its own bureaucratic objectives, and its own allegiances to yet higher and more remote authority.

Of course, some central, regional and district administrative control and leadership are essential to any fully effective primary care system, and even at practice level administrative skills are essential. The proviso is important, because the whole medical tradition, and especially the tradition of general practice, is (in its middle-class way) anarchic, contemptuous and intolerant even of obviously necessary administration; 'if they would only leave us doctors and nurses alone to get on with the job, we could do twice the work in half the time'; an ignorant and condescending attitude to health service administration of which we should be ashamed. But the hatred and mistrust of bureaucracy felt by so many doctors, and particularly by GPs, has real foundations. The withering effects of bureaucracy on initiative have been obvious in our own Public Health and School Medical Services, and in many under-funded but over-administered public primary care services abroad. The counterweight to bureaucracy is not cocksure autonomy for clinicians, but participative democracy: the only people besides ourselves who can really know the nature of our work are the populations we serve, and they are the only people who could and would defend us and themselves from bureaucracy in a planned and accountable service.

Just as doctors in the USA are ending up as salaried employees of for-profit medical corporations because of their obstinate refusal to accept a socialized health service,[27] British GPs could end up as Poor Law doctors serving a pinchpenny bureaucracy rather than the needs of their patients, if they refuse to develop real partnership with their patients in a people's service.

That puts the conclusion before the evidence. The next two chapters examine the real components of accountability to patients.

NOTES

1. Nussey, S.S., Pilkington, T.R.E., Saunders, K.B., 'Where will this month's medical school intake go?', *Lancet 1986*; ii:977. See also *Lancet* editorial 'Medical student numbers and medical manpower', *Lancet 1987*; i:723-4.
2. Allsop, J., May, A., *The emperor's new clothes: Family Practitioner Committees in the 1980s*, London: King's Fund, 1986.
3. NHS Act 1977. Regulations. London: HMSO, 1986.
4. Shaw, G.B., *The Doctor's Dilemma: a tragedy*, London: Constable, 1907.
5. Anon. 'The insurance medical service week by week: payment for keeping records', *British Medical Journal 1935*; ii:suppl. 174.
6. Pereira Gray, D., 'General practitioners and the independent contractor status', *Journal of the Royal College of General Practitioners 1977*; 27:746-51.
7. *The best of health: charter for the family health service*, Labour Party, 150 Walworth Road, London SE17 1JT, 1986.
8. Smith, R., 'The wasted opportunity of the election', *British Medical Journal 1987*; 294:1438-9.
9. House of Commons Committee on Social Services. 'First Report Session 1986-7: Primary Health Care', Paper 37-I. London: HMSO, 1987.
10. Secretaries of State for Social Services, Wales, Northern Ireland & Scotland, 'Primary health care: an agenda for discussion', (Cmnd 9771). London: HMSO, 1986.
11. Marinker, M., 'Developments in primary care', in *A new NHS Act for 1996?*, London: Office of Health Economics, 1984.
12. Maynard, A., Marinker, M., Pereira Gray, D., 'The doctor, the patient, and their contract. III Alternative contracts: are they viable?', *British Medical Journal 1986*; 292:1438-40.
13. Hart, J.T., 'Community general practitioners', *British Medical Journal 1984*; 288:1670-3.
14. Mant, D., Anderson, P., 'Community general practitioner', *Lancet 1985*; ii:1114-7.
15. Royal College of General Practitioners, 'Quality in general practice',

Policy Statement 2, London: RCGP, 1985.
16. Crombie, D., *Personal communication*, 1987.
17. The front line of the health service; College response to 'Primary health care: an agenda for discussion', *Report from general practice 25*, London: RCGP, 1987.
18. Marinker, M., Pereira Gray, D., Maynard, A., 'The doctor, the patient, and their contract. II. A good practice allowance: is it feasible?', *British Medical Journal 1986*; 292:1374-6.
19. Bosanquet, N., Leese, B., 'Family doctors: their choice of practice', *British Medical Journal 1986*; 293:667-70.
20. McKee, I., 'A proposal without merit', *The Physician 1986*; 839.
21. Bourne, S., Bruggen, P., 'Secrecy and distinction awards', *British Medical Journal 1987*; 295:393.
22. Hasler, J., 'Supporting good practice', *Journal of the Royal College of General Practitioners 1986*; 36:394-7.
23. The GMSC is the most important body representing GPs in negotiation with government. Its composition is extremely complex, but understanding of it is essential to anyone who wants to understand the politics of the medical profession. An excellent account is given by Steve Watkins in his book *Medicine and Labour: the politics of a profession*, London: Lawrence & Wishart, 1987.
24. 'Promoting better health', Cmnd 249, London: HMSO, 1987.
25. Marsh, G.N., Channing, D.M., 'Deprivation and health in one general practice', *British Medical Journal 1986*; 292:1173-6.
26. Anderson, D., 'The great health collision', *The Times*, 26 November 1987.
27. Starr, P., *The social transformation of American medicine*, New York: Basic Books, 1982.

Chapter 7
ACCOUNTABILITY
FOR AND TO INDIVIDUALS

Within the Osler paradigm, doctors have generally accepted accountability in two directions; to their professional colleagues collectively, and to their patients individually. In each case, accountability has been at two levels: a formal level of official complaint, disciplinary action or litigation; and an informal level of custom and expectations.

Because in Osler's time doctors had so little influence on the outcome of illness, accountability for outcome was not possible. Even the traditional Hippocratic rule 'primum non nocere' (above all, don't harm) was not enforceable; desperate fear condoned desperate remedies; so doctors were encouraged to add substantial risks from treatment to the uncertain but often serious risks of illness. The dangers of surgery were obvious, but less well remembered are the often highly toxic medicines in everyday use well into the 1940s. Strychnine, lead, arsenic and mercury were common ingredients of pills, medicines and ointments used for a wide variety of conditions for which no treatment of experimentally proven effect was available. Doses were supposed to be safe, but chronic lead and arsenic poisoning were common in sufferers of multiple sclerosis, motor neurone disease, migraine, trigeminal neuralgia, hysteria and other chronic disorders for which they were often prescribed. When I was a medical student in 1950 'pink disease', an often fatal disorder of infants, was proved (after prolonged and acrimonious controversy in the medical journals) to be chronic mercury poisoning from teething powders, prescribed by doctors or bought over the counter from chemists.

When the Osler paradigm was developed, transactions between doctors and patients were largely illusory. Then as now, they were seldom consciously deceptive. The chief therapeutic agent, and the chief product of a medical consultation, was hope, and doctors and patients collaborated more or less equally in producing and sustaining it. There was a tacit social agreement that the alleged centre of the medical process (attempts to alter the course of illness) could not be subjected to serious direct criticism, because then there would soon be no profession left to criticize. Credulity was an important part of the medical process, valued by patients as much as by doctors, and this was the principal justification for the very tight definition of medical privilege and exclusion of competing skills. Instead, criticism was focused on the medical process rather than its outcome. The most dependable defence was strict adherence to conventional process, not only clinical process but also the ways in which doctors dressed, spoke and behaved. Outrageous social behaviour and barefaced fraud were the main targets; not what doctors did, but how they did it.

This refusal to look objectively at the clinical centre of medical failure and success, at the overall gains or losses in long-term health and happiness, is still with us. Despite massive evidence that effective medical knowledge is very incompletely applied, this hardly figures in the personal accountability of doctors for their daily work. Instead, we maintain systems for chasing exceptional offenders accused of exceptional crimes, while leaving the effectiveness of our daily work unmeasured and largely unknown.

Accountability to Professional Bodies and Administration

Professional accountability in Britain is to the General Medical Council (GMC), representing a mixture of lay and professional establishment opinion, with its own disciplinary powers to suspend or expel doctors from their profession, outside the ordinary legal system. Similar European bodies, like the Ordre des Medecins in France and Belgium, combine these powers with representation of the real or imagined interests of doctors in negotiation with the State, reinforcing the power of established doctors to restrict social innovation within the profession. In Britain this negotiating function has always been carried out by the BMA, distantly flanked by the minuscule MPU, without disciplinary powers or compulsory membership.

In 1983, 920 doctors out of about 60,000 in all forms of practice were reported to the GMC for suspected misconduct. Only 40 of these were ultimately referred to the Professional Conduct Committee. The most that can be said for the GMC is that it sets an outer limit to professional negligence or incompetence, but this is so remote from everyday success or failure that it is of little interest to doctors concerned (as the vast majority are) with the effectiveness of ordinary care.

Formal complaints by patients about doctors either in hospitals or general practice are infrequent. The Royal Commission on the NHS[1] recorded that of about 200 million patient contacts with GPs in 1978, only 1,465 led to formal complaints to Family Practitioner Committees. Complaints about doctors in hospitals were more frequent, but of six million in-patient treatments and nine million new out-patients in that year, less than 1% led to written complaints. In 1983 there were about 19,600 written complaints about hospital care, about one in 2,000 episodes of treatment.[2] Less than half of these were complaints about clinical management.

The NHS remains a popular service, and those who work in it are still generally well thought of. However, in a retrospective analysis of 500 consecutive deaths in my own practice from 1964 to 1985, I was able to identify avoidable factors in 45%, of which 59% seemed mainly attributable to the acts and omissions of patients, 20% to misjudgements by myself and my GP colleagues, and 4% to misjudgements and errors by hospital doctors, though it was difficult to get as much information about the last category as I had about myself and my colleagues.[3] I have no reason to believe these figures are unusual, so evidently few events deserving (hopefully constructive) criticism lead to any formal complaint. I do not, of course, suggest that they should, but a mature science should be founded on self-criticism and mutual criticism, in which doubt rather than faith is the accepted norm, not in order to pillory malpractice, but to advance the practice of scientific medicine. Our existing machinery of criticism is almost entirely irrelevant to this aim, and lags far behind the real moral position already attained by most doctors.

In hospitals, where doctors are salaried and their work is at least nominally co-ordinated within teams and between specialties, NHS administration has in practice little to do with maintaining standards of medical care, except in this negative and exceptional sense of fielding complaints. Even then, accountability of consultants is unconvincing. In an editorial in the *British Medical Journal*,[4] a teaching hospital consultant has described and explained the problem:

> In hospitals administrative staff are accountable to general managers and nurses to the District Nursing Officer, but the accountability of doctors is not clear. Hospital doctors in training are answerable to their superiors, but after being appointed consultant. . . a doctor has a secure job and does not appear to be accountable for the quantity or the quality of his work.
>
> There are several reasons for this. One is historical: years ago consultants gave their services free to charitable institutions, which could hardly complain when the consultant was not in constant attendance. The influence of this tradition persists, and some consultants still think that their main clinical job is simply to be available for consultation to junior staff. Another reason is that consultants—unlike senior nurses—have a mixture of clinical and administrative responsibilities, which are closely interlinked. It is difficult for an employer to make a consultant accountable for administration while deferring to him on clinical matters, and the question of clinical accountability is a sensitive one.

Even more in general practice than in hospitals, most complaints concern style rather than clinical management, probably because in this area patients have more confidence in their own judgements. Klein[5] reviewed complaints to Family Practitioner Committees (FPCs) in 1973. Nearly 35% were about GPs' or their receptionists' manners and remarks, 22% were about delays in visiting or problems about appointments and only 11% were about diagnosis or treatment. He noted that whereas doctors seemed mainly to fear and organize to defend themselves against accusations of clinical incompetence, patients actually complained mainly about how GPs, hospital doctors and their office and nursing staffs treated them as people, though they may rightly have believed that rudeness and secrecy may have serious clinical consequences.

Litigation

Litigation by patients and their relatives for medical malpractice, though rising, remains uncommon in the NHS. An estimate for 1983 was that only about 5% of formal complaints resulted in writs for damages, of which 30–40% were successful.[2] This is in striking contrast with the USA, where in 1986 18.3 claims were made for every 100 insured physicians, and sums awarded in compensation were vastly greater than in Britain. The reasons for these differences are complex. In a careful analysis, Quam, Dingwall and Fenn[6] pointed out that:

In principle the National Health Service seems likely to reduce claims in at least four ways: there is no direct cost to the patient for extra medical care to remedy an injury; access to care is guaranteed throughout life; there is no direct financial relation between doctors and patients; and the system of referral restrains specialists while encouraging loyalty between patients and their general practitioners.

However, they go on to warn that all these supportive features could be lost.

. . . unless the level of National Health Service resources is seen to be adequate to ensure reasonable access and treatment, so that there is no need to litigate for funds to purchase care. . .

and that:

The present constraints on National Health Service funding may,

by their pressure on medical personnel, also precipitate an increase
in the number of incidents capable of leading to claims. . . Fatigue
is not a legal defence against an allegation of negligence. Similarly,
if junior doctors take on work beyond their level of skill and
experience they cannot rely on this as a defence. There is only one
legal standard of care: if a doctor is not sufficiently experienced to
perform a particular procedure he or she should not undertake the
work. Obviously, it is difficult to insist on this when faced with
pressing clinical needs, but then the risk of litigation must be
evaluated as a cost of a system which requires young doctors to
work long hours with limited senior cover.

Whether lawyers accept it or not there are different clinical
standards in general practice (particularly industrial working-
class practice) on the one hand, and in hospitals on the other,
and many GPs as well as young doctors in hospitals work
long hours isolated from peer criticism. All evidence suggests
that the relative immunity from formal complaint and
litigation of British doctors, and particularly of British GPs,
has depended on the gratitude and loyalty of the public and
its low expectations in a free but always overworked and
underfunded State service. Recent evidence from the Social
and Community Planning Research (SCRP) surveys[7] on
public satisfaction with the NHS, shown in Table 7.1, gives
no ground for complacency.

Table 7.1 Public satisfaction with the NHS

Survey year:	1983	1984	1986
Very satisfied	11%	11%	6%
Quite satisfied	44%	40%	34%
Neither satisfied nor dissatisfied	20%	19%	19%
Quite dissatisfied	18%	19%	23%
Very dissatisfied	7%	11%	16%

In the same study, dissatisfaction (quite or very dissatisfied) in 1983[8] rose from 21% of those with annual
incomes under £5,000 to 34% of those with incomes over
£10,000; 13% of all respondents were dissatisfied with the
GP service, compared with 7% for hospital in-patient services
and 21% for hospital out-patient services. Patients, particularly younger and richer patients, are becoming more critical,

and possibly more litigious.

Accountability to Colleagues

More perhaps than anything else, medical students learn to respect clinical competence, a term frequently used by doctors but difficult to define. In the sense in which it is usually understood, it need not include several features essential to effective medical care. We all understand what is meant by describing a doctor as clinically competent, but so rude and unsympathetic to patients that this competence cannot be effectively expressed. Competence always includes knowledge of the biological aspects of disease, and the technical means of dealing with it, but understanding of people, even as necessary vehicles for disease, is a desirable but not essential extra.

Clinical competence is the currency in which all kinds of intraprofessional negotiations and conflicts are conducted. A woman doctor in the USA quoted by Good[9] expresses this idea of currency very perceptively:

> I think for a long time I tried to increase my competence, or my vision of myself as competent, or other people's visions of me as competent, at the expense of other physicians' competence. I think that's what a lot of doctors do. It's like there is only so much competence in this world. If I have more, they have less; if they have more, I have less.

Clinical competence, in other words, is like other kinds of wealth and power. There must be winners and losers; we all love winners, nobody likes losers. Forget about our profession as a band of brothers and sisters in service to mankind, it's just another part of the universal war of every man against every man. Incompetent doctors are, like incompetent patients, simply rubbished.

In this view medicine is predatory, and the most successful doctors can be judged only by others who have shed blood in the same way. In 1984 Dr David Kinzer[10] reiterated an opinion he first published in 1959, that the needs of physicians are best understood as resembling fighter pilots in the Second World War:

> Relating to my combat experience flying dive bombers and fighter planes, the success or failure of our performance was measured in one-to-one situations. No dive-bombing run on an enemy ship or dogfight with an enemy plane was like any other. It was always a very lonely experience. The carrier we took off from and, we hoped, would land back upon was always, during these moments, a remote and almost irrelevant entity. . . An explicit reality here is that the missions of the pilot and the carrier were not the same, nor are the missions of the hospital and the clinicians on its medical staff. This distinction is important. The carrier (or the hospital) is an organization whose only reason for being is to provide a support system for the missions of its pilots (or physicians). Whether the mission is a dogfight or a critical trauma case, it is still the prime responsibility of the pilot or the attending physician. The organization, with its technical hardware, supply system, and support personnel, has only a backup role.

This view is typical of the way in which junior hospital doctors see themselves and their work. Mizrahi and colleagues[11] studied 207 US hospital internists in residency training over a period of three years, using questionnaires and in-depth interviews to study their attitudes to accountability. Here are some typical statements, which could equally be heard from equivalent British resident staff:

> As time goes on you don't criticise as much because you know that you may have made the same mistake in the past. On the other hand you realise that you're not going to change people if you criticise them. All you're going to do is make them angry at you.

> I remember my first patient who died that I felt in some way responsible. . . If I had done something differently maybe it would have made a difference. As a third year medical student, the patient had a bloody stool and my intern told me he was a 'crock' and not to be concerned.

> Practically the first week I was on as a third year medical student, the chief resident told me a particular patient was a 'SHPOS' [Sub-Human Piece Of Shit]. I was there alone that night when he decided to crump [die]. . . If I hadn't been told he was SHPOS I might have gotten on the situation sooner.

> I can't say I have a whole lot of allegiance to anyone. I'm pretty

much a loner. I feel accountable to myself and I feel accountable to try to do the best I can for the people I'm taking care of.

I'm accountable to me. Because it's my job and I have chosen to do this to the best of my ability.

Mizrahi found that these completely doctor-centred views of accountability failed to convince even the doctors themselves:

Notwithstanding this shared elaborate repertoire of denial, discounting and distancing, it was found that profound doubts and even guilt remained for many housestaff. . . For many the case was never closed, even as they terminated formal training. . . The housestaff ultimately sees itself as the sole arbiter of mistakes and their adjudication. Housestaffers come to feel that nobody can judge them or their decisions, least of all their patients. . . They have developed a strong ideology justifying their jealously guarded autonomy. In the graduate medical socialisation process, they have learned to believe that because they perceive themselves as their own worst judges, they should be their only judges. Because of the insularity and isolation of the housestaff subculture in a position of high prestige, with the power to make life and death decisions, they see themselves as singularly responsible for their actions and disparage any attempt by others to insert themselves into the process of accountability.

Kinzer and Mizrahi's junior hospital doctors are talking about the USA, but what they say is easily recognized by doctors everywhere; the Osler paradigm of socially isolated, gentlemanly privilege is international. From their first day in medical school, doctors learn to see themselves as hunters, who know diseases as beasts in the jungle, and can shoot from the hip, hopefully hitting the disease more often than the patient, but accepting that hunting accidents are in the nature of the game and are bound to happen. It may be dangerous for patients, but it's also dangerous for doctors. In a study of 170 junior house officers in British Hospitals, Jenny Firth-Cozens[12] found that 50% reported emotional disturbance arising from stress, mostly overwork and loss of sleep. 28% showed evidence of depression on psychiatric criteria, 19% drank alcohol heavily and 6% had suicidal thoughts. The study was prompted by two deaths from suicide in junior house officers.

Apart from crisis situations, the fantasy of doctors living dangerously as hunters, rescuing helpless and ignorant patients from attack by predatory diseases which doctors alone can recognize and understand, is an absurdity; but it is ideally designed for a service which abandons caring to concentrate on salvage.

The Patient's Role in Diagnosis

Conan Doyle, a good middling doctor unable to make a living in Osler's time, modelled Sherlock Holmes on an impressive teacher at his own medical school. Holmes was a stunning solo performer, creating a convincing diagnosis from whisps of this and crumbs of that, evidence available to the slower minds of his witnesses and to Dr Watson, but transformed by the great detective into creations entirely his own.

How Conan Doyle's ideal managed to stage his apparently convincing performances only medical students familiar with the theatre of teaching consultancy can know. For most performers, some prior investigation and several rehearsals are necessary, with a spotlight blinding the captive audience to the equally essential contributions of the patient, nurses and junior medical staff. The solo consultant who can produce a dazzling diagnosis while making everyone else look a fool is as much a fictional character as Sherlock Holmes himself.

Consultation of a patient with a doctor for a newly presented complaint usually consists firstly of a diagnostic process ('What's wrong with this patient?'), then of a plan for treatment ('What can be done to put it right?'). Objective studies of both these parts of a consultation show that patients as well as doctors must make active contributions of their own, if diagnosis is to be relevant to the patient's problems and treatment is to be effective.

The diagnostic process usually has three stages: a history (what the patient says, mainly in response to a more or less systematic interrogation); physical examination; and laboratory, x-ray or other technical investigations. A group in Oxford[13] studied the relative importance of each of these to diagnosis by getting consultants to make a provisional diagnosis successively at each stage (after the history, after examination and finally after routine technical tests), and then comparing the proportion who reached the final diagnosis (made retrospectively at follow-up three months later) at each point. In 80 newly-referred medical out-patients, the final diagnosis was reached after reading the GP's letter and taking the history in 66 (82%); physical examination added 6 (7%) and technical investigations added 7 (9%). Listening to the patient is not only more productive than these other more technical and perhaps more impressive processes, but is also essential to guide them in an intelligent direction; experienced doctors already have one or more hypotheses before they examine their patients to confirm or refute them, and their choice of technical tests similarly depends on hypotheses generated chiefly by the history.

'Listen to the patient,' said the great French 19th Century neurologist Jean-Martin Charcot, 'he is telling you the diagnosis.' Of course, patients cannot usually give a relevant history unaided, but the huge importance of their active, intelligent contribution only becomes obvious when because of cultural or language barriers, no history is available. Diagnosis and subsequent medical management then become veterinary rather than human, crude mechanistic inter-ventions of value only in crises, when the patient's role always tends to become passive.

It is doubtful whether Charcot fully understood the truth of his own aphorism. He is said to have refused ever to examine patients in a public teaching hospital unless they were stripped naked; only then, with a patient dumb with fear and shame before a hundred or more students, would he condescend to proceed with his examination. The social assumptions of Osler's time made this conduct normal; sick people having free treatment in teaching hospitals were expected to speak only when spoken to, answering 'yes' or 'no' to cross-examination by the doctor, venturing no opinions of their own. Even when I was a clinical student in 1948–52 little of this had changed. Patients today are probably less willing to submit to such arrogance, but the problem is still recognizably there. Useful diagnosis is not just professional recognition of a biological process incomprehensible to the laity, but a useful analysis of interdependent problems which always (not sometimes) have multiple biological, psychological and social causes, all of which must be understood if we are to find effective solutions. To the extent that patients are discouraged from sharing in the definition of their medical problems, diagnoses will be made which are irrelevant to real lives, however biologically true they may appear to be.

A Clinical Example

As the antithesis of swashbuckling episodic battles with acute or end-stage disease, let me give an example of the sort of case where years, even decades of work are required, with less dramatic but probably more important results.

I have been responsible for primary medical care for Hopkin Morgan (the name is, of course, fictitious) since 1961, when I was 34 and he was 36. He's a big man, a big soccer player in his youth, and a big coal miner who rarely missed a shift until a runaway tram gave him a compound fracture in one leg in 1964, and killed the man working beside him. A routine medical examination in 1960 had shown a blood pressure of 194/126 mmHg, but when this was repeated a couple of weeks later it had fallen to 168/94, still well into the top 1% of the distribution of blood pressure for a man of that age, but not high enough to justify treatment with the antihypertensive drugs available at that time. His blood pressure was not checked again until 1966, when two readings reached 200/120 and 170/120. He has at least nominally been on treatment with antihypertensive drugs ever since, and Fig. 7.1 shows in very simplified form what has happened since then to his weight and blood pressure, in relation to some other events.

Until his compound fracture he had no apparent medical problems. As there is no record of his blood pressure before 1960, there is no way of knowing how long it had been raised, but it was first recognized as a medical problem in 1966, though it was not causing symptoms. Evaluating his other risks for coronary heart disease, I found a blood cholesterol of 8.2 mmol/1 (318 mg/dl), a figure almost as exceptionally high as his blood pressure. The only good news was that he was a lifelong non-smoker. I also found persistent protein in his urine, suggesting some sort of kidney damage which might be causing his high blood pressure, so I referred him for investigation at a teaching hospital in 1967.

There he was found to have kidney damage from a raised level of blood uric acid, which can also cause kidney stones and gout (painful uric acid crystals in a joint, usually the big toe), though he did not yet have either of these. His kidney damage was severe enough to cause raised levels of metabolites excreted through the kidney, with blood urea concentrations averaging 52 mmol/1 (313 mg/dl). He was very overweight: six feet tall and weighing 103.4 kg. Like most miners, he was also a heavy beer drinker, getting through about 5 gallons a week according to his own probably modest estimate. Finally they confirmed an even higher blood cholesterol level of 9.5 mmol/1 (373 mg/dl).

In 1967 he therefore had the following inter-related medical and medicosocial problems, shown as reversible and for the most part measurable risk factors, together with their likely outcomes:

CURRENT PROBLEMS	PREDICTABLE OUTCOMES
Persistent disability from major compound fracture	Employment problems and loss of earnings
Very high blood pressure 200/120 mmHg Very high blood cholesterol 9.5 mmol	Early coronary heart disease, heart failure, and/or stroke
High blood uric acid	Kidney stones and kidney damage potentially leading to kidney failure, joint damage from gout

High alcohol intake	Social damage at home and at work, obesity, further rise in blood pressure, further rise in blood uric acid
Obesity	Greater pain from old fracture, further rise in blood pressure, more joint damage, possibly diabetes

It is interesting to note how many of these outcomes were also potential causes, suggesting that early efforts put into control (Anticipatory Care) might yield disproportionately high dividends. His medical needs, his and my joint medical tasks, were optimal control of these risks to minimize or avoid these outcomes. He has now reached 62 years of age without angina, a heart attack, heart failure or stroke, and he has never had any important psychosocial problems from his heavy drinking. He has always had a strong, friendly personality, and his level of drinking, though a serious health hazard, is a cultural norm in a coal-mining community. His liver function, initially impaired (gamma glutamyl) transferase 250 units, about 200 units above the conventional upper limit) is now virtually normal (59 units). He did get repeated attacks of urate kidney stones in 1969 and 1970, but none since then, and his kidney function has been well preserved (blood urea in 1986 was 11.4 mmol/1).

On the other hand, his employment and other social problems were serious. After about a year off from his injury, no light work was available and he had to do heavy manual work in the coal washery which gave him a lot of severe pain. In 1970 his wife began to be seriously handicapped by chronic obstructive airways disease and emphysema, with three short admissions to hospital over the next five years. Eventually she became dependent on portable oxygen, and Hopkin gave up his work to look after her at home. She died in 1975. As you can see from Fig. 7.1, weight control was poor and in 1980 he developed diabetes, bringing a new set of risks of coronary heart damage, stroke, kidney damage, and eye damage. His diabetes has been well controlled on diet only, with glycosylated haemoglobin consistently below 9%.

Quality of blood pressure control was poor; his target pressures of 160/90 mmHg were rarely achieved. There were serious problems of non-compliance with medication, at first because he didn't understand the importance of good control and because I didn't understand his antipathy to taking many different tablets. At one point in his wife's long illness both he and she were suicidally depressed. There are many more important things in life than control of blood pressure or compliance with doctors. Like many patients, he tried to simplify his medication, with predictably bad results; but using other ideas of his own, he set up a rigorous exercise programme, walking five or ten miles a day over the mountains with his dog, which probably contributed a lot to his generally favourable outcome.

Overall, the story is a success. It's hard to find any point in it with scope for fighter pilots, or where I might not have done better if I had listened more to the patient, or perhaps if he had listened more to me. If there were any fighter pilots around, they were probably on the orthopaedic team which mended his fracture, though I doubt if this is the way the best orthopaedic surgeons view their work. For the staff at our health centre it was a steady unglamorous slog through a total of 310 consultations. For me it was about 41 hours of work with the patient, initially face to face, gradually shifting to side by side. Professionally, the most satisfying and exciting things have been the events which have *not* happened: *no* strokes, *no* coronary heart attacks, *no* complications of diabetes, *no* kidney failure with dialysis or transplant. This is the real stuff of primary medical care.

The Patient's Role in Treatment

Patients share in implementing treatment even more obviously than in diagnosis. No tablets work if they are put in the

Fig. 7.1

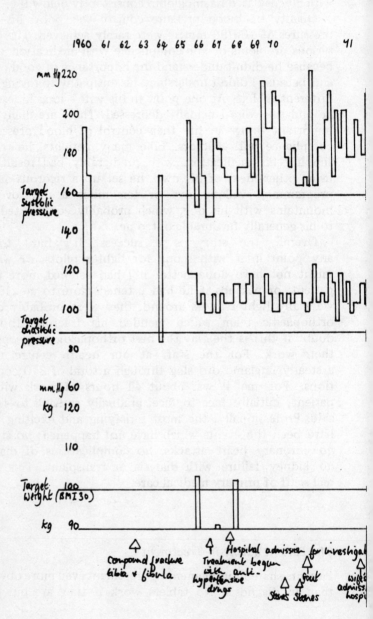

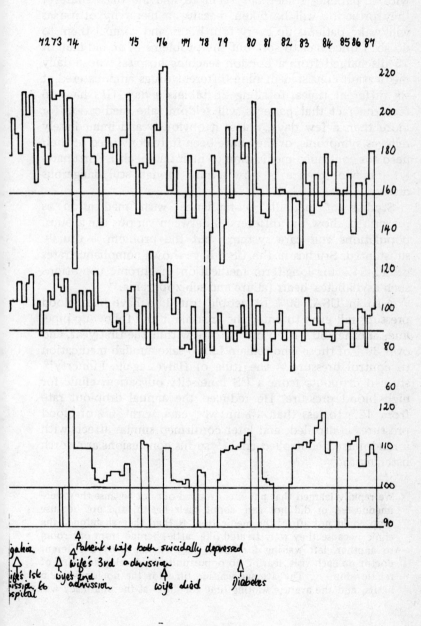

toilet instead of the patient. Hospital doctors dealing mainly with in-patients sometimes seem to imagine that whatever they prescribe will be taken, because a hierarchy of nurses will wake patients up every four hours and compel them to do so. I once had to sort out the problems of an old man of 75 discharged from a London teaching hospital whose daily medication consisted of nine different drugs administered at six different times, totalling 28 tablets a day. GPs have to face the fact that patients will seldom take medication for more than a few days, unless it obviously and immediately relieves symptoms, or they have been fully convinced of their need for continued medication to maintain health. Fortunately, blind obedience is now a rare though still dangerous disease.

Studies of patients' compliance with medication as prescribed show big differences between various age-groups, populations and care systems, but the problem is usually substantial. Studies in the USA have shown compliance rates of 41–54% for long-term medication of chronic conditions such as diabetes, heart failure and schizophrenia.[14]

Also in USA, 50% of people found to have high blood pressure fail even to enter the treatment and follow-up pipeline, another 50% drop out of care within the first year, and over 30% of those who remain fail to take enough medication to control pressure;[15] the Rule of Halves again. Finnerty[16] studied dropouts from a US inner-city outpatient clinic for high blood pressure. He reduced the annual drop-out rate from 42% to less than 4% in two years, with 85% of blood pressures controlled, and later confirmed similar effects with a randomized controlled trial,[17] so his conclusions are worth listening to:

> We rapidly learned that patients dropped out not because they were uneducated or did not care about their health, and not because they could not afford the medication. Rather, they abandoned the clinic because they were treated like cattle, herded from one room to another, left waiting for hours, then examined by a different doctor on each visit, leaving no opportunity to develop any kind of relationship. . . The average waiting time for the doctor was 2.5 hours, and the average waiting time for drugs at the pharmacy was

another 1.8 hours. . . In contrast. . . the average time actually spent with the physician was only 7.5 minutes.

Finnerty's solution was to reorganize the clinic by developing an effective appointments system (average time spent by patients in the clinic fell from 4 hours to 20 minutes), and by ensuring continuity of staff-patient relationships. This turned out to be more important than staff qualification:

> Most important was the assignment of every patient to his or her own paramedic whom he would see on every visit. The paramedics frequently came from the same neighbourhood as the patient. . . chosen not so much because of [their] prior experience or education but because of [their] friendly and sympathetic personality and ability to identify with the patients.

Perfunctory care has perfunctory results. If we want patients to take their treatment seriously, doctors must show that they take it seriously too, which means negotiating agreement on a plan of management. This must include education of patients in the reasons for, and the advantages and disadvantages of treatments recommended and of other options if there are any, and education of doctors on the real-life constraints within which patients have to apply their remedies. Where doctors develop a continuing relationship with patients, listen to them, and encourage them to share in devising realistic treatment plans, patient compliance can be excellent. Studying their own patients in general practice, Porter[18] in 1969 and Drury[19] in 1976 found medication compliance rates of over 80%. Ettlinger and Freeman[20] likewise found over 80% compliance overall, and 91% compliance in patients who felt that they knew the doctor who prescribed the tablets well, compared with 44% in patients who did not.

How Doctors see Patients as a Resource

Doctors who still operate within the Osler paradigm nevertheless concede that patients are generally under-used as sources of information, that someone (perhaps some sort of attached social worker) should find out more about their social circumstances so as to avoid the more nonsensical consequences of treating diseases rather than people, and that the necessary education of patients in the nature of their treatment should involve at least an appearance of listening to their opinions; but all these are still seen as add-on, luxury features, subordinate to a general scheme in which doctors must be active and well-informed, but patients may be and usually are passive and ignorant.

Most doctors believe there are big differences in intelligence between patients, that this limits the information patients can accept and recall, and that experienced doctors are able to discriminate between patients who can make good use of discussion of their problems at a reasonably adult level, and those on whom such efforts are wasted.

There is some evidence on how these beliefs work out in practice. Joyce and co-workers[21] studied 54 patients attending a hospital clinic for rheumatoid arthritis and similar disorders, complaints for which communication (listening and explaining) are often the main help available. Among other things, the doctors rated the patients as more or less articulate. They found that patients rated as more articulate were told more about their condition, and told it more often, than those rated as less articulate, though the proportion of information they retained and understood was the same. In other words, the doctors thought they could identify the better learners, and then gave them more information, though logically one would imagine that slow learners need more rather than less teaching time; retention of the information was not better in those rated by the doctors as more articulate. All doctors I have discussed this with agree that all of us at least initially had this attitude; we may have learned it from schoolteachers, who also traditionally give most attention to their aptest pupils, also believe they can predict learning capacity, and are also frequently proved wrong by rapid progress in many pupils once they have left school.

Similarly, doctors tend to think they can predict compliance. They are wrong; studies have shown that apart from extremes of age, no sociodemographic variables are consistently associated with either compliance or non-compliance.[22,23] Doctors are poor predictors of patient behaviour. French physicians who tried to predict who would continue and who would lapse treatment with digitalis and diuretic tablets for heart failure were wrong in 50% of cases, suggesting that their forecasts were no better than random choices.[24]

Are Doctors Interested in what Patients know and think?

Influenced particularly by Balint's modification of the Osler paradigm, which appears to emphasize patients' own perceptions of their problems, progressive GPs since the 1970s have been confident that they are moving rapidly towards a more shared, less unequal relationship with their patients, both in defining medical problems and in devising solutions, which should ensure at least an informal level of accountability to patients which might be more effective than a formal structure.

Careful work by David Tuckett[25] and his group has shown conclusively that this is not so. Little if any change has in fact taken place in the overt behaviour of doctors, whether or not they believe such a change to be desirable. Their aim was to explore the extent to which ideas can be shared in medical consultations, because of general agreement by progressive GPs that giving information is often the only available help in a consultation; because patients need information to follow advice and assist them in making difficult choices; because many patients already act as experts in their own self-care (e.g. people with diabetes, asthma, epilepsy, multiple sclerosis) and more should do so; and because patients should be regarded as individuals who interpret and try to make sense of what happens to them.

Their study material was 1,302 tape-recorded consultations by two groups of GPs. The first was a study group of eight, selected because they were recognized trainers responsible for teaching consultation skills, who had attended lengthy RCGP courses in the Balint tradition, deliberately aimed at changing doctors' behaviour. Some of these GPs had conducted and published research and others had senior university teaching appointments. The comparison group consisted of another eight GPs chosen randomly from lists of NHS GPs in the same areas as the study group. Very detailed studies were made of a random sample of 69 consultations, and of another 405 consultations selected because they included problems likely to require sharing of information.

Their original intention was to look at expected differences in the way these two groups of GPs (one theoretically convinced of the need for mutually shared information, the other with traditional ideas of active doctors and passive patients) actually behaved. In fact there were virtually no differences. All the doctors in both groups appeared in practice to see transmission of information and ideas as an almost entirely one-way process, and none of them sought patients' ideas about how their problems were caused or defined, or how they might be remedied.

This uniformity of behaviour, despite real differences in attitude and intention which have seriously divided GPs for many years, suggests that virtually all doctors are in fact working within constraints of which they are as yet scarcely conscious (the Osler paradigm). Patients, however assertive they may normally be, also accept these constraints within consultation, so that their own information and intelligence is not used.

Many people will regard this as a rather trivial discovery, hardly warranting the £250,000 of Health Education Council money it consumed. It has long been fashionable to attribute most problems in medical care to the arrogance of doctors and their refusal to share power with the public they serve, in fact this is a central point of the Liberal Critique. Tuckett's group agrees, but modifies this in critically important ways which make it constructive and helpful rather than divisive and defeatist in its effect:

> The pattern of consultation we have observed. . . may, in part, be the product of more or less conscious attempts to maintain hierarchical relationships. But these in turn may result from still

more fundamental causes. Virtually all of the doctors whom we studied and with whom we later worked gave us the impression that they were very devoted to the welfare of their patients. In recent years medical practitioners, especially in the UK, have devoted an enormous amount of time and effort to self-evaluation and self-criticism. Many doctors also spend a great deal of time voluntarily trying to improve their skills. . . The need to maintain or create hierarchical relationships can be caused by other factors than the pursuit of power. For example, the innate conflicts and anxieties built into being a doctor may all too easily produce the need to stay in control. The doctor's consulting role carries special responsibilities and anxieties and is inherently difficult. He must deal on a day-to-day basis with his own and his patients' uncertainties, experiences of disaster, failures, helplessness, blame, panic and anxieties, as well as with the unconscious feelings that go with them. Actions must sometimes be taken quickly and routinely without adequate knowledge and with the awareness that a mistake can be fatal. Inevitably decisions will sometimes be hard to justify in cooler moments. The role also involves conflicts arising from social reality: for example, the doctor must mediate the demands of different patients, allocate scarce resources, mediate between the patient and his family and social network, mediate between the needs of his patients and those of himself, etc. To cope with the role both institutional and personal methods of coping have been developed: including, perhaps, tunnel vision, emotional withdrawal, being busy, being obsessed with one or more technical aspects of medicine and being omnipotent in his behaviour. The Apostolic Function [Balint's term for the effect on an illness of the doctor's own personality] is a similar defence.

All these fundamental reasons applied even more in the past, when so much of medical care was hopeful illusion, maintained by patient and doctor who colluded in production not of effective care, but of often wilfully blind optimism and evasion of reality. All this has been a part of the Osler paradigm, escape from which requires understanding, not acts of will. Doctors still have to shoulder a great deal of threatening uncertainty, which few experienced people, either doctors or patients, would suggest can at all times be borne equally by both sides; it is still a necessary part of the job for most doctors most of the time to reserve to themselves a burden of uncertainty in diagnosis and prognosis, sharing this with the patient only after a narrower and more tolerable range of possibilities has been defined; otherwise they will

add even more to the patient's own load of uncertainty and
fear. Doctors are socially useful workers, a point sometimes
overlooked by some of their academic critics.

Are Patients Consumers or Producers?

Patients, and where there is a freely available health service,
the public at large, are often referred to as consumers of
medical care. Even the groups which are most hostile to
medical dominance generally see the remedy for this in a
strengthening of the rights and power of consumers, and see
themselves as part of a national or even international
consumers' movement. Doctors chastened by the Liberal
Critique are eager to concede this; they see limitation of the
hitherto unchallenged authority of doctors as care-providers,
and extension of the choices open to patients as consumers,
as entirely progressive steps. The idea originated naturally
from the private consultation as an essentially commercial
transaction, in which doctors created a commodity which
patients bought to consume for their personal benefit. Where
no commercial transaction took place, for example when
Sir William Osler examined a poor patient with an interesting
disease at Johns Hopkins or the Radcliffe Infirmary, or later
a National Health Service patient was treated free by her GP
(what we might call 'public' rather than 'private' consultations), the rights and powers of patients were diminished and
the authority of the doctors increased, because both rested
on the unenforceable customs of charity rather than the
clearly defined property rights of sale. Beggars can't be
choosers, and accountability in a charity service arises only
in extreme cases of breakdown. Patients' rights appeared to
be maximized when they were paying consumers within a
essentially commercial transaction.

The Osler paradigm was most apt where patients paid for
their care, and were able to choose their doctor and insist
on treatment of a quality consistent with its price. Private
practice set the optimal level of quality with which State
Charity was supposed to stand comparison, and was supposed
to be what everyone would want if they could afford it. For

doctors influenced by the Liberal Critique this was a slightly uncomfortable conclusion, because they knew very well that marketed medicine is no more trustworthy than marketed motor cars or any other commodity. *Caveat emptor*, above all when the seller seems to know everything and the buyer almost nothing. *Sed quoque caveat vendor*; a commercial sale may present a threat to the integrity of the seller as much as to the pocket of the buyer. The relation between all vendors and consumers is inherently adversarial, and liberal doctors remain fundamentally uncomfortable with the consumer-provider relationship.

However, we have seen that medical problems can only be realistically defined by a joint effort between at least two kinds of skilled people: patients skilled in observing their own past history, present symptoms and the social settings within which problems arise and must be solved; and doctors (or other health workers) skilled in interpretation of this information, and able to construct from it a set of realistic diagnostic and therapeutic options. We have also seen that once medical problems are appropriately defined, there cannot be a realistic plan for their containment or solution without the same kind of joint effort, from doctors (or other health workers) who know what kinds of solutions to look for, and from patients who know how they might be applied within the constraints of their real personal lives.

This is a production process, in which various consumptions (tablets, x-rays, doctors' and patients' time, etc.) may be necessary, but in which something new is present at the end of a consultation which did not exist at the beginning; a defined set of problems, together with tentative plans for their solution. This view is bad for medical sales. If doctors are to sell their skills as a commodity at the best price, they must discount or even conceal (first of all from themselves) skills contributed by the purchaser. If patients are customers they must be encouraged to think they can buy better health from doctors as a package, but may therefore be less willing to accept that they are going to have to do most of the work. Why buy a dog and bark yourself?

Commercial transactions have almost vanished from British

general practice since 1948, yet this conception of patients as consumers not only survives, but is gaining influence. How can this be explained? The idea has certainly gained new strength from the rapid growth of private medical care as the NHS has become less and less able to bridge the gap between public demand and State supply, though little of this has as yet occurred at GP level. It has also been reinforced by the strength of the consumerist movement in general, which, starting in the USA in the 1960s, has provided a popular platform for superficially radical and democratic ideas, without challenging (in fact powerfully reinforcing) the fundamental requirements of capitalism: private investment for the market rather than public investment for human needs, and denial in practice of all creativity which cannot be expressed in commodity terms.

The weakness of this view becomes obvious as soon as we look at the real medical problems of real people. Who was responsible for maintaining the health of Hopkin Morgan? I was, he was, and so were a lot of other people who helped me (orthopaedic surgeons, renal physicians, radiologists and radiographers, laboratory technicians, nurses, etc.) and him (his wife, sons, daughters, mates at work and drinking companions). We were not always successful, and all of us may sometimes have counter-produced; but his present state of health is a social product of work done well or badly by many people, but usually starting from GP and patient in joint consultation. This process can be commercialized, albeit with difficulty. It is possible to break it down to make some of the more suitable fragments into commodities for sale, but not without damage; a jointly produced value which might have been shared and developed further must be divided into a sold profit for the vendor and a bought possession for the consumer, who then owe one another nothing. The episode of diagnosis and treatment becomes isolated, transient and superficial. The transaction damages and limits the value it claims to sell.

All aspects of medical science are advancing, and inevitably this includes high-technology salvage in medical crises, in which the patient is indeed almost entirely passive and dependent on professional skills. In these primitive conditions, the Osler paradigm works. Such care could easily become a commodity for sale if society were sufficiently de-civilized to allow a market in life and death to operate, a possibility which our leaders of public opinion have now made thinkable. But acute care is not the main line of advance of either medical science or medical practice. Most of its effective techniques are already well understood and for the most part fairly well delivered, and many of the most superficially impressive new techniques don't work in practice. Though the component techniques of (for example) intensive coronary care are impressive when taken one by one in isolation, careful studies in Australia, USA and Scandinavia of death rates from coronary heart attacks in hospitals offering different levels of technical sophistication show that those offering continuous monitoring, specially trained nursing staff for coronary care and emergency resuscitation, a staff cardiologist, and a cardiac surgical service are no more effective than hospitals without these facilities.[26-30] Whatever benefits there may have been from more sophisticated technology since the late 1960s are evidently already available at nearly all hospitals, and special units with their very elaborate and expensive care have not improved outcome. More than half the deaths from coronary heart attacks occur during the first two hours after onset of symptoms, but the average delay between onset and arrival at hospital is at least three hours in most parts of Britain, mostly because of delay by patients in sending for a doctor or ambulance, probably because they don't want to believe the pain has a potentially lethal cause (the process of denial). By the time most patients get to hospital, many of them might as well be looked after at home if family and nursing support are good.[31,32]

Future advance in medical care will only develop on a mass scale through prevention or limitation of organ damage by strategies which depend on changes in human behaviour, or on interventions arising from the revolution in molecular biology which will be prompted by findings from population screening rather than presented symptoms. Much of this could be achieved by improved living conditions for the whole population, better education, full participation in society and better customs of eating, working and playing freed from commercial pressures; but we will also need the precise individual targeting and support which could be available from professional health workers, if they were helped to escape from the Osler paradigm by a socially-oriented NHS which set targets and measured their attainment. Of course we need public health campaigns directed at the whole population, but the real test of useful change is whether we are giving effective help to the most vulnerable groups in immediate danger of irreversible organ damage, people with chronic disorders such as asthma, diabetes, high blood pressure, schizophrenia or epilepsy, and the honest present answer has to be that for the most part we are not. Previous chapters of this book have documented the evidence of incomplete care, with many patients still undiagnosed, and many more who have entered the care system but then dropped out because it is not geared to their needs.

Riddle's Five Steps for Effective Care of Chronic Disease

In his paper 'A strategy for chronic disease', Matthew Riddle,[33] an American specialist in diabetes, gave a perceptive review both of what's wrong with medical care now and what needs to be done to put it right. The example he gives concerns diabetes, but applies equally well to every other chronic disorder:

> diagnosis and treatment [of diabetes] is not the major problem. . . We first make recommendations concerning diet and physical activity. If plasma glucose remains high, we prescribe oral drugs or insulin. But here begins the larger problem. These interventions must be more or less permanent and demand daily attention by the patient. They may require major changes in behaviour and the pattern of daily life. Thus, they are not treatments in the usual sense, administered by an expert to a passive beneficiary; they are new ways of living. A major and sustained change in behaviour is easy to discuss but hard to achieve. . .
>
> Research presses on at great cost, with substantial yield. . . We

have new tools and better models of the old ones: purer insulins, accurate disposable syringes, glucose-oxidase strips, home glucose analysers and, on the way, the first generation of hang-from-the-shoulder, open-loop artificial pancreases.

All these innovations are helping, yet they are not enough. They are, I think, slightly off the target. For one thing, more sophisticated specialists, systems and gadgets will bring more sophisticated forms of disaster. . . But my main concern is that we are juggling the parts without assessing the whole. . . We need a new strategy.

Management of diabetes is a process which can be divided into five steps. All the steps must be completed if management is to be as satisfactory as possible. They have a logical sequence. Completion of the later steps reinforces the earlier ones, so management improves with time. Each step must be recognized as part of the overall plan, not over-valued for itself.

1. Acquisition by the health professionals involved of an adequate base of information about the disorder.
2. Acceptance by the patient of primary responsibility for coping with the disorder and maintaining health.
3. Learning by the patient of the physiology, complications, and details of treatment.
4. Negotiation between patient and health professionals of general goals and specific objectives for management acceptable to both.
5. Assessment of success in meeting the objectives using quantitative measures understood by both patient and health professional.

. . . a systematic approach to chronic disease should become a central part of our medical heritage, together with the scientific method for research and the responsibility of the healer for the acutely ill. This five-part strategy may be a start.

Medical care that is effective and available to all who need it, rather than illusory and promoted on the market or distributed charitably as an appearance of care without verified effect, is a social product in which patients as much as doctors need to become central performers. Escape from the tradition of doctor-centred consultation requires more than the narcissistic self-criticism of Balintry in practice, however patient-centred it may appear in theory.

It requires first of all that doctors insist on having enough time to do their work properly, while also insisting that this quality of service must be available to the whole population as a human right. Effective consultations, which maximize inputs from patients and outputs in relevant action consistently applied, cannot be done within the 5 minute, 5 x 7 inch format of Lloyd George industrial practice. Unhurried, friendly, thoughtful consultation is not a luxury for the future, but a present necessity for effective care, and it's time both patients and GPs insisted on having it.

Secondly, doctors and patients must recognize the limited clinical effectiveness of the Osler paradigm, so that they no longer see the doctor-centred, episodic technical fix as the core of good practice, to which patient-centred ideas may be bolted on as an afterthought.

The alternative paradigm is anticipatory care democratized at the design stage to include both active outreach from caregiver to patient, and active responsibility of the patient for definition and solution of problems. The only valid test of its capacity to deliver medical science more effectively than the Osler paradigm will be its effect not on individual cases at anecdotal level, but on the morbidity and mortality of populations, which leads us to the next chapter.

NOTES

1. Report of the Royal Commission on the National Health Service, para. 11.12. Cmnd 7615, London: HMSO, 1979.
2. Capstick, B., *Patient complaints and litigation*, Birmingham: National Association of Health Authorities in England & Wales, 1985.
3. Hart, J.T., Humphreys, C., 'Be your own coroner: an audit of 500 consecutive deaths in a general practice', *British Medical Journal 1987*; 294:871-4.
4. Drife, J.O., 'Consultant accountability', *British Medical Journal 1987*; 294:789-80.
5. Klein, R., *Complaints against doctors*, London: Charles Knight, 1973.
6. Quam, L., Dingwall, R., Fenn, P., 'Medical malpractice in perspective. I. The American experience. II. The implications for Britain', *British Medical Journal 1987*; 294:1529-32, 1597-1600.
7. Jowell, R., Airey, C., *British social attitudes: the 1987 report*, Aldershot: Gower Publishing, 1987.
8. Jowell, R., Airey, C., *British social attitudes: the 1984 report*, Aldershot: Gower Publishing, 1984.
9. Good, M-J.D., 'Discourses on physician competence'. In, Hahn, R.A., Gaines, A.D. (eds.), *Physicians of Western medicine*, 247-67. Boston, Mass.: D. Reidel Publishing, 1985.

10. Kinzer, D.M., 'Physicians as fighter pilots', *New England Journal of Medicine 1984*; 311:206.
11. Mizrahi, T., 'Managing medical mistakes: ideology, insularity and accountability among internists-in-training', *Social Science & Medicine 1984*; 19:135–46.
12. Firth-Cozens, J., 'Emotional distress in junior house officers', *British Medical Journal 1987*; 29:533–6.
13. Hampton, J.R., Harrison, M.J.G., Mitchell, J.R.A., Prichard, J.S., Seymour, C., 'Relative contributions of history-taking, physical examination and laboratory investigation to diagnosis and management of medical outpatients', *British Medical Journal 1975*; ii:486–9.
14. 'Keep on taking the tablets: a review of the problem of patient non-compliance', OHE Briefing no. 21, London: Office of Health Economics, 1983.
15. Sackett, D.L., Snow, J.S., 'The magnitude of compliance and non-compliance'. In, *Compliance in health care*, ed. Haynes, R.B., Taylor, D.W., Sackett, D.L., p. 11. Johns Hopkins University Press, Baltimore, 1979.
16. Finnerty, F.A. Jr., Mattie E.C., Finnerty, F.A., 'Hypertension in the inner city. I. Analysis of drop-outs', *Circulation 1973*; 47:73.
17. Finnerty, F.A. Jr., Shaw, L.W., Himmelsbach, C.K., 'Hypertension in the inner city: II. Detection and follow-up', *Circulation 1973*; 47:76–8.
18. Porter, A.M.W., 'Drug defaulting in general practice', *Journal of the Royal College of General Practitioners 1969*; 17:170.
19. Drury, V.W.M., Wade, O.L., Woolf, E., 'Following advice in general practice', *Journal of the Royal College of General Practitioners 1976*; 26:712–8.
20. Ettlinger, P.R.A., Freeman, G.K., 'General practice compliance study: is it worth being a personal doctor?', *British Medical Journal 1981*; 282:1192–4.
21. Joyce, C.R.B., Caple, G., Mason, M., Reynolds, E., Mathews, J.A., 'Quantitative study of doctor–patient communication', *Quarterly Journal of Medicine 1969*; ns 38:183–94.
22. Menard, J., Degoulet, P., Hong, A.V. et al., 'Compliance in hypertension care'. In, *Mild hypertension: recent advances*, ed. Gross, F., Strasser, T., p. 349. New York: Raven Press, 1983.
23. Haynes, R.B., 'A critical review of the determinants of patient compliance with therapeutic regimens'. In, *Compliance with therapeutic regimens*, ed. Sackett, D.L., Haynes, R.B., p. 26. Baltimore: Johns Hopkins University Press, 1977.
24. Mushlin, A.I., Appel, F.A., 'Diagnosing patient non-compliance', *Archives of Internal Medicine 1977*; 137:318.
25. Tuckett, D., Boulton, M., Olson, C., Williams, A., *Meetings between experts: an approach to sharing ideas in medical consultations*, London: Tavistock Publications, 1985.
26. Reznik, R., Ring, I., Fletcher, P., Berry, G., 'Mortality from myocardial infarction in different types of hospitals', *British Medical Journal 1987*; 294:1121–5.

27. Bain, C., Siskind, V., Neilson, G., 'Site of care and survival after myocardial infarction', *Medical Journal of Australia 1981*; ii:185-8.
28. Bloom, B.S., Peterson, O.L., 'End results, cost and productivity of coronary care units', *New England Journal of Medicine 1973*; 277:72-8.
29. Hofvendahl, S., 'Influence of treatment in a CCU on prognosis in acute myocardial infarction', *Acta Medica Scandinavica 1971*; 519s:1-78.
30. Christiansen, I., Iversen, K., Skouby, A.P., 'Benefits obtained by the introduction of coronary care unit: a comparative study', *Acta Medica Scandinavica 1971*; 189:285-91.
31. Mather, H.G., Pearson, N.G., Read, K.L.Q., et al., 'Acute myocardial infarction: home and hospital treatment', *British Medical Journal 1976*; i:925-9.
32. Hill, J.D., Hampton, J.R., Mitchell, J.R.A., 'A randomized controlled trial of home-vs-hospital management for patients with suspected myocardial infarction', *Lancet 1978*; i:837-41.
33. Riddle, M.C., 'A strategy for chronic disease', *Lancet 1980*; ii:734-6.

Chapter 8
ACCOUNTABILITY
FOR AND TO GROUPS

Doctors are rarely accountable for the average quality of their work in terms of outcome. They have to answer for exceptional events, unexpected disasters lying outside the normal range of experience, but rarely for assessment of average process, and virtually never for average outcome. If disasters don't occur, or don't reach the ears of authority, quality of work is assumed to be satisfactory. Even if it is so obviously unsatisfactory as absolutely to demand enquiry, that enquiry will use process rather than outcome measures.

For example, the expected mortality of a planned operation for repair of inguinal hernia in a man of 65 is between 3 and 6 per 1,000 operations.[1] Death from such an operation is exceptional for an individual, but since not even the best surgeons have an operative mortality of zero, some deaths will always occur. The quality of a surgical unit (allowing for the average age and state of health of the patients) can't be judged fairly or usefully from the litigation, press criticism, or individual complaints it appears to provoke. Intelligent judgement depends on comparing average results in different centres, and then asking why differences are what they are. Fear of litigation is unlikely to improve the outcome of operations if the real fault is overwork and fatigue among junior staff, a shortage of nurses, or a high proportion of patients in poor health.

Hospital teams with enough pride, interest and confidence in their work to review their results and expose them to peer criticism at clinical meetings or in serious medical journals provide most of the evidence we have on the effectiveness of medical care. These generally show steadily improving outcomes, not because of pressure from litigation and complaint, but because the advance of medical science generates motivation of its own, initially at centres of innovation, later among pioneers at the periphery. Useful studies are based not on exceptionally good or bad individual results, but on the outcome of care in groups large enough to eliminate the confusing effects of chance, and the variable age, sex, and other factors relevant to survival which make individual outcomes so unreliable as a guide to the quality of care.

No public service has ever had much interest in suspecting, identifying, or advertising its own limitations, but scientists do generally accept that the advance of knowledge depends on precise recognition of their ignorance. GPs as graduates in medical science have been slow in accepting this self-critical stance because of their autonomous status as entrepreneurs in a public service. However, just as there are no zero-risk surgeons, there are no zero-risk GPs. All medical interventions entail some risk, however small, of going wrong. This risk must be multiplied if interventions are applied indiscriminately in hasty 5-minute consultations, where the prescription pad may be used more to speed throughput than to change outcomes intelligently. If thoughtful medical interventions chosen and aimed accurately at selected targets are effective, then their inappropriate omission will also increase risk. If doctors are required to be perfect, they're damned if they do and damned if they don't. Many will maintain the greatest possible ignorance about the real results of their work by avoiding objective measurements and denying their value. They can remain comfortable with entrepreneur status, accountable to no one providing they satisfy their customers. Once these customers are sufficiently well informed to make more accurate judgements, however, the always fallible GP may find it better to abandon the omniscience of medical trade, and promise only what can really be delivered; the best we can do jointly with the people we serve, with incomplete information and nearly always less time than we need.

A scientific approach to measuring quality must be realistic rather than legalistic, and can only begin if GPs are allowed and encouraged to search for their own errors. Good doctors are those who are prepared to measure, or let others measure, how bad they are; or, more constructively, are prepared to accept that their work can be convincingly improved only if they are prepared to start by measuring its outcomes, errors and omissions. This in no way contradicts the rule that medical care should not be judged only by what is most easily measured (for example, the proportion of patients whose blood pressures have been measured or who have had cervical smears). Many very important qualities, like friendliness, approachability, and readiness to listen, are difficult to measure and tend to be ignored in plans for evaluation of care; but this does not mean that they can't, with imagination and some readiness to ask the patients, be quantified just as much as any other medical process. In practice, however, rude and inaccessible doctors simply will not attain good indices even on the simplest measures of performance. Regardless of status, bad doctors are those who refuse to measure, or to allow others to measure, their outcomes, errors and omissions. And these measures must be repeated; doctors whose poor performance is improving are better than those whose good performance is stagnant or deteriorating.

Perfection for Some of the People Some of the Time, or our Best For all of the People all of the Time?

About 20 years ago a newly appointed consultant visited one of my patients at home. Before his appointment, his specialty did not exist in South West Wales: he brought essential skills for the first time to a total population of nearly a million people. We were both enthusiasts for better clinical medicine, so after the visit we took 10 minutes off for a beer, an exchange of gossip, and for me to congratulate him on the dramatic improvement in the quality of care available to my patients in his specialty. Everything he said suggested contempt for doctors who pursue fees rather than science and public service, so I was amazed to hear he had chosen to work part-time, and after only a year in post had already developed substantial private practice. 'Why on earth do you do it?', I asked. His answer (rather shamefaced; he was not yet completely comfortable in his new role) was the typical defence within the Osler paradigm: 'I feel I owe it to myself to practice really good medicine at least one session a week; without that I'd lose my self-respect.'

It's difficult to deliver a specialized service to about half a million people with inadequate resources; still, we previously had no service at all in that specialty, so we (the GPs and the population) were more grateful than critical. It is clever, but not nearly so difficult, to see a few who can afford to pay (in another country we would call it a bribe) for more time, more thought, and more courtesy—in fact, better care.

The test of quality applied in the Osler paradigm is a capacity to excel under ideal conditions, mainly more time. The constraints of practice are seen as unchangeable; the good doctor in the Osler paradigm gets out of bad circumstances as soon as he can, to work better in good ones. Bad practice because of circumstances which preclude good practice is seen as a problem for doctors, not patients, with doctors' not patients' solutions.

The test of quality for the New Kind of Doctor we need is measured outcome for the registered whole population at risk, whether that be the 500,000 or so served by a neurosurgeon at a tertiary hospital, the 100,000 served by a cardiologist at a District Hospital, the 10,000 served by a group of five GPs at a health centre, or the 2,000 served by one GP with nursing and office staff. Simple ultimate outcomes, for example death rates standardized for age, sex, social class and locality, can rarely be applied to populations of less than 10,000, and even then only over periods of 5 years or more, because of chance variability where numbers of events are small. But intermediate outcomes, group average blood pressures in hypertensives, group mean glycosylated haemoglobins in diabetics, changes in the proportions of smokers in different age and sex groups, changes in the hospital-admission rate in child asthmatics, the number of fits in epileptics, and so on, have predictable effects on more serious outcomes and are certainly feasible, particularly now that we have the huge data-handling capacity of micro-computers.

The justification offered for excellent care for a few is that it sets standards for the many. If that is true, it can have a place within the new paradigm, for the average quality of care, measured as average outcome, will rise. Important new ideas often start from individual cases, and the condescending attitude to anecdotal experience often adopted by non-clinical medical scientists is usually though not always unjustified. However, in choosing subsets of the population for innovative and exceptionally excellent care to pioneer general advances, it seems odd to select these according to their ability to pay fees, since fee-payers are not typical of the general population and usually present fewer problems in care. Scientific medicine, which now incorporates epidemiology (the study of disease in whole populations) throughout its fabric, cannot be practised with integrity in a commodity health market.

This argument is becoming of critical importance. In hospitals, more and more doctors and nurses are being forced to work without enough time, without enough staff, without enough space, tolerance, courtesy, or thought for anything but how to cope from one day to the next. The easy answer, permitted in the Osler paradigm, is to get out; out into some part of the NHS which still has adequate resources, out into private practice or agency nursing, out into one of the many hundreds of for-profit private hospitals and nursing homes now going up all over the country—to 'help' the ailing NHS, as well of course as their owners and shareholders, or out of your own country altogether, to seek your fortune abroad if there are still any richer countries that will let you in. Beds in private nursing homes and hospitals in England and Wales rose from 25,300 in 1971 to 33,500 in 1981 and 51,000 in 1985, while available NHS hospital beds fell from 526,000 in 1971 to 450,000 in 1981 and 421,000 in 1985. Private hospitals are concentrated around London and the South East, the very areas most subject to NHS cuts.

This process already exists in general practice to the extent that industrial practice remains generally constrained by high demands and low expectations, which some (but by no means all) GPs seek to evade rather than to change, but we are far from a frank division into a two-tier service, with private practice of high quality in the Osler paradigm and a threadbare public service. However, few doubt that in one form or another this is the future foreseen by the New Conservatives, probably by the same process of cutting off resources necessary for new advances which now operates in hospitals. The most probable development is tax-relief for private medical insurance premiums for private GP care. Like private care by hospital specialists, this will be justified by claims that it relieves pressure on the NHS: and the real effect will be exactly the same, that NHS doctors who effectively write their own timetables without official supervision will have even less time to do NHS work which (they say) is already too rushed to be done well. GPs who do not choose or are unable to enter this minority market will pose an embarrassing question to those who do; precisely what is it that they will give to their private patients, which they do not give to their NHS patients? If private and NHS care are the same, the transaction is fraudulent; if they are not the same, they are clearly doing less than their best for NHS patients. The BMA in 1858 believed that because disease affected people of all social degrees, the same medical skills should be available for everyone; the BMA must still believe this in 1987, for otherwise it has to concede a division in the profession of the same nature as the division in society.

In the new paradigm, the test of a good doctor is that we do the best we can, verified by measurement, for all our patients, in the circumstances we find: and also that if necessary we do our best to change those circumstances. The best doctors won't look for easier circumstances somewhere else, but join with their patients in changing conditions which preclude good practice, if necessary by blowing the whistle by full use of the newspapers and television. We have the social authority to do that, and no right not to do it, for no one else can. Loyalty to the populations we serve must become more important than our own value in the international professional market.

Doctor-centred Studies of General Practice

Mainly through initiatives from the RCGP and its members, much descriptive data has been collected ever since the 1950s on many aspects of the patients GPs see and what they do for them. Notable examples are the 1951, 1971–2 and 1981–2 National Morbidity Surveys organized jointly by the OPCS and Donald Crombie's RCGP Research Unit in Birmingham,[2,3,4] Wright's study of general practices in the South West of England,[5] W.O. Williams' study of general practices in South Wales,[6] and the study of 208 GPs in Manchester by David Metcalfe's group.[7] These surveys follow the general pattern of enquiry long established in hospitals; their starting point is doctors and the patients they see, and though the size, age and sex distribution, and sometimes the social class composition of their base populations are available, the underlying assumption has to be that states of public health can be studied by looking only at the people who demand care, with little information about those who do not, or (more often) who demand care that is not relevant to their principal causes of ill-health.

These studies show great diversity between GPs in their rates of consultation, organized follow-up, home visiting, prescribing, laboratory and x-ray investigations, nursing referral and hospital outpatient referral, and in their average consultation time per patient. Very high workload is typical in some areas such as South Wales, which are still generally under-researched because their GPs seldom volunteer to take part in surveys. We always know less about what happens in Toxteth, Clydebank and Gateshead than we do about the Thames valley. At high workloads (whether caused by big lists, high levels of sickness and distress, or both) GPs' work seems to be constrained to a more uniform pattern of short consultation times. Metcalfe's[7] study of 189 GPs in Manchester showed that below a list size of 2,000, GPs released from these absolute constraints of workload were extremely diverse in their behaviour. This diversity was apparently related to personal characteristics of the doctors rather than to the age or social composition of the populations they served, confirming in detail the more general conclusions of the three National Morbidity Surveys.

The BMA has asked for a target average list size of 1,700 per GP, justifying this by the need for more time if preventive work is to expand and clinical standards are to improve. Metcalfe found no evidence that the extra time released by lower list size led to more preventive work or more of any other indicator of clinical activity of personal care below a threshold of about 2,500. GPs with smaller lists apparently suited themselves, and expansion of preventive work, better clinical standards, or more personal care seem not to have commanded more of the extra time available than GPs' other interests. Obviously there will have been exceptions to this, but they did not reach statistical significance.

One conclusion to draw from these studies seems to be that GPs as a social group are no more to be trusted as their own sole judges, and should no more trust themselves, than police, popes, prime ministers, presidents or patriots in the marine corps and secret service. There are big differences in health and therefore in potential primary care workload between local populations, depending on their age, occupational and social class composition, the availability of other sources of care, and their morbidity as reflected in local Standardized Mortality Rates. These differences should be reflected in the way GPs work, a reflection which should become closer as list sizes decrease and GPs have more time to show imagination in tackling local health problems, but evidently this is not happening.

The need for smaller lists should not be in doubt, but if GPs are to have fewer patients for the same pay as the BMA demands, the public has the right to expect more time given as better and more personal care. It should not be pocketed by GPs as compensation for conveyor belt work which has remained perfunctory through custom and low expectations long after the pressure of work which originally caused it has gone, while they seek equally mundane but better-paid part-time work outside their practices and even outside the NHS.

More constructively, we might conclude that without defined health objectives, it is hardly surprising if GPs wander off in all directions. Why not develop feasible local target figures for (for example) ascertainment and control of diabetes, high blood pressure, epilepsy, asthma or any other measurable and reversible health impairment? No doubt there would still be a healthy variety of answers, but at least we would know what questions are being asked.

Patient-centred Studies in General Practice

Data obtained from GPs who volunteer to take part in national studies such as the National Morbidity Surveys must inevitably be biased away from practices that are more overworked, less well organized, or have a smaller social conscience, a problem which has still not been acknowledged by some of the principal authors in this field.[8] The studies listed above started with GPs counting the patients they saw, perceiving their population at risk (if at all) only as a residual denominator, the ones they didn't see. Only data obtained from random samples of the general population can give us generalizable information about the quality of care in general practice as a whole.

Few studies have sampled patients randomly from the general population, looking at the GPs the patients happened to have, and thus observing general practice through the public it serves. Data of this kind have for some years been gathered routinely by the General Household Surveys of the OPCS,[9] based on recall of events over the two weeks previous to interview, but their sample sizes are small and detailed studies of particular problems, for example the care of diabetics or people with chronic lung disorders, are not possible with them.

Ann Cartwright and her colleagues from the Institute for Social Studies in Medical Care have provided the most complete, detailed and reliable series of studies of how general practice relates to its populations, starting in 1964 with

Patients and their doctors,[10] still the best source of data about the nature of British general practice, and ending rather weakly with *General practice revisited*[11] in 1977. Like the General Household Surveys, these studies do not connect with its clinical content, and are therefore easily dismissed in the Osler paradigm as relevant only to the psychosocial fringe of practice, rather than its clinical care. Two of Ann Cartwright's studies are exceptions to this; *Life before death*[12] and *Life after a death*[13] looked at what happened to patients during the year before their deaths (randomly sampled from registered deaths in the general population) and to their bereaved spouses afterwards. These two studies are sited well within clinical territory and should be required reading for every medical and nursing student and every medical and nursing teacher, but judging from the few references to them in the general clinical literature, they seldom are.

Clinical Epidemiology and Audit in General Practice

As we have seen at length in Chapter 5, GPs with registered lists of people for whose primary medical care they are responsible are able, unlike all other clinicians, to measure both what they do and what they don't do. The inefficiency, ineffectiveness, and for most of the time unreality of the Osler paradigm of episodic salvage can only be fully exposed, and the paradigm fully superseded, on its own territory of clinical practice, and by measuring health outcomes rather than clinical processes.

Both Osler himself and Clifford Allbutt recognized the superiority of public health and preventive measures over episodic care,[14] but could not in practice bring it to the centre of their clinical teaching because teaching hospitals had no clearly defined source populations, follow-up was erratic, and generally they were producing doctors for self-employed private practice rather than for Public Health Service, and inevitably adapted their teaching accordingly. Less thoughtful than they were, true believers in the Osler paradigm today are not seriously concerned by its ineffectiveness at a psychosocial level, because they see psychosocial problems as optional features at the periphery of their work, bolted on or omitted according to the style and interests of individual clinicians, who can retain their reputations for clinical competence whether or not they accept them. If, however, it can be shown that within the Osler paradigm even the best GPs, who measure their work against a known population base and publish in the medical literature, are unable to deliver effective clinical care to more than about half the people who need it, it can be recognized as an obstacle rather than an aid to effective anticipatory care, though it will remain an effective albeit incomplete method for handling salvage in symptomatic disease.

Bearing in mind that all clinical audit and population-based research in general practice is voluntary, unpaid and very time-consuming, the proportion of practices which have done work of this kind, and the rate at which this proportion is growing, are impressive and compare well with other nations and care systems. Until paid and protected sessional time is made available in all practices for internal clinical audit and planning, it will not involve more than a small minority of enthusiasts, but the rate-limiting factor is already more the social and economic structure of NHS general practice than the attitudes of GPs, which have already in many cases outgrown its entrepreneurial form.

Death of the Medical Officer of Health: Did he fall or was he pushed?

At present, no one is really responsible for local health in concrete terms. If the NHS were organized to enable and encourage primary care teams to take responsibility for the health of their local registered populations, and to make them accountable to those populations, a critical mass of medical and nursing opinion would already be available to make a serious start on a national scale; but it is not there now.

From 1918 to 1974, Medical Officers of Health (MOsH)

were employed by and answerable to elected Local Government authorities for supervision of all aspects of local health other than personal medical care, including enforcement of laws controlling quality of housing and some occupational risks, as well as monitoring of water supplies and sewage disposal. They built up and led teams of sanitary workers, nurses and salaried doctors, varying from very small units performing minimum statutory functions in some smaller areas, to huge organizations with many specialized medical and other departments in large cities. Though the BMA fiercely resisted all proposals for personal preventive work by salaried public health medical officers, failure of GP entrepreneurs to develop planned ante-natal care, to give help in birth control, to help young mothers by systematic personal advice in child-rearing, or to achieve more than sporadic immunization for diphtheria, led to development of Local Authority clinics which did provide these things. In the early years of the NHS these clinics continued to develop, and many salaried medical officers serving them developed valuable skills in preventive and educational work and in early diagnosis and supervision of handicap.

MOsH had wide discretionary powers and considerable professional independence (they could not be sacked by their employing authority, for example), and where both MOsH and local government really wanted to develop an effective public health service, achievements before the NHS were remarkable in some areas, recently reviewed rather optimistically by Sir George Godber.[15] Unfortunately for each vigorous pioneer there were at least ten others who sank into bland bureaucratic optimism, well described by Webster:[16]

> . . . MOsH as a whole developed a reputation for minimising the problems with which they were confronted. Their scientific judgement was clouded by pressures from the centre to present an optimistic impression of the nation's health, or by local reluctance to incur additional expenditure. . . With so few positive virtues the image of the MOH was shaped by negative factors. To other doctors the MOH was an officious and bullying bureaucrat, presiding over an empire of clinics and institutions. . . delivering services of disproportionately small benefit considering the costs involved.

In fact most MOsH still looked to the Osler paradigm, reconciled to their peripheral position in relation to clinical medicine by a relatively well-paid, undemanding and secure job. Between the wars they took on functions as local hospital administrators which had nothing to do with public health or prevention. When the NHS came in 1948 and they lost this part-time role they found, in Webster's words, 'no alternative worth contemplating'. When MOsH were abolished in the NHS reorganization of 1974 few noticed their disappearance, and fewer still were prepared to defend them.

The 1974 reorganization, later reinforced by the Griffiths Report on NHS administration, created a unified administrative machinery modelled on the administration of corporate private industry. Business executives with corporate industrial experience were brought in, whose example Community Physicians were expected to follow. Local control by elected councillors from Local Authorities was greatly reduced, compared with their previous powers to appoint, support and receive information from MOsH, a de-democratizing tendency which is now (1987) almost complete.

The background to and consequences of this development have been excellently reviewed by Jane Lewis.[17] Detailed public health functions such as control of water supplies and sewage disposal went to engineers, social services escaped from their absurd subordination to a medical leadership which was rarely either interested or informed about the skills of social casework, most GPs were running their own ante-natal clinics and some were running their own baby clinics, leaving only co-ordinating and leadership functions to the MOH. Co-ordination and leadership of staff they did not employ and over whom they had only a moral authority amounted nearly always to virtually nothing.

Such residual energy as still remained in the dying MOsH was bequeathed to their successors, Area Community Physicians, who retained an advisory role to local government for environmental hazards and occasional epidemic disease, but for practical purposes no doctor now had personal responsibility for reporting on or doing anything about the health of local communities. In fact, just when

epidemiology was showing that powerful environmental and
social causes underlay the modern epidemics of (for example)
coronary heart disease, lung cancer and maturity-onset
diabetes (susceptible to environmental and social control and
requiring planned environmental and social policies and
monitoring which only a public health service could provide)
the traditional Public Health machine was being dismantled,
its principal staff corps of MOsH being bribed into abdication
by profitable early retirement or lucrative posts as Community
Physicians ranked as consultants, and theoretically supposed
to co-ordinate the work of hospital specialists, but without
any real power to do so. The underlying assumption was that
the nation was now too healthy to benefit much from public
health measures and the monitoring of groups; future
advances would come from a powerful system of individual
clinical care within the Osler paradigm, which scarcely
existed in the 19th Century when the public health idea
was born.

As for the grand new conception of the Community
Physician, like Mozart's Arabian phoenix, everyone has
heard of it but few have seen it. As always, there are
exceptions, but their efforts seem to have been more an
embarrassment than a source of pride to most of their
colleagues. I have met Community Physicians doing excellent
work, excellently trained at the London School of Hygiene,
but they were Catalans practising in Barcelona. Though the
theoretical training of community physicians in Britain is
second to none, it is in practice impossible for most of it to
be put into practice in the NHS, a system managed for
economy rather than planned to conserve and restore health.
The Public Health Alliance[18] launched in 1987 by Dr David
Player after he was deposed as director-general of the Health
Education Council because of his outspoken opposition to
socially divisive government policies, is campaigning for a
redefinition of Public Health in much the same terms as those
advocated in this book. This could be an important rallying
point, particularly if it becomes associated with progressive
movements in primary care.

Origins of the British Public Health Tradition

The Public Health tradition in England was founded on four perceptions by those with the wealth and power to implement policies:

That as industry concentrated population in cities, the health of the rich could not be insulated from that of the poor, requiring control both of communicable disease (above all, cholera), and of its most immediately obvious causes.

That as labour skills became more sophisticated and valuable, ill-health in the labour force became a potentially avoidable burden on the costs of production.

That military manpower depended on a reserve of fit young men.

That charitable care for the poor could endorse the rule of the rich, thus stabilising a divided society.

This is not the authorized 'on and on and up and up' version of history taught in medical schools, typified by Sir George Newman,[19] who traced the origins of the British Public Health Service to

. . . the expansion and interpretation of Humanism and an ever-extending Education of the people as a whole. . . the benevolence and altruism of the medical profession; the evangelical revival of Wesley and the Methodists; the humanitarian ideals of Elizabeth Fry, John Howard, Samuel Romilly, and Wilberforce; 'the greatest happiness of the greatest number' of Bentham; the broad common sense and understanding of Percival, Ferriar, Haygarth and the medical officers of the Poor Law Commission; the 'socialism' of Owen, Cobbett, Place and the Chartists; the co-operative movement; Lord Shaftesbury, Chadwick, Simon, and Florence Nightingale; the far-seeing economy of employers; Mill and the Utilitarians; and the promoters of national registration and insurance.

A bland list of good people with good intentions, borne irresistibly upward by the justice and common sense of their cause; that was not how history happened, nor how it was felt by those it happened to.

More than by any other man, the British Public Health system was conceived and brought to birth by Edwin Chadwick, who started as personal secretary to Jeremy

Bentham. His ideas developed while he was secretary to the
Poor Law Commissioners, during implementation of the Poor
Law Amendment Act of 1834, when he became arguably
the most hated man in England. The New Poor Law was
consciously designed to reduce the burden of rates on landowners, and to herd surplus labour from the countryside
into the new industrial towns by eliminating all alternatives
except the workhouse, and then ensuring (by the 'doctrine
of less eligibility') that survival inside the workhouse would
be more unpleasant than starvation outside. It therefore
had the support of both the old landed gentry and
aristocracy, and the new rising class of industrialists. The
Act, which was largely Chadwick's creation, was ruthlessly
utilitarian in the Bentham tradition. Because it was directed
at the propertyless classes, it was a collectivist intervention,
contradicting the *laissez-faire* individualism of the propertied
middle class. The stoutest efforts of revisionist historians
have failed to scrub out the horror of the workhouse, which
has permanently tainted all efforts at authoritarian reform.

Having failed to legislate pauperism out of existence with
the Poor Law, Chadwick turned to ill-health as one of its
causes. In 1838 he persuaded the Poor Law Commissioners to
support a survey of the condition of the people in industrial
cities, mainly relying on the Medical Officers of the Poor Law
Unions (mostly part-time GPs) as his reporters. Their findings
appeared in his Report on the Sanitary Condition of the
Labouring Population of 1842. Few men of 50 were still well
enugh to work; in Manchester the average age at death was
38 in the families of professionals and gentry, 17 in the
families of labourers and artisans. Chadwick's comments on a
radical workers' meeting show how his interest in the health
of the working class derived from his perception of the
utilitarian interests of employers. He observed that

> the bulk of the assemblage consisted of mere boys, and that there
> were scarcely any men of mature age to be seen amongst them.
> Those of mature age and experience. . . generally disapproved of the
> proceedings of the meetings as injurious to the working classes
> themselves. These older men, we were assured by their employers,
> were intelligent, and perceived that capital, and large capital, was not

the means of their depression, but of their steady and abundant support. They were generally described as being above the influence of the anarchical fallacies which appeared to sway those wild and really dangerous assemblages.[20]

Chadwick's chilly utilitarianism was in a class by itself, but more sympathetic reformers shared the same ultimate social allegiance. William Farr, Britain's first Registrar General and founder of social statistics, sympathized with the popular battle against the workhouse, but looking back from the 1870s concluded that despite its abuses, the Poor Law was 'an insurance of life against death by starvation, and of property against communistic agitations'.[20]

The highest incidence of disease was everywhere associated with absent or foul water supplies, open drains and filth of every description. It was common for corpses to remain for several days before burial, in all weathers, in the single rooms inhabited by most families. In a supplement on burial of the dead, Chadwick proposed the appointment of Medical Officers of Health whose first task would be to verify deaths, ascertain their cause, and thus build up an information system on the state of public health and what was being done about it. The Health of Towns Act of 1848 laid down the legal basis of all subsequent public health work, revolutionizing the structure of towns, introducing universal safe water supplies and drainage, legal control of housing standards, and the safe distribution of food.

Chadwick successfully overcame the opposition of private water companies, slum landlords, and the innumerable local profiteers from corrupt and inefficient Local Authorities which were still elected by a small propertied class, mainly of landowners. The odium in which he was held by the working class gave him a relatively free hand from the most powerful economic and political interests, but pursuit of the causes of ill-health, even in the name and interest of the Establishment, was bound eventually to lose the support of the comfortable classes once the two fears of revolution and cholera had receded. Chadwick's enemies combined against him in 1854, when the government's Bill to continue his Central Board of

Health, organizing centre for the defeat of cholera by cleaning
the slums, was defeated in parliament. No mass support was
available from the poor, who saw him as oppressor rather
than liberator. *The Times* gloated over this easy isolation of
an authoritarian reformer:

> We prefer to take our chance of cholera and the rest than be bullied
> into health. . . It is a positive fact that many have died of a good
> washing. All this shows the extreme tenderness with which the work
> of purification should advance. Not so thought Mr Chadwick. New
> mops wash clean, thought he, and he set to work, everywhere washing
> and splashing, and twirling and rinsing, and sponging and sopping,
> and soaping and mopping, till mankind began to fear a deluge of
> soap and water. . . The truth is, Mr Chadwick has very great powers,
> but it is not so easy to say what they can be applied to. Perhaps a
> retiring pension, with nothing to do, will be a less exceptionable
> mode of rewarding this gentleman, than what is called an active
> sphere.[20]

And that is what he got; a pension and no further public
employment for the last 36 years of his life. Chadwick's
downfall has been attributed to his obstinate, intransigent
and uncompromising personality, but that has been said of
every energetic reformer who tried to enlighten the ignorance
of wealth enthroned. His rise and his influence in fact
depended on these same uncomfortable qualities, together
with more courage than the Poor Law Commissioners, who
initially refused to publish his Report on the Sanitary
Condition of the Labouring Population because of its criticism
of powerful interests, finally letting it appear only under
Chadwick's own name, leaving him with sole responsibility
for it.

Limits of Authoritarian Reform

The same theme has arisen many times in the subsequent
history of public health reform, in Britain and in every other
country. Reform imposed from above, addressing fears of
the rich rather than felt needs of the poor, succeeds only so
far as the affluent are willing to pay for even a part of the
cost of maintaining the health of the labouring class.

Historical experience suggests that at the top, social conscience depends more on the sound of hammering at the
gates than on spontaneous altruism. Once the fears of cholera
and revolution receded in the 1850s, Chadwick the
authoritarian reformer had no friends.

The workhouse legacy remained, to provide most of the
buildings and the attitudes inherited by the NHS in 1948.
Listen to this interview about life in Wandsworth workhouse,
from the Report of the Royal Commission on the Aged Poor
of 1895:[21]

Q. We have now to ask you about the aged poor; those about sixty.
A. They have to go and pick oakum for eight hours a day, twisting
little pieces of corded string for eight hours a day until the people
nearly become imbecile; they do not know what to do.

Q. Up to what age are they kept at this work?
A. They are kept at this from sixty-five until—well, there were some
there seventy. There was one man there seventy-nine, at least he
said he was.

Q. And they were all alike, worked for eight hours a day?
A. Eight hours a day; they have a quarter of an hour to go out and
smoke a pipe. . .

Q. Did you find the work severe?
A. No, not severe; monotonous. You did not know what to do. You
could not go out to write a letter, or to read, or to do anything:
you had no time of your own; in fact it was a place of punish-
ment, not relief. . .

The thoughtless cruelty of the workhouse system was still
forcibly separating elderly married couples when I qualified
in 1952. The entire system of gentrified ignorance,
hierarchical snobbery and judgemental condescension, run by
starched matrons and soaked in a pervasive stench of carbolic,
which typified all health service institutions, gave way slowly
and reluctantly, not because of a wave of reforming enlighten-
ment, but because working-class people with a little money
in their pockets and a health service they had voted for and
was theirs by right would no longer tolerate it, and the
supply of genteel unmarried women with few alternatives to
a life of dedicated ingrowing virginity dried up. Of 42,000

residential places in 1949, one year after the NHS began, all but 2,000 were in former workhouses.[22] Even in the early 1960s, hospitals for long-term care of the chronic sick and elderly were mostly in a state of undiminished squalor. Here is a description of geriatric wards by Peter Townsend:

> This ward is reached up twenty steep stone steps. . . On the wind-swept landing are twelve WCs in two rows of six, with no doors, no wooden seats, and divided from each other only by iron bands three feet high. The stone floors were saturated with urine and one man could be seen groping with his trousers in a confined space. . . The beds are iron-framed and are only two feet apart, each man having a bedside chair and sharing a locker with one other. There are no wardrobes, bedmats, or other amenities. In the day-room part, where the men both sit and eat, there are 41 armchairs crowded close together. All the walls and ceilings are grimy with dust.[23]

The health of poor people remained apalling. Nearly two-thirds of young men volunteering to fight in the South African war were physically unfit to bear arms. Lord Rosebery, leader of the Liberal Imperialists, observed that:

> An Empire such as ours requires as its first condition an imperial race, a race vigorous and industrious and intrepid. In the rookeries and slums which still survive, an imperial race cannot be reared.[24]

If this appears, perhaps surprisingly, to anticipate events about 30 years later in Germany, listen to Lord Rosebery's fellow-imperialist, Lord Haldane, in his rectoral address to the students of Edinburgh university in 1907; after calling on them to recognize the new significance of the State in establishing and maintaining world supremacy, citing the examples of Scharnhorst, Clausewitz, von Moltke and Bismarck, he went on to say:

> When a leader of genius comes forward the people may bow down before him, and surrender their wills and eagerly obey. . . to obey the commanding voice was to rise to a further and wider outlook, and to gain a fresh purpose.[24]

I quote Rosebery and Haldane to emphasize the imperial,

authoritarian mood of the time which was one important influence, though not of course the only influence, on early conceptions of the Welfare State.

The government was frightened enough to set up an Interdepartmental Committee on Physical Deterioration in 1904 which initiated school medical inspections, school meals, free school milk, leading later to sporadic beginnings of maternity and child welfare, and public nursing and health education services during the next two decades. For the first time, unevenly and incompletely depending on the social attitudes and resources of Local Government and the resistance of established GPs, a body of salaried doctors began to deliver personal preventive care.

Lloyd George, more in touch with reality than Lord Rosebery, presented a new idea to a Liberal Party frightened by the recent birth of the Labour Party:

> . . . if a Liberal government tackles the landlords, and the brewers, and the peers, as they have faced the parsons [over the Education Act], and tries to deliver the nation from the pernicious control of this confederacy of monopolists, then the Independent Labour Party will call in vain upon the working men of Britain to desert Liberalism that is gallantly fighting to rid the land of the wrongs that have oppressed those who labour in it.[25]

With such motives, it is no surprise that despite democratic rhetoric, Lloyd George looked to Bismarck for his model in setting up his health and insurance service. Beatrice Webb and the Fabians differed less from this tradition than their socialist beliefs might suggest. They were authoritarian, indifferent and often hostile to the working-class movement, supported the South African war when all other socialists opposed it, and opposed the creation of an independent Labour Party.

The Webbs' Minority Report on the Poor Law has correctly been seen as a principal origin of the British Welfare State as it eventually emerged. For example, far ahead of its time, it proposed a comprehensive personal medical service through State-salaried doctors, who could devote themselves

. . . in practice as well as in theory, to searching out disease, securing the earliest possible diagnosis, taking hold of the incipient case, removing injurious conditions, applying specialised treatment, enforcing healthy surroundings and personal hygiene, and aiming always at preventing either recurrence or spread of disease in contrast to mere 'relief' of the individual.[26]

However, the report was actually written at Luton Hoo, stately home of Sir Julius Wember, with his 54 gardeners, 30 house servants, and 10 electricians; here is what Beatrice Webb wrote, in the same Report, on the disposal of the undeserving poor:

Besides. . . the helpless deserving poor for whom Homes for the Aged have to be provided, there exists, we regret to say, no inconsiderable class of old men and women, whose persistent addiction to drink makes it necessary to refuse them any institutional provision. For this class, indeed, the Aged Poor of Bad Conduct, out of all the pauper host, it might well be urged that the. . . General Mixed Workhouse, with its stigma of pauperism, its dull routine, its exaction of such work as its inmates can perform, seems a fitting place in which to end a misspent life.[27]

Their friends and as they believed principal allies were the radical imperialists of the Liberal and Conservative parties, Lord Milner, R.B. Haldane, Joe Chamberlain, and Robert Morant, men with big social and imperial visions, firmly entrenched on the radical wing of the ruling class, many of them anticipating the later ideas of Fascism. The Fabians' point of departure (their various destinations were a different matter) can best be understood as one response to an epochal change in the ideas of the ruling class itself, a process described by Hobsbawm in his essay 'The Fabians reconsidered':[28]

. . . laissez-faire economic liberalism. . . had the force of natural law: a world in which, as in Newtonian physics, prices like water found their natural level, wages, like stones, when unnaturally raised must come down, and pint pots did not hold quarts. It was an orthodoxy which made virtually no provision (at least in the all-important field of production) for state interference, whose effects. . . must be ruinous. Politically it rested on the peculiar compromise of 1832 by which the old political rulers applied the manufacturers' policy (except in certain fields affecting the social status of a landowning aristocracy), on the absence of a working-class electorate and of any labour movement disposed to, or capable of, seriously challenging social stability. On the military. . . side it rested on the stability of the 1815 balance of power, which left Britain in control of the seas and with a deciding voice in international affairs. The electoral reforms of the 1860s, the unifications of the USA and Germany, the emergence of Japan, and the Great Depression after 1873 undermined all these three pillars.

In consequence the set of theoretical beliefs which dominated mid-Victorian Britain, like the Whig–Liberal–Radical alliance which provided its almost unbroken parliamentary majorities from 1846 to 1874, broke down. A shift from individualist to collectivist thought reflects the necessary intellectual adjustment. . . this was an intellectual problem of liberalism, for no other coherent body of doctrine was available. There were, for practical purposes, no socialists and such conservatives as essayed thinking rather than feeling were, at least in their economic and legal theories, liberals. Hence, not only did the great majority of middle-class (or any other) native socialists of the 1880s revival [of socialism] begin their intellectual lives as Liberal–Radicals, but—more paradoxically—[they] were initially influenced by] the systematic borrowing of the Prussian attitude to the State. . .

The need to find some alternative to laissez-faire, the readiness to define any such alternative as socialism, and the capacity. . . to separate socialism from the working-class movement, therefore provided a very apt background for the Fabians' peculiar version of it.

The apparatus of the British welfare state, its public medical services and its machinery of Public Health, were completed in outline in the heyday of imperial power and on the brink of its decline. In Britain today the guardians of received wisdom seem to find it difficult to separate the idea of military and economic dominance (imperialism) from the idea of civilization. As our ruling class learns, slowly and reluctantly, to accept third-rate military and economic status, it embraces and rationalizes successive retreats from the civilized social commitments it accepted in the heyday of imperialism.

Bold conceptions of Public Health and organized public responsibility are no longer of interest. The Public Health idea today is an orphan, unsupported by real resources though potentially more powerful than at any time since the mid-19th Century. In the 1960s it was widely believed that mass prevention (which can and should include personalized anticipatory care on a mass scale) had been superseded by technically sophisticated personal salvage. This belief is now wholly discredited among informed people, as a social policy if not as a strategy for their own personal survival. Epidemiology, the study of the natural history of disease in populations, and its response to treatment and to environmental and social change, originally concerned almost entirely with infectious disease, has developed into a powerful research weapon concerned with all forms of disease and all ways of combating it, and Britain has been a pioneering nation in epidemiology as a research discipline.[29],[30] The systems of data collection required to support a national epidemiological information service, so that intelligent planning decisions could be made in a Health Service positively oriented to the solution of health problems, have been earlier and more fully and comprehensively developed in Britain than anywhere else in the world. All British medical students now have some undergraduate training in epidemiology. There is now wide support, particularly among GPs, for integration of personal clinical care into an overall pattern of anticipatory care on a population scale. The conclusions of the Cumberlege Report,[31] driven through by a Conservative lady curiously oblivious of the traditional relations between GPs and their favourite Party, set out simple and practical guidelines for planned community care. The only real objections to the Cumberlege proposals by GPs have been anticipated difficulties in sharing management decisions with nursing officers, which must appear at least equally great when viewed from the other side of an intolerable divide which simply has to be bridged if we are to see any progress at all, and the fact that registered GP populations are more scattered than the neighbourhoods which Cumberlege correctly identifies as the obvious focus for care. Granted a little patience and flexibility on both sides, the work of primary care teams could be integrated with little difficulty, as most GPs do in fact wish already to set reasonable limits to the areas within which they are prepared to visit.[32,33]

The registered list system which began with the clubs, consolidated by Lloyd George in 1912, and universalized by the NHS in 1948, make local organization of population-based anticipatory care an easier undertaking than in countries where people generally do not have their own personal doctors or any well-established tradition of referral to hospital-based specialists. But though epidemiology and the Public Health idea are used to question and discount the value of so-called curative clinical medicine, and thus to disarm informed resistance to the growing lag in application of advances in personal medical care, they are not used to provide the structures of a Public Health service truly concerned with the health of the public.

An Orphan Agenda: The Black Report

The Black Report[34] in 1979 showed clearly that Britain still had public health problems of fundamentally the same nature as in the 19th Century, equally susceptible to environmental and social change in their broadest sense, though somewhat more accessible to personal clinical salvage. The Report concluded bluntly that in terms of better health and reduced disability and premature mortality, the biggest returns on social investment would come from the following main courses of action:

A. Within the health and personal social services:
   1. That government should adopt three principal health objectives:
      To give children a better start in life.
      To encourage good health among a larger proportion of the population by preventive and educational action.
      To reduce the risks of early death in disabled people, to improve their quality of life whether in the community or in institutions, and as far as possible to reduce the need for these.
   2. That allocation of resources be based on need, using

Standardized Mortality Ratios (SMRs) for allocation at Regional level, and other indicators of health care and social needs at District level.

3. That resources within the NHS and personal social services be shifted toward community care, particularly to antenatal, postnatal and child health services, and home-help and community nursing services for the disabled.

4. That the quality and geographical coverage of general practice be improved, particularly in areas of high morbidity and poor social conditions. The distribution of GPs should be related not only to population but to medical need as indicated by SMRs and other indicators, and GP payment by capitation should be modified accordingly.

B. Measures to be taken outside health and personal social services:

1. Abolition of child poverty should be adopted as a national goal for the 1980s, with an immediate increase in child benefits to 5.5% of average gross male industrial earnings (£5.70 at 1979 prices), progressive introduction of larger increases for older children, an immediate increase in maternity grant to £100 (1979 prices), and an infant care allowance.

2. Provision of free school meals to all children as a right.

3. A staged introduction of a comprehensive disablement allowance for people of all ages, beginning with the totally disabled.

4. Government, unions, and employers should agree on minimum conditions at work, and the Health and Safety Executive and Employment Medical Advisory Service should be more active in preventive health work.

5. Local Authority spending on housing should be substantially increased, and LAs should widen their responsibilities to provide all types of housing need. Public and private housing policies should be co-ordinated. Special housing for the disabled should be improved by joint funding schemes by Local Authority housing and

social service departments.

6. The health implications of public policies in many different fields should be considered by interdepartmental machinery at Cabinet office level, with local counterparts.

7. A Health Development Council should be established with an independent membership to play a key advisory and planning role in relation to a collaborative national policy to reduce inequalities in health.

Everything possible was done first to limit the circulation of the Report, and then to discount its conclusions. Secretary for Social Services Patrick Jenkin contributed a foreword to the Report, in which he said:

> . . . the Group has reached the view that the causes of health inequalities are so deep-rooted that only a major and wide-ranging programme of public expenditure is capable of altering the pattern. I must make it clear that additional expenditure on this scale which would result from the report's recommendations—the amount involved could be upwards of £2 billion a year—is quite unrealistic in present or any foreseeable economic circumstances. . .

Subsequent authoritative reviews including new evidence,[35],[36] which have broadly confirmed its conclusions, have also been ignored and discounted by central government. The only academically respectable supporters for the government view are Prof. Raymond Illesley and Julian Le Grand,[37] who still argue that widening health inequalities are a statistical artefact, and that class-based measures of inequality are no longer useful. Interested readers must make up their own minds, comparing the evidence offered by these authors with the material in Wilkinson's book,[36] bringing together a wide range of expert authors, and the rebuttal by Nicky Hart,[38] statistician to the Black Report.

In contrast with the complacency of central government, there have been many local area-based studies by District Health Authorities and City Councils (for example Bristol,[39] Glasgow,[40],[41] Manchester,[42] Sheffield,[43] Merseyside,[44] Newcastle,[45] Belfast,[46] and six different areas of

London[47-52] which have used the 'Black approach', well reviewed by Betts.[53]

Since 1979, government actions relevant to this agenda have included:

A rise in the number of people claiming means-tested supplementary benefit from 4.6 million in 1979 to 7.1 million in 1983, and in those entitled to benefit but not claiming from 2.1 million in 1979 to 3.3 million in 1983. By 1983, about 9 million people,[54] and about 28% of all children[55] were living in families with incomes at or below Supplementary Benefit level.

Levels of child benefit have risen only at the same rate as inflation, even this is now in doubt, and there is now wide discussion of an end to unselective child benefit as a right. The aim seems to be to make all social benefits subject to means tests.

Of a total of £4.17 billion cuts in income tax since 1979, the richest 1% got 44% and the poorest 25% got 3%.[54]

A tax on employees for their employers' contributions to workplace nurseries, although only 20% of British 3-year-olds have any nursery provision, compared with 42% in the Netherlands and 88% in France.[56]

Abolition of maternity grants as a right, replacing them with a means-tested benefit. Abolition of maternity allowances for about 25% of mothers who received it before 1987.[57]

Annual construction of new Local Authority houses for rent fell from about 140,000 throughout the 1970s to 43,000 in 1985. Private sector housing construction stayed about the same as in the 1970s at 154,000 a year. Demolition of slum houses fell from 64,000 a year in the early 1970s to 12,000 in 1985. The number of homeless families recognized by Local Authorities rose from 83,000 in 1981 to 109,000 in 1985. The number of houses repossessed by building societies because of mortgage arrears rose from 2,500 in 1979 to 16,800 in 1985.[58]

Regional allocation of resources, already in operation at the time of the Report, has continued, but allocations at District level have generally not been related to other indicators of need. Allocation of resources to community rather than hospital services has increased by about 1-2%. Child health services have not been developed actively in any direction, and home help services have been reduced, in some areas drastically; in my village we now have 8, where we once had 16. Community nursing services have been expanded significantly, more or less in line with a reduction in hospital beds and shortening of the average duration of in-patient care. Nothing has been done to increase the number or quality of GPs serving areas of high morbidity, or to modify GP pay to encourage selective improvement in care. Of 16 other more detailed recommendations made for action within the NHS and Social Services, only one or two seem to have led to any widespread action.

The Black Report, though a well-documented and scholarly argument chaired by a President of the Royal College of Physicians, has been rejected on political grounds, with little attempt to marshall any serious scientifically-based argument against it. Equivalent studies in Sweden, where even con-servative groups are more humane,[59] have been much more fully developed with wider research, and are now being implemented. There are real problems about the further development of the liberal welfare state within capitalist economies, even where humane political traditions are much tougher than in England,[60] but the Scandinavian experience shows that disintegration of the NHS, and abdication from previous public health commitments, is not inevitable; it is a clear political choice today, as was the creation of work-houses in the early 19th Century.

Official Attitudes to Information

The decennial reports on occupational mortality of the OPCS, the main source of data on disease in relation to social class, have increasingly been discounted by the OPCS itself, and are now issued in such a way and at such a price (micro-fiched tables without summarized commentaries, at a total cost of £55) that they are accessible only to a few scholars, not to the public at large or its elected representatives.[61,62] The Health Education Council, which under Dr David Player began to take its independent role seriously, has been sacked and reconstituted as the Health Education Authority, subject to the DHSS and with more docile nominees.[63,64] After giving partial and hesitant support to experiments in GP microcomputers, the DHSS has abandoned general practice data collection to commercial firms offering powerful free microcomputers with sophisticated software, in return for data which can then be sold to pharmaceutical companies, an extraordinary admission that commercial interests which derive most of their profit from the NHS need to take planning decisions based on evidence, while those leading a public service can continue to grope in the dark.

The definition of unemployment used for compiling official statistics has been changed several times since 1979, each time in a way that reduces the official figure, publication of health and health service statistics generally has been delayed and reduced, production of national and local propaganda material glorifying the government's record on health services at public expense has increased steadily, and health service employees have been disciplined for drawing public attention to shortcomings in the service. Unlike the USA, Britain has no tradition of open government in the sense of legal requirements to expose its work to un-restricted public criticism, but we have had a strong tradition of systematic statistical monitoring of social trends and free criticism within the politically less dangerous circle of scholarship. Even this is now being steadily eroded; unlike its predecessors, who had enough wisdom and social confidence to value informed academic dissent, the New Conservatism sees no advantage for itself from informed criticism, nor danger from secret government.

British Public Health was imposed on the rest of society by ruthless men acting for a brutal but confidently advancing class. Public Health measures were done always to, sometimes for, but never by the people; yet they were done, with energy, confidence, and faith in the idea of social progress, and a concept of civilization which demanded a decent minimum of social investment. All this is now being abandoned.

In the absence of central action to develop a real rather than rhetorical public health programme, the initiative has been left to whatever parts of the periphery are prepared to assert some self-respect and autonomy: Health Authorities

of exceptionally independent mind, Local Government
Authorities with enough imagination to reach beyond their
now very restricted responsibilities for health, and general
practice, at the levels of Family Practitioner Committees
and of GPs themselves. Enough of these exist to develop
several models for more effective planning and care, but these
do not constitute a national policy; in fact without exception
the pioneers who have built up these projects are hostile to
current Government policies.

The GP as Community Physician

David Mant[65] and I[66] have both suggested that the MOH
function could and should be performed by GPs, each group
practice being responsible for individual and group health
surveillance in its own registered population. GPs are in touch
with a known local population, and groups of GPs generally
serve somewhat loosely defined neighbourhoods. Though
these do not as a rule coincide with the tightly defined
patches suggested as planning units by the Cumberlege
Report on community nursing, there is already a tendency
for GPs to rationalize the boundaries of their practices to
reduce travelling time, and with flexibility and good will
there is no reason why GP groups should not eventually serve
the neighbourhood units of 10,000 or so envisaged by
Cumberlege.[31] This happens to be roughly the size of the
average electoral ward, so the possibilities exist (ignored in
the Report and specifically rejected by Julia Cumberlege
when I wrote to ask her about this) of creating locally
elected machinery of accountability.

Primary care teams can obtain intimate knowledge of local
health hazards and are then well situated to initiate community action to control them. Mant[65] lists five principal
Public Health tasks which could be undertaken by GPs:

Monitoring the state of the practice health; an annual report with
local data set in context with regional and national statistics, with
a commentary drawing attention to particular problems and
suggestions for tackling them.

The drains function; surveillance of local environmental hazards and infective disease.

Planning tasks; varying 'from the bizarre (medical care in the case of nuclear war) to the pedestrian (how many chiropodists are needed?)'. These would include liaison with social services, education departments and voluntary agencies; maintenance of chronic disease and handicap registers; and 'a saintly patience and a freedom from other practice commitments in order to cope with the tedious bureaucracy of local government'.

Auditing the effectiveness of preventive programmes; monitoring screening and immunizations, and recording prevalence of disease risk factors in the community.

Evaluating population effects of medical intervention. Mant suggests local randomized controlled trials to evaluate practice diagnostic and treatment procedures. In the light of my own experience of running several such trials in my own practice, he seems to underestimate the limitations of small numbers in population units of 10,000 or so, and the time, skills and resources required for valid trials. However, a national network of Public Health practices would be able to undertake powerful nationally or regionally administered multicentre trials.

Some of these elements have always been included in the work of GPs in many fairly remote communities in Norway and Northern Sweden (Distriktslekke), and in most of Scandinavia this is a tradition which is already beginning to be seen as a portent for the future rather than a survival from the past.

In my own practice in Glyncorrwg, socially isolated and with a 'Public Health' orientation in the whole staff developed over 25 years, we have had experience of action (sometimes triumphant, usually successful, occasionally a failure) under all of Mant's headings. Examples have included public discussion of and sometimes action on repeated fatal or near-fatal road accidents at the same danger points; licenced Public Houses which serve more alcohol to people who are already drunk, to children of 14, and at 2 o'clock in the morning; shopkeepers and school bus drivers who sell cigarettes one at a time to children; tipping of vegetable peelings and other food refuse into the river where they maintain the rat population; derelict industrial buildings which have been the site of serious accidents to children; and a large leak of raw sewage into a river used by children for bathing. This last case was interesting. It occurred in the late 1960s, when we still had a Medical Officer of Health. Until he was shown a coloured photograph of faeces flowing from the broken pipe he refused to accept that any real problem existed; even then his immediate response was that it was against the law for children to swim in the river!

These are all examples of negative action, but our Health Centre Committee has also made positive proposals and organized public pressure for their adoption, for example development of jogging and cycling tracks away from main roads, and real rather than rhetorical provision of facilities for mothers to stay with their children in hospital. Positive screening procedures for detection of high blood pressure, smoking, obesity, diabetes, airways obstruction, alcohol problems and cervical cancer have been applied to the whole population at risk for more than 15 years, and these policies have been backed by the Patients' Committee. The practice has worked closely with the preschool playgroup and with teachers in the local primary school to integrate brain-damaged children and to compensate positively for inadequate parenting.

Primary care teams can review local causes of death, drawing attention to practical lessons which can be learned from them in a way that was never possible at the impersonal, large-population level of traditional Public Health. We have done this in Glyncorrwg, circulating the results to the local population as well as publishing them in the national medical press.[67] Clinical targets can be set for local communities which are comprehensible to local people, and for which action lies within their imagination, for example the elimination of measles and cancer of the cervix, or reduction of the population of smokers to 25% of all adults aged 20-64.

Annual Reports

Annual reports by GPs are not a new idea. In Northern Ireland, Ballymoney Health Centre, which serves about

13,000 people, published its 17th annual report in 1986, of particular interest because it literally looks back to the Dawson Report of 1920.[68] The Dawson Report set out a conception of health centres on a cottage hospital model, with autonomous GPs and specialists jointly providing care in much the same way that actually occurred in small towns in the USA in the '40s and '50s. It was used by the BMA to head off proposals for salaried service, which soon evaporated as post-war plans for a land fit for heroes were discarded. It was then virtually forgotten until the 1966 Package Deal, with its extensive programme for health centre building, when renewed interest in health centre building required more respectable origins than the Socialist Medical Association's wartime campaigns for health centres based on salaried team practice.

Dr Burns' team at Ballymoney Health Centre is based on one of the few surviving GP hospitals, and its report has the traditional form of a hospital report, extended to include an account of work done by GPs, practice nurses, health visitors, community nurses, social workers for the elderly, physiotherapists, dieticians, a radiologist, a psychologist, in its various special clinics (ante-natal, cervical cytology, immunization, family planning, eyes, well babies, speech therapy, chiropody, dental, child psychiatry, geriatrics, well men and paediatric surveillance), and of undergraduate and postgraduate educational activities. An annual medical meeting is held with a visiting speaker, and an annual obstetric meeting with a visiting expert assessor to discuss the statistical results of the year's work.

Apart from its obstetric review, the report does not relate its work quantitatively to its population base, but this could be done if one member of staff with some epidemiological training (not necessarily a doctor) were made responsible for developing and using an information system. Though this would have revolutionary implications, it would probably be acceptable to the apparently conservative (but also very progressive) group of doctors who account for 9 out of 13 members of the Health Centre's Committee of Management (the others are a dentist, the director of nursing services,

the District Administrative Officer and the Health Centre
Nursing Superintendent). In 1984 the 8 GPs at the centre
worked with 4 trainee GPs, 5 office staff, 3 practice nurses,
3 health visitors, 4 community nurses, 1 social work assistant, 5 physiotherapists, 1 community midwife, 2 speech
therapists, 2 chiropodists, 1 dentist, 1 dental therapist, 1
community dietician and 1 psychologist. The Osler paradigm
remains firmly in place, with no direct input from any
member of the public. Addition of population-oriented
statistics could introduce a necessary element of criticism
and change into what has been a pattern only of incremental
reinforcement of things as they are, and this is likely to
happen as the group moves into organized screening for
hypertension and other coronary risk factors. Ballymoney is
of great interest as an impressive example of the best that
has been achieved (under unusually favourable conditions)
within the old paradigm, and therefore the least that should
be achieved by any new alternative.

In contrast are annual reports describing the work of
radical teams moving consciously towards objectives defined
in terms of population need as well as demand. Dr Brian
McGuiness has been producing annual reports since 1977 at
the Weaver Vale practice at Runcorn, with an obvious effort
to relate local to national data. Other examples are: Dr Martin
Walsh's team at Birley Moor, the first health centre built in
Sheffield, serving 11,000 patients; Dr John Robson's team at
South Poplar Health Centre (Chrisp Street) serving 8,900;
my partner Brian Gibbons' reports on work at the
Blaengwynfi medical centre serving 2,000; and my own
reports on the Glyncorrwg Health Centre serving only 1,700.
Two teams I know of have also produced printed newsletters
aimed mainly at the populations they serve. Dr Laurie Pike's
group at Handsworth in Birmingham, and Dr Cyril Taylor's
group at the Princes Park Health Centre in Toxteth, Liverpool.

There are large differences in style between these reports,
some with a traditionally dry statistical approach resembling
the old MOH reports and apparently aimed mainly at professional colleagues, others with a simpler, more self-critical,
anecdotal or campaigning approach aimed chiefly at involving

the local population. In practice the active readership (that
is, those who talk to members of the team about what they
have read) for all these documents seems still to be almost
entirely within medical and perhaps nursing peer groups.
No one, so far as I know, has had much response from
patients, apart from uncritical praise for making the effort.
Perhaps in the eyes of local people, any attempt to take
accountability seriously is such a huge step forward that they
see little to criticize in either approach. This judgement
seems to me to be probably right; at the point we are now
at, any attempt by doctors to give an organized account of
their work, however traditional or even complacent in
form, should be welcomed. We should be careful not to
apply to our colleagues the sort of destructive criticism made
wearily familiar by medical sociologists over the past two
decades, few of whom seem able to imagine what it is like to
be responsible for actually providing care, rather than acting
as a full-time chairborne critic.

Logically it is difficult to deny the need for an annual
report on any public service, though in fact few schools (for
example) have done this until recently. Having produced
such a report, who is it for? In Glyncorrwg we have sent
copies of all our reports to the local Community Physician
and Family Practitioner Committee, but have never received
any comment, positive or negative, from either. I suspect
they have no idea what to do with them. Though annual
reports certainly should be circulated to local Community
Physicians and FPCs in the hope that they will be taken
into account in local planning (assuming such planning
really exists) their principal target audience should be patients
themselves, the neighbourhood population.

There are problems about designing an annual report
detailed and comprehensive enough to meet the requirements of Community Physicians and FPCs (if these had a
serious and positive planning function) yet sufficiently
simple and short to encourage local people to read it, express
their own opinions, and supplement it with their own experience. My own conclusion is that these two functions can't
be combined; it would be better to produce two reports, a

comprehensive one in a fairly traditional style for peer review by medical and nursing colleagues, and a popular version concentrating on one or two key issues for change in the coming year, though obviously both should be made freely available to anyone who is interested.

Annual Meetings

Whatever the difficulties, and these are bound to be great where there is no tradition of community accountability and participation, the logical way to present an annual report to the local population is at or immediately before an annual general meeting open to all registered patients, and the logical way to act on its findings is to use that meeting to elect a patients' committee.

Relatively few annual reports seem to be presented to open meetings of patients, and when they are, turnout and response are generally disappointing. Practices which attempt this have tried to attract larger audiences by inviting outside speakers, ideally local hospital specialists prepared to discuss their work directly with the population they serve. This was very successful in Aberdare, only a few miles from my own practice. Our experience in Glyncorrwg is that few consultants are willing to do this, but when they are, we have big turnouts and none of the destructive criticism specialists seem to fear. Because all doctors have so much autonomy, there are big differences between different localities, and it is dangerous to generalize from local experience, good or bad. Consultants in many areas seem to be more willing to meet the communities they serve on a more equal footing.

Patients' Committees

Patients' committees, or patient participation groups, began in a few centres in England and Wales in the mid-1970s, reaching a total of perhaps 80–100 groups by 1986; 63 of them have been surveyed by Ann Richardson and Caroline Bray.[69] Some are composed entirely of delegates representing organized groups such as pensioners and the Red Cross, others of a mixture of delegates and self-appointed volunteers. All surviving groups seem to have begun on the initiative of GPs; the only exception I know of, in which patients took the first initiative, collapsed fairly quickly. All groups in which GPs do not attend regularly have collapsed.

Ours in Glyncorrwg was elected at an open community meeting of about 60 out of 1,000 adults at risk in 1975, with reserved places for some groups which I thought needed to be represented; mothers of young children, a local teacher, local healthworkers, a pensioner, a shift-worker, and so on. In practice, it probably makes little difference whether such groups, without statutory rights or powers, are elected or more or less self-appointed. Those which survive more than three or four years become autonomous groups of interested local people, not subject to real popular control, but certainly having a viewpoint different from doctors, though this will seldom be pressed to the point of conflict. Ours meets once a month, discussing and taking decisions on such problems as frequency of GP visits to the housebound elderly, provision of sleeping accommodation and meals for mothers accompanying their children in hospital, collection of data on patient opinion about the practice and on the effects on patients of prescription charges, training in resuscitation, campaigns for a local swimming pool (which failed) and for safe cycle and running tracks away from main roads and against closure of the local ambulance station (which succeeded), hospital waiting lists, and a more or less permanent process of explanation and discussion of how the NHS is supposed to work, how it actually works, and how it might work in the future.

In 1986 the Labour Party's National Policy Committee on Health and Social Services nominally accepted annual reports, annual meetings, and elected patients' committees with an advisory function, as necessary reforms for general practice. It is doubtful whether these aims were really accepted, understood, or even remembered by the relevant shadow ministers, and they were not included among the twelve key points listed in the Labour Party's Charter for Health which was supposed to be the basis of its campaign on health in the

1987 general election. I don't know of any moves to include these reforms in the policies of other political parties, though they are consistent in principle with the official aims of all of them, even the Conservative Party. A majority of the National Committee for Patient Participation Groups remains opposed to legislation to establish groups as a civic right, on the grounds that GPs as independent contractors can't be told what to do. The logic of this escapes me; it takes two sides to make a contract, and there is no reason why a new contract should not be negotiated which would include this provision. Most GPs who have initiated groups seem to see them as having very limited advisory functions, without any wider potential for organized accountability. Many soon come to function mainly as (usually very effective) fund raisers for equipment the government considers itself too poor to provide.

A more or less universal experience is that patient participation groups steadily increase workload for GPs and others on the team, at least by adding yet another evening meeting once a month, much more by finding new tasks which need to be done and old tasks incompletely done. Justified fear of this additional workload, more than reflex despotism, may account for the general reluctance of GPs to encourage such committees, even when they approve of them in principle.

The rate of formation of new patient groups is only slightly greater than the rate at which old ones collapse, and few that I know of claim to have a really vigorous life with a wide local population base and an assured future, even if the initiating GPs were replaced by more average ones. Several vigorous, progressive, and otherwise successful group practices in central urban areas of great social need have failed to create viable patient participation groups, despite dedicated efforts sustained over months or years. The problems seem to be the same everywhere in the industrialized capitalist world; Mullan[70] reports similar experiences from community-oriented groups in USA. My guess is that progress would be quicker if we gave higher priority to organizing special interest groups addressing practical tasks, for example diabetics and hypertensives and their spouses, child asthmatics and their families, and other chronic disease groups who face immediate material problems at all levels in the NHS, giving an immediately credible, concrete and practical agenda for patient participation, which might later be extended to more general participation.

Despite this generally rather negative experience, the principle of organized, representative patient participation in the work of primary care teams is of critical importance if we are to move seriously into planned anticipatory care of local populations with minimal bureaucracy, fear of which is the main argument advanced by GPs against salaried service or any other form of regular positive accountability.

Local Public Health: Amateur or Professional?

Substantial protected time is essential for any serious commitment to a Public Health function for general practice. In Glyncorrwg this work has taken the equivalent of about two full sessions (8 hours) of working time each week, one hour of which has had to be at evenings or weekends. There would be some economies in a larger unit, but judging from my experience a serious government policy would require an absolute minimum of three sessions a week for each Public Health professional to service a group practice serving a population of 10,000.

This work could be done either by a doctor or by a fully qualified nurse, but each would need both specific training and remedial education. Selection of candidates should be based on evidence of capacity for informed confidence and sustained enthusiasm, and ability to transmit these to the whole primary care team, from doctors to office staff and cleaners. Training should as far as possible be by people who have experience of this work themselves; academics whose field experience is limited to research surveys will know more about statistical handling of data, but they are seldom credible to GPs or nurses who already have a lot of coping experience with less structured, more demand-sensitive work in real communities, and the first task of trainees will be to become credible advocates of a Public Health function in their probably sceptical home teams. The main statistical skills required are awareness of common sources of error in data collection, elementary trial design, simple sampling methods, and some idea of appropriate sample size, all based on examples of real work done by similar workers under similar conditions to those already experienced by the learners. Other essential skills are ability to organize contact with the local population, to run public meetings and produce local health education literature, awareness of the strengths and limitations of various levels of NHS administration and Local Government in local terms, and ability to use and eventually contribute to local, national and international medical and nursing literature with simplicity, boldness and imagination.

There is no way this can be done both well and quickly; we are talking about an agenda for the next hundred years. The Public Health movement of the 19th Century took about 100 years to become legislatively complete and ideologically exhausted, but nobody denies that it was effective. There is no reason why even now, in an economic and political climate more discouraging than at any time since the 1930s, a start should not be made everywhere by those GPs, Community Physicians, community nurses and Nursing Officers who understand the need for it, with or without material support from higher administration. Excellent work has already been done in Oxford by just such a combined force, together with an imaginative and pro- gressive Local Authority.[71] More than a start is not possible without support from a radically new central government policy, but with the acceleration added every week by the literature of medical science and examples of work already begun in cities like Oxford and Sheffield, once this idea begins to roll it could become an irresistible force from below.

Salaried Service

David Mant[72] concluded that the immediate limiting factor on implementation of the GP community physician idea was the hostility of GPs to salaried service, without which planned and protected work in sessional time is difficult. GPs accustomed only to the breakneck pace of their junior hospital posts and of general practice, particularly industrial general practice, are generally unable at first to understand and therefore respect the slower and apparently inefficient pace of sessional work in Public Health and School clinics. They have learned to measure their work not by health outputs achieved, but by their own exhaustion in meeting demand. If GPs are to move seriously into anticipatory care and prevention, most will need a remedial education which is difficult to obtain as self-employed entrepreneurs.

If GPs remain independent contractors, they cannot share fully the loyalties, understand the anxieties, or perceive the full possibilities of a team composed of other salaried office workers, community nurses, health visitors, midwives, and the many other health workers who for the most part do not now exist, but are badly needed—community dieticians, physiotherapists, sports instructors and more or less specialized lay counsellors of every kind. They may satisfy themselves that, as first among equals, they accept the team, but does the team really accept them? Doctors have hitherto had too much autonomy, all other health workers have had too little. What seems boldness and enterprise to GPs may look like arrogance and recklessness to salaried staff, and what seems only prudent recognition of administrative reality to community nurses, looks to GPs like unimaginative servility. There is some truth in both perceptions, suggesting that what we may need is a team in which all are salaried but all have greater confidence and autonomy.

Apart from simply leaving things as they are (always the most popular answer), there are five possible solutions for this problem of primary care teams which exist on paper but do not function. First, there is the Cumberlege solution; forget about the GPs, who are and will remain independent entrepreneurs, and construct a new neighbourhood-based team of salaried health workers employed by the Health Authority, led by nurse-practitioners, who will do the job on their own. There may be an underlying assumption that

GPs will eventually join the team, once they recognize their own isolation. This scenario is probably not viable: because it has given no serious thought to the existing content of primary care, and little to the training requirements for nurse-practitioners; because of a growing excess of doctors and shortage of nurses; and because there is not even potential majority support for such a development, either among the public, the politicians or any of the health professions. However, some enterprising Nursing Officers are beginning to set up (for example) diabetic clinics in health centres with only passive acceptance by GPs, possibly a first step in the Cumberlege scenario.

Secondly, Prof. Dennis Pereira Gray once proposed that health visitors and community nurses should be independent contractors like GPs. This is scarcely a serious option (it has never had any significant support or even interest from health visitors or community nurses themselves), but there is a real need for greater professional autonomy for all health workers, though this need not be inconsistent with salaried service. As a practical proposal it seems to have lapsed.

Thirdly, and at present most importantly, there is a trend slowly to increase the proportion of primary health workers employed by GPs under the 70% wages-reimbursement scheme. Just over 50% of staff-time available under this scheme is actually taken up, and the quickest and easiest way to expand primary care teams under present legislation would be for all GPs to employ staff to their full entitlement.[73] As a short-term solution this is attractive to the minority of GPs who show active concern for the effectiveness of their population care, because it bypasses the sometimes considerable difficulties of obtaining lasting agreement from Health Authority Nursing Officers on stable allocation of nursing staff and imaginative job-definitions permitting real team autonomy in setting objectives and deciding on means to attain them. Like other Health Authority staff, nursing officers have been accustomed to leading their troops from behind, and are not always sensitive to the needs and the mood of nurses in the frontline. However, both GPs and nursing officers have hitherto been accustomed to defensive action against disease by reactive care, rather than the pro-active offensives against disease implied by population-based anticipatory care, so both have much to learn about how actually to work in teams, rather than write and speechify about them; there is no evidence I know of on whether GPs or Community Nurses prove more adaptable, but I wouldn't bet on the doctors. As this learning process proceeds, it seems unlikely that progressive GPs will want to be employers of the teams they want to integrate into. Pressure for employ-ment of practice nurses, rather than agreement with Health Authorities on attachments, will in the future reflect either a business orientation among GPs, or failure of Nursing Officers to approach their work realistically. Either way, it is an attractive short-term solution, but is probably not a good formula for sustained progress.

The fourth option is for Community Physicians to give a lead by employing facilitators and deploying more attached community nurses to group practices in which one GP is paid sessionally to accept responsibility for planning and evaluation of anticipatory care and prevention in the group. This system is already operating in the Oxford region with great success. This principle of giving protected time by sessional employment, ultimately controlled by the District Community Physician who must be satisfied by evidence from clinical audit that progress is being maintained, is easily reproducible in all Districts and would certainly be more immediately acceptable to GPs than salaried service. The only obstacles to it appear to be that it would require money, energy and imagination, all three of which seem to be in very short supply. Certainly in my own Health Authority the Oxford experience has so far been greeted with a deafening silence, and this seems to be typical though not universal. We need to hear a lot more from Scotland, where every dimension of primary care seems to be a generation ahead of England and Wales; the Scottish Home and Health Depart-ment maintains a large-scale GP computers scheme using standardized software, over half of Scottish GPs are using A4 records, and big prevention and anticipatory care schemes such as the Good Hearted Glasgow project are based on attached Community nurses rather than GP-employed nurses.

The fifth and final option is that GPs should accept salaried service, probably under a Primary Care Authority fusing the present community functions of District Health Authorities and FPCs, as recommended by the Cumberlege Report and the Royal College of Nursing. The BMA and the RCGP have persistently refused to encourage serious and informed discussion of salaries within their membership. In the only articles ever to appear on the subject in the *British Medical Journal* in the past 30 years (a well-documented paper in favour by John Robson,[74] and a wholly undocumented one against by BMA under-secretary Michael Lowe[75]), Lowe did not refer to any real experience with salaries anywhere (not even to the fact that all hospital medical staff are salaried) but relied entirely on abstract argument. There is now considerable experience of salaried service by GPs in many countries with social systems and economies broadly similar to our own, including France,[76] Norway,[77] Sweden,[78] Finland,[79] and Spain.

The idea that GPs could be paid by salary naturally occurs to salaried junior hospital staff because all their consultant and nursing colleagues are salaried. They generally forget this as part of their professionalization into the GP role. This probably accounts for the hilarious events at the National Trainee GPs' Conference in Swansea in 1986. I was an invited speaker on planned anticipatory care in general practice, and referred in passing to my opinion that effective care was limited by a business approach and would eventually require a salaried GP service. Later that day an amiable doctor employed as a full-time negotiator by the BMA spoke to the trainees about pay structure, and a number of voices from the floor raised the issue of salaried service. One young man who seemed to speak for many said he was excited by the opportunities of primary care, more so than by anything else he had seen in his medical training, but he was repelled by the need also to be a business entrepreneur; he was trained in medical science, not business; had he wished to be a businessman, he would not have gone into medicine; why should he not be paid a salary to work as a community

medical generalist, just as his consultant colleagues were
paid salaries to be hospital specialists? Someone suggested
that a vote be taken; the chairman, overtaken by events,
agreed, and in no time at all Independent Contractor Status
was laid out on the floor, apparently breathing its last. By a
large but uncounted majority the trainees had voted for
salaried service, so far as I know the first politically unselected gathering of GPs or would-be GPs ever to do so.

At the inevitable dinner that evening I met the BMA man,
who was most friendly. 'Well, that was one for the books!',
he said. 'What was the majority then?', said I, for the chairman never told us. 'Oh, a good two to one at least; I wonder,
would you care to come and speak to our quarterly meeting
of negotiators sometime in the new year? I'll drop you a line
in a week or two.' When not being trampled by mobs of their
own rousing, BMA officials are intelligent and flexible men,
readily adaptable to changing circumstances. Of course I
never heard from him again, the BMA knowing well enough
that one swallow doesn't make a summer. The dignified
journals, the *British Medical Journal* and the *Lancet*, ignored
the incident; the free journals paid for entirely by advertising,
generally referred to by GPs as 'the medical comics' (*Pulse,
GP* and the like) but far more widely read than the heavies,
ran angry editorials claiming that the meeting had no elected
delegates, was over-run with suspect enthusiasts who had
taken the trouble to go to a national meeting rather than the
sound average chaps who let other people do their thinking
for them, and was probably swept off its feet by emotional
speeches. The chairman and secretary of the national committee of trainee GPs wrote a solemn letter to all these
journals disavowing the display of subversion at its annual
meeting, and claiming (without any evidence) that a large
majority of trainees stood foursquare behind independent
contractor status. At the 1987 national Trainees' Conference
the next generation of aspirant medical politicians went one
better, resolving that the prevous year's conference had been
stampeded by impassioned speechmaking into an un-
constitutional and unrepresentative vote, a decision head-
lined in one of the comics as 'Trainees were duped'. Why the

1987 Conference was more representative than 1986 they did not explain.

In sober fact, it was a straw in the wind. Unwillingness of GPs to accept the accountability inherent in any salaried service is only one of the obstacles to such a development, and from international experience, particularly in Scandinavia and Spain, not the most important. Salaried service starts where GPs are badly needed but cannot otherwise be found, and in those circumstances recruitment is not difficult if salaries are realistic. The question has been raised several times in relation to inner city practice in Britain, and other areas such as the South Wales valleys where there are exceptional loads of sickness and great difficulty in recruiting young doctors with good training and an imaginative interest in clinical medicine rather than small business. The possibility has been ignored in the 1987 White Paper, probably to ease negotiation of its terms with the BMA.

A more serious obstacle is the increased cost of a salaried rather than independently contracted service, not only because of the cost of the salaries themselves (including payment for work outside normal hours), but because once general practice stops being limited by what GPs can afford out of their own pockets, they are likely to press harder for extension of its scope and resources. Rational planning for health objectives is also likely to lead to a larger, certainly more labour-intensive service. Such a service would probably be more cost-effective, but it would also be more costly. One admittedly subordinate reason for the intransigent opposition of the BMA to GP salaries is its historically justified suspicion that such a service would be even more underfunded than at present; that it would increase responsibilities, while grudging the means to carry them out. Salaried service under a Conservative government, a not unimaginable consequence of a two-tier service if things continue as they now are, would certainly present serious dangers of this sort.

Bureaucracy and Sloth

However, the main reason given by GPs and their professional organizations for opposition to salaried service is their fear of bureaucracy and loss of initiative. Though these reasons are often advanced to conceal opposition on entirely different grounds (people who are able to run public services as private businesses are on more comfortable tax-scales with some scope for evasion, and enjoy all the other spin-offs of small business), they are real and deserve to be taken seriously.

The claims are that a salaried service in general practice would necessarily have the following four consequences:

Individual GPs would no longer accept personal responsibility for the care of individual patients, or for continuity of care, but pass these responsibilities on to an anonymous administration. Care would become more impersonal and therefore less efficient as well as less human.

Being paid at a flat rate unrelated to registered patient numbers, GPs would no longer have an economic incentive to be pleasant or conscientious in their care, and there would be a general decline in professional behaviour.

24-hours a day, 365 days a year cover would require a big expansion in medical staffing, which is not feasible.

Clinical objectives would be set, and their attainment verified, by a non-clinical bureaucracy of medical officers, with a career structure leading up and away from personal responsibility for patient care, towards chairborne and probably nepotic hierarchy.

There is some historical justification for all these fears, both from British and foreign experience, but not much. Salaried primary care in Britain has not yet been permitted (by the medical profession) to have the clinical scope of general practice; fusion of the preventive and curative traditions has not only not been encouraged, for most of our history it has not been allowed. There has never been any evidence that work done in British Maternity and Child Welfare Clinics, School Clinics, or Family Planning Clinics is inferior in average quality to equivalent work done by GPs. The fact that these clinics were all set up because GPs generally were not doing consistent work in these fields testifies otherwise. Continuity of care and personal responsibility is a real problem under any system, and is generally recognized to have got worse in many large group practices. This is to a large extent a function of increasing unit size, and the reasonable demands of GPs and their families to lead a more normal life, with recognized hours of work and arrangements for deputizing. Some large group practices discourage continuity of care and thus evade personal responsibility for their patients, a trend which is deplored by a majority of their colleagues and much resented by most patients. Bureaucracy can develop both in independent contractor status and in salaried systems; whether it actually does so depends on attitudes of care givers, above all of senior doctors who usually dominate the team. If they want personal lists and personal responsibility they can have them, with measurable improvement in the quality of patient care. Though theoretically implied by the present contract, personal responsibility for care has never been enforced. I can see no reason why personal responsibility could not be included in the job-definition of salaried GPs, with possibly greater continuity than there is now in many group practices. There can be problems of unequally divided labour where one doctor is more sought after by patients than another, but these will arise under any system. They should be solved by seeking causes and putting them right, not by pooling and thus depersonalizing the work, as is often the case in group practice today.

Any salaried service in British general practice would have to begin from the traditions and styles of work already customary with independent contractor status, and in the end we shall probably reach it simply by building up the salary elements (Basic Practice Allowance, Seniority Payments, Area Inducement Payments and so on) in the present contract (which account for about half of current GP earnings), diminishing capitation and fees-for-items-of-service payments, better enforcement of a more clearly defined contract, and development of properly trained and properly paid planning teams in the Family Practitioner Committees.

Some growth in bureaucracy is certain, because general practice is at present almost completely unplanned and unmonitored, both these functions are essential to effective work, and there is no way they can or should be done wholly by GPs or nurses on their own. Like any other industry, there is a minimum level of administration at every level in the NHS essential for optimal performance. Contrary to the assumptions of virtually all fieldworkers, the NHS is not, by world standards, over-administered, and there is no evidence that NHS administration contains more deadwood than either consultant or general practice. All of us can think of people with secure tenure in all three fields who would do patients a service by retiring in name, as they have done long ago in fact. It is true that implementation of the Salmon Report on the staff structure of nursing has led to a career structure which penalizes continuing responsibility for patient care by forcing nurses to choose between poorly-paid clinical and better-paid administrative careers, but the logical conclusion from this is to stop modelling NHS staff structure on the undemocratic traditions of corporate industry, and start paying more attention to the unique opportunities in health services to combine administrative responsibility with continued clinical experience.

Malignant growth in bureaucracy is a possibility, but if (and only if) GPs develop regular and organized contact with their registered populations as groups as well as when they consult individually, we have a powerful weapon with which to keep it under control. We should also remember that many Community Physicians now miscast as economic managers with few opportunities for imaginative work, could develop in new and positive ways in a system of population-based anticipatory care.

The last word on salaries should be left with perhaps the world's most expert observer of health care systems, their effectiveness, and their practical feasibility, Prof. Brian Abel-Smith of the London School of Economics:[80]

Under any system of payment it is the ethics and social commitment of the doctor which matter most of all. Where standards are low in these respects no financial structure can induce doctors to be what they are not. But where standards are high, salaried payment best indicates to the public the ethical stance of the doctor as a servant of the public, as a priest of medicine.

It is a pity the BMA has hitherto had so little confidence in the ethics and social commitment of its members. If we ever do have a salaried service, we shall need negotiators with well-informed and imaginative ideas on the subject; there is little evidence of that now.

Epidemiology is Accountability: Accountability is Democracy

British general practice already has the solution both to verifiably effective medical care, and to socially responsible professional autonomy. Because it has registered populations, it has denominators for its clinical numerators, and a listed local electorate of a size permitting participative democracy. It has the solution but has not recognized it, and has therefore been unable to use it. Within the Osler paradigm general practice has perceived only the care of complaining individuals, not the care of populations, and commodity production by experts for patients whose only active contribution is to demand medical action, which otherwise does not occur.

The basic population units of general practice, around 2,000–10,000 people centred in neighbourhoods with increasingly well-defined boundaries, could in an organized system of anticipatory care be basic units both for monitoring of national health and the effectiveness of care, and for democratic control of the NHS, a popular counterweight to bureaucracy. The methods of epidemiology take into account and demand the co-operation of all the people in a population; one person, one vote. Rescued from academic isolation, epidemiology could become a new field for participative democracy.

Until this is understood, the medical profession will continue to provide politicians with all the excuses they need to keep health at the top of their agenda in rhetoric, while leaving it last in practice.

NOTES

1. Neuhauser, D., 'Elective inguinal herniorrhapy versus truss in the elderly'. In, Bunker, J.P., Barnes, B.A., Mosteller, F. (eds.), *Costs, risks and benefits of surgery*, pp. 223–39. New York: Oxford University Press, 1977.
2. General Register Office. Morbidity statistics from general practice 1955–6 (vols I–III). London: HMSO, 1958.
3. RCGP, OPCS, DHSS. Morbidity statistics from general practice 1971–2: second national study. Studies on medical and population subjects no. 36. London: HMSO, 1979.
4. RCGP, OPCS, DHSS. Morbidity statistics from general practice 1981–2: third national study. Series MB5 no. 1. London: HMSO, 1979.
5. Wright, H.J., 'General practice in South West England', *Report from general practice no. 8*, London: RCGP, 1968.
6. Williams, W.O., 'South Wales study on morbidity', *Report from general practice no. 12*, London: RCGP, 1970.
7. Metcalfe, D., 'No excuses'. In, Pereira Gray, D.J. (ed.), *The Medical Annual 1985*, pp. 184–204. Bristol: John Wright, 1985.
8. OPCS General Household Surveys. Introductory Report 1973, annually thereafter to 1984. London: HMSO, 1973–84.
9. Hart, J.T., 'General-practice workload, needs, and resources in the National Health Service', *Journal of the Royal College of General Practitioners 1976*; 26:885–892.
10. Cartwright, A., *Patients and their doctors*, London: Routledge & Kegan Paul, 1967.
11. Cartwright, A., Anderson, R., *General practice revisited: a second study of patients and their doctors*, London: Tavistock, 1981.
12. Cartwright, A., Hockey, L., Anderson, J.L., *Life before death*, London: Routledge & Kegan Paul, 1973.
13. Bowling, A., Cartwright, A., *Life after a death: a study of the elderly widowed*, London: Tavistock, 1982.
14. Seipp, C., *The ambiguities of greatness: Sir William Osler, 1849–1919*. Unpublished MS 1981. Health Services Research Centre, University of North Carolina, Chapel Hill.
15. Godber, G.E., 'Medical Officers of Health and health services'. *Community Medicine 1986*; 8:1–14.
16. Webster, C., 'Medical Officers of Health—for the record', *Radical Community Medicine, 1986*; autumn:10–14.
17. Lewis, J., *What price community medicine? The philosophy, practice and politics of Public Health since 1919*, Brighton: Wheatsheaf, 1987.
18. 'Rethinking public health: the Public Health Alliance', *Lancet 1987*; ii:228. The address of the Alliance is c/o The Health Visitors Association, 50 Southwark Street, London SE1 1UN.
19. Newman, G., *The rise of preventive medicine*, London: Oxford University Press, 1932.
20. Quoted in Watson, R., *Edwin Chadwick, Poor Law and Public Health*, London: Longman, 1969.
21. Royal Commission on the Aged Poor, 1895, XV, 15,409–31.

Quoted in Hobsbawm, E.J., *Labour's turning point 1880-1900*, London: Lawrence & Wishart, 1948.
22. Ryan, M., 'The workhouse legacy', *The Medical Officer*, 11 November 1966; 270-1.
23. Townsend, P., *The last refuge: a survey of residential institutions and homes for the aged in England and Wales*, London: Routledge & Kegan Paul, 1962.
24. Simon, B., *Education and the Labour Movement 1870-1920*, London: Lawrence & Wishart, 1974.
25. Quoted in Morton, A.L., Tate, G., *The British Labour movement 1770-1920*, pp. 223-4, London: Lawrence & Wishart, 1956.
26. Murray, D.S., *Why a National Health Service? The part played by the Socialist Medical Association*, London: Pemberton Books, 1971.
27. Mackenzie, N., Mackenzie, J., *The first Fabians*, London: Weidenfeld & Nicholson, 1977.
28. Hobsbawm, E.J., *Labouring men: studies in the history of Labour*, London: Weidenfeld & Nicolson, 1964.
29. Jefferys, M., 'The transition from Public Health to Community Medicine: the evolution and execution of a policy for occupational transformation', *Society for Social History of Medicine Bulletin 39*, December 1986, 47-63.
30. Terris, M., 'The changing relationships of epidemiology and society: the Robert Cruickshank lecture', *Journal of Public Health Policy 1985*; 6:15-36.
31. DHSS, 'Neighbourhood nursing—a focus for care'. Report of the community nursing review (Cumberlege Report), London: HMSO, 1986.
32. Jarman, B., Cumberlege, J., 'Developing primary health care', *Journal of the Royal College of General Practitioners 1987*; 294:1005-8.
33. Williams, E.I., Wilson, A.D., 'Health care units: an extended alternative to the Cumberlege proposals', *British Medical Journal 1987*; 37:507-9.
34. Townsend, P., Davidson, N., *Inequalities of health: the Black Report*, London: Penguin, 1979.
35. Fox, A.J., Goldblatt, P.O., Jones, D.R., 'Social class mortality differentials: artefact, selection, or life circumstances?', pp. 34-49 in, Wilkinson, R.G. (ed.), *Class and health: research and longitudinal data*, London: Tavistock Publications, 1986.
36. Wilkinson, R.G., 'Income and mortality', pp. 88-114 in, Wilkinson, R.G. (ed.), *Class and health: research and longitudinal data*, London: Tavistock Publications, 1986.
37. Illesley, R., Le Grand, J., 'Measurement of inequality in health'. Discussion Paper no. 12, London: Suntory-Toyota Centre for Economics and Related Disciplines, 1987.
38. Hart, N., 'Class, health and survival: the gap widens', *Radical Community Medicine, Spring 1987*; 10-17.
39. Townsend, P., Simpson, D., Tibbs, N., *Inequalities in health in the City of Bristol*, Bristol: University of Bristol, 1984.
40. Howe, G., 'London and Glasgow: a spatial analysis of mortality

experience in contrasting metropolitan centres', *Scottish Geographical Magazine 1982*; 119-127.

41. West of Scotland Politics of Health Group, *Glasgow, health of a city*, Glasgow: WSPOHG, 1984. Available from John Boswell, 469 Tantallon Road, Glasgow G41.
42. Manchester Joint Consultative Committee (Health), *Health inequalities and Manchester*, Manchester: MJCC, 1985.
43. Thunhurst, C., *Poverty and health in the City of Sheffield*, Sheffield: Sheffield City Council, 1985.
44. Ashton, J., *Health in Mersey: a review*, Liverpool: Department of Community Health, University of Liverpool, 1984.
45. Leinster, C., *Primary health care*, Newcastle: Newcastle Inner City Forum, 1982.
46. Ginnety, P., Kelly, P., Black, M., *Moyard: a health profile*, Belfast: 1985.
47. Golding, A., *Health needs and social deprivation*, London: Camberwell Health Authority, 1984.
48. Curtis, S., *Intra-urban variations in health and health care: the comparative need for health care survey of Tower Hamlets and Redbridge, London*, London: Queen Mary College, 1984.
49. Betts, G., *Health in Glyndon: report of a survey on health in Glyndon Ward*, London: Greenwich Community Health Council, 1985.
50. Catford Community Health Project, *Wells Park health survey*, London: WPHP, 1986.
51. Tower Hamlets Health Campaign, *Taken bad: the state of health in Tower Hamlets*, London: THHC, 1985.
52. North East Thames RHA, 'Patient census study: social factor analysis'. Management services report no. 1249. Also ditto, 'Further analysis of patient census data with respect to social development'. Report no. 1259. London: NE Thames RHA, 1983.
53. Betts, G., 'Area-based studies of health', *Radical Community Medicine Spring 1987*; 22-31.
54. Becker, S., MacPherson, S., 'Poverty reaches record levels', *Labour Research, July 1986*; 75:15-18.
55. Townsend, P., 'Why are the many poor?' *International Journal of Health Services 1986*; 16:1-32.
56. 'The fall and rise of workplace nurseries', *Labour Research*, December 1985; 74:309-311.
57. 'Fowler's second stab at social security', *Labour Research*, February 1986; 75:17-19.
58. Central Statistical Office, *Social Trends 1987*, no. 17. London: HMSO, 1987.
59. Dahlgren, G., Diderichsen, F., 'Strategies for equity in health: report from Sweden', *International Journal of Health Services 1986*; 16:517-37.
60. Therborn, G., Roebroek, J., 'The irreversible welfare state: its recent maturation, its encounter with the economic crisis, and its future prospects', *International Journal of Health Services 1986*; 16:319-38.
61. Editorial. 'Lies, damned lies, and suppressed statistics', *British

Medical Journal 1986; 293:249–50.

62. Editorial. 'The occupational mortality supplement: why the fuss?', *Lancet 1986*; ii:610–12.

63. Editorials: 'Inequalities and the new Health Education Authority', *British Medical Journal 1987*; 294:857–8. 'A poor start for the Health Education Authority', *ibid.*, 664.

64. Editorial. 'A mockery of health promotion', *Lancet 1987*; i:489.

65. Mant, D., Anderson, P., 'Community general practitioner', *Lancet 1985*; ii:1114–7.

66. Hart, J.T., 'Community general practitioners', *British Medical Journal 1984*; 288:1670–73.

67. Hart, J.T., Humphreys, C., 'Be your own coroner', *British Medical Journal 1987*; 294:871–4.

68. Ministry of Health, Consultative Council on Medicine & Allied Services, 'Interim Report on the Future Provision of Medical & Allied Services (Dawson Report)', Cmnd 693, London: HMSO, 1920.

69. Richardson, A., Bray, C., *Promoting health through participation: experience of groups for patient participation in general practice*, London: Policy Studies Institute, 1987.

70. Mullan, F., 'Community practice: the cake-bake syndrome and other trials', *Journal of the American Medical Association 1980*; 243:1832–5.

71. Health Education Authority & Oxford City Council, *Healthy Oxford 2000: a healthy city strategy*, Oxford City Council, 1987.

72. Mant, D., 'Community medicine and general practice', *Radical Community Medicine, autumn 1986*; 28–30.

73. Hart, J.T., 'Practice nurses: an under-used resource', *British Medical Journal 1985*; 290:1162–3.

74. Robson, J., 'Salaried service—a basis for the future?', *British Medical Journal 1981*; 283:1225–7.

75. Lowe, M., 'No future for a salaried service', *British Medical Journal 1981*; 283:1227–8.

76. Porter, A.M.W., Porter, J.M.T., 'Anglo-French contrasts in medical practice', *British Medical Journal 1980*; 280:1109–12.

77. Bentsen, B.G., 'A revolution in primary care of Norway', *Scandinavian Journal of Primary Health Care 1985*; 3:53–4.

78. Law, J., 'Swedes stick to salaries', *Medeconomics*, October 1986, 69–70.

79. Scally, G.J., 'Taking primary care seriously: the Finnish experience', *Public Health, 1984.*

80. Abel-Smith, B., *Value for money in health service: a comparative study*, London: Heinemann, 1976.

Chapter 9
THE NECESSITY OF COMMUNITY

No word has been more fashionable over the past twenty years than 'community'; Community Care, Community Nurses, Community Physicians, Community Health Councils, even the poll-tax is beautified as the Community Charge. No ministerial speech is complete without some reference to it, and the urgency of returning tasks and responsibilities to it, previously supposed to have been undertaken by hospitals and welfare agencies. All this seems to assume that everywhere real communities still exist, with the qualities and resources necessary for care.

Do Communities Still Exist?

Population data from national or regional statistics tell us very little about real communities. They have to be studied each in their own right. Coal mining and heavy industrial communities all over the world have long been generally accepted as the supreme example of social cohesion and self-organized mutual aid, which strengthen in adversity. Like other industrial communities, their traditions of mutual help have derived from shared work experience and a necessary unity developed in struggle with ruthless employers. The taproot of this tradition has now been cut by the collapse of the industries from which it grew. Is it now so well established that it has other social roots, and can survive long enough to resume growth in whatever new kind of society is to follow, or will it disintegrate into a demoralized,

261

declassed, socially irresponsible rabble?

Glyncorrwg is the community I know, and is as good an example as any of a community previously employed almost entirely in heavy industry, which has now almost completely lost such employment. In 1966 we did our own occupational census. Of 554 men aged 16–64, only four were of unknown occupation, and 92% had employment of some kind. Exactly half (278) worked for the National Coal Board (69% of them underground), 34 (6%) were steelworkers, 159 (29%) were employed in other manual work mostly dependent on the coal and steel industries. For the rest, 45 (8%) were unemployed or disabled and permanently unemployable in local industries, or in long-term institutional care; only 21 (4%) were self-employed shopkeepers, farmers and professionals. It was a population typical of many others dependent on heavy industry, with almost no middle class and more than its share of chronic sickness and unemployment, but prosperous compared with the terrible years from 1926 to 1941, when local male unemployment rates reached 80% in some villages of the Afan Valley. Few women had paid employment outside their homes, many had large families with eight or ten children, shotgun marriages were commonplace and single parent families almost unknown. The village had its own vigorous social, cultural and commercial life, with three working men's clubs, four pubs, a church and five competing chapels, branches of the Labour and Communist Parties, one cricket, three soccer and two rugby teams, a betting shop, a cafe, a hairdresser, a newsagent, an ironmonger, two drapers, three sweetshops and four grocers.

Since then the industrial base for employment in all the South Wales Valley communities has been almost completely destroyed. The three coal mines in the Afan Valley were all closed between 1968 and 1970, and by the end of the great strike of 1985-6 all the remaining mines in the adjoining Ogwr, Garw and Llynfi valleys were closed. We now have about 30 men in Glyncorrwg who still travel long distances to work in surviving pits; 93% of the jobs in coal have disappeared. The Port Talbot steelworks has reduced its workforce from 15,000 in 1965 to 4,500 in 1987.

In 1986 I carried out another employment census in the practice. Of 368 men aged 16–64, only 178 (48%) were in full-time employment, including 20 students; 22 (6%) had part-time work or were on government job-creation or training schemes with incomes at subsistence level, 114 (31%) were claiming unemployment benefit, and 53 (14%) were certified as unfit for work. As in 1966, the large number certified unfit reflected not only high sickness rates, but also the serious local employment problems of people with any disability; when there are a hundred applicants for any good job, and with a Disabled Persons Employment Act which has never been seriously enforced by any government, employers have no need to take people with problems. Realistically, therefore, the extent of unemployment can be measured only by including those certified as unfit for work as well as those claiming unemployment benefit, giving us a total of 45% without jobs of any kind, or 50% if we include those on job-creation schemes at subsistence wages.

One small factory was built in Glyncorrwg in the late 1960s, assisted by national policies for redistribution of industry, to provide some alternative employment, mostly for women. Three different enterprises have come and gone, though the last has now been here for 8 years and looks as though it may stay. Collapse of our local economy led to the Upper Afan Valley having the fifth highest rate of out-migration in the UK in 1971, with a fall in total population from 9,480 in 1966 to 8,640 in 1971, and a continued decline to just over 7,000 in 1987. Of all the South Wales mining valleys, the Upper Afan has probably suffered the most, so 35% of out-migrants still moved away to other valley communities resembling their own and facing the same ultimate future; 56% moved to towns in the South Wales coastal belt, with better economic prospects; mainly because of prohibitive housing costs there, only 8% emigrated to England.[1] Collapse of basic industry, together with competition first from supermarkets, later from hyper-markets, has almost wiped out the small shops, and accelerated the decline of religious, political and cultural groups. The church and 4 chapels cling to dwindling congregations, one pub still survives, but we now have only the newsagent and 2 grocers' shops.

In Glyncorrwg at least, the answer is that community does still exist; but as in most places where community was strongest and at its best, its continued development or even existence is seriously threatened by destruction of what was always its principal root, male employment in industry.

Changes in the Status of Women

These are the losses, but there have also been gains. There has been a historic shift in the lives of women, and because so much care in the community has been borne by women, this has important implications for community care.

Women's lives have changed through changes in family structure, control of fertility and increase in paid employment. Family size has declined throughout this century. The army of unmarried women who previously gave lifetimes of underpaid or completely unpaid service to aged parents, the chronic sick and the surplus children of their married brothers and sisters, has disappeared. Young mothers have one or two brothers and sisters where their parents had eight or ten. The small nuclear family, established as a social norm in the 1930s, is now a minority phenomenon. Only 26% of all British households now consist of a married couple with one or two children, and only 5% of the total workforce consists of an employed man with a wife and two children at home. Between 1961 and 1980 the proportion of one-person households doubled, from 4% to 8%, and the proportion of one-parent families with dependent children also doubled, from 2% to 4%.[2]

Oral contraception began to be widely used in the early 1960s. Legal termination of pregnancy became available under the Abortion Act of 1967, and by 1969-72 was performed at an annual rate of 7.8 per 1,000 women aged 15-44 in Glamorgan and Monmouthshire, the centres of South Wales industrial valley populations, compared with a live birth rate of 82 per 1,000.[3] Together with widespread acceptance of male sterilization by vasectomy, rapid though still incomplete progress has been made towards two inter-dependent social goals: that every child born should be a wanted child, and that no woman should have to continue with a pregnancy she can't cope with.

Attainment of these objectives could have important effects on the health of both women and children, and there is some evidence that for children at least this may already have occurred. In 1921-25, before the 1926 strike and inter-war years of mass unemployment, infant mortality in the South Wales valleys was 2% higher than the rate for England and Wales as a whole; by 1931-35 it was 22% higher, and by 1961-65 25% higher, than the England and Wales rate; but in the period 1971-72 it fell dramatically to a level 4% below the England and Wales rate, and has stayed there ever since. Levels of income, and every other index of social advantage, have all worsened in the South Wales valleys relative to the UK as a whole, in line with renewed mass unemployment and destruction of our industrial base, but nearly all the valley communities happen to be served by hospitals which have adopted liberal policies in applying the Abortion Act in the NHS, in contrast to areas such as Cardiff and Birmingham.

The third big change for women has been their rapid recruitment to paid employment, mainly in light industries attracted to the valleys by regional employment policies. Whereas labour activity rates for men in the South Wales valleys fell from 81% in 1961 to 72% in 1971, for women they rose from 27% to 33% (still well below the UK average).[4] For the first time since the conscription of young women to work in munitions factories during the war, they have their own money in their pockets. The effect in both eras has been the same; women's expectations and confidence in their own strength have risen. But whereas during the war there was a simultaneous rise in the expectations and confidence of working class men, jointly expressed in the 1945 election which gave birth to the NHS, women are now moving forward while men are in retreat.

Community Care of the Sick

These complex, contradictory trends are important, not only because of the destructive effects of mass unemployment on the capacity of industrial working class communities to preserve their traditions of social discipline and mutual support which have always been the most important foundation for the work of doctors and nurses, but also because so much of that support at a personal or family level has depended on women's unpaid and unregulated labour. It is estimated that about one and a quarter million people in Britain care for sick, disabled, or elderly people living at home,[5] and at least three-quarters of these carers are women;[6] wives, mothers, daughters, grand-daughters, nieces, mothers-in-law, sisters-in-law, daughters-in-law and women friends and neighbours. This has been the true basis of community care for 24 hours a day, to which GPs and Community Nurses have been visiting adjuncts.

This informal community care structure is, in general, effective and efficient. Wilkes,[7] reporting GP experience in Sheffield generally similar to ours in Glyncorrwg, found that in 1972 55% of cancer deaths were still occurring at home, 10% in long-stay geriatric units of various kinds, and the remaining third in hospitals. About half of these patients were thought by their GPs to have no significant pain, suffering or distress. About one-third did have problems, but only for 6 weeks or less. Only 15% had problems for more than 6 weeks, and only 12% made heavy demands on GPs. With important reservations, this generally optimistic view was confirmed by Cartwright, Hockey and Anderson's large study (through surviving relatives) of the last year of life of 785 randomly-sampled people who died (40% at home, 6% in long-stay units, 54% in hospital) over the age of 15.[6] Only 9% were bedridden or mainly confined to bed for a year or more, 3% for 6 months but less than a year, 8% for 3 months but less than 6 months, and another 15% for less than 3 months. As Wilkes concluded, 85–90% of terminal illnesses were being coped with well enough to present no obvious problems to GPs attending.

Even so, he described the other 10–15% (of patients and their carers) as suffering 'deplorable neglect', and that is a lot of people. The task is more difficult than many attending GPs or even Community Nurses appreciate. In Cartwright's study,[6] 32% of patients nursed at home were incontinent of urine during the last year of their lives, but 53% of them never discussed this problem with either GPs or Community Nurses attending; 28% were incontinent of faeces, but 40% of them never reported it; and even of the 20% who suffered double incontinence of both urine and faeces, 26% failed to present this as a problem to doctor or nurse. Only 11% died without any previous symptoms, and 63% had symptoms for a year or more before death. At some point in their last year 66% had pain, 36% were mentally confused, 36% were depressed, and 30% vomited or felt sick; altogether 69% had symptoms recalled by relatives as very distressing, but only 47% of these symptoms were ever reported to GPs attending.

Almost one-third (30%) of main carers ('brunt-bearers') were in full-time employment before they took on their caring role, and a quarter of these had to give up work, 40% of them for a year or more. One-third of brunt-bearers were themselves over 65, and 14% said that the burden of caring had affected their health. In the Sheffield study,[7] 14% of terminal cancer patients dying at home were being looked after by relatives who were themselves aged over 70.

In the Cartwright study,[6] 9% of deaths occurred in people who remained in institutional care for the whole of their last year of life. Of the other 91%, 61% were admitted to hospital at some time during their last year, and 78% had been seen as hospital outpatients. The proportion helped at some time by various kinds of community worker are shown in Table 9.1.

Relatives, friends and neighbours gave nearly all the social care and help at night, most of the help with housework and self care, and much of the nursing care. Wives, husbands and daughters were the most likely people to provide all kinds of care (self-care, nursing care, help at night, social care and housework), except financial assistance.

Table 9.1 Help from various kinds of community worker received by non-institutionalized people during their last year of life

GP (all contacts)	96%
(home visits)	88%
Community Nurse	33%
Any church worker	29%
Other Local Authority or voluntary worker	12%
Chiropodist	11%
Other nurse	8%
Home help	5%
Special laundry service	2%

Community Care of the Elderly

Care of the aged involves even more people than care of the dying, and with less help from the NHS and other social agencies. These informal carers cannot go out to work, their family lives are disrupted for months, years or decades, they may be socially isolated and exhausted, and often they are sick or old themselves. Increasingly, the caring generation comes from small families of only one or two brothers or sisters, often dispersed across Britain or to Canada or Australia, while the proportion of very old people or severely handicapped younger people who survive because of successful medical interventions increases their burden.

Dee Jones[8] studied 1,066 people over 70 living in their own or their relatives' homes or in local institutions for the elderly in Cardiff in 1984. Nearly one-third (32%) needed help with one or more of 15 daily tasks basic to daily living such as washing all over or cutting their toenails; of these, 11% were in old people's homes and 8% had help from statutory services only. All the other 81% (273 old people in need) depended wholly or partly on care from relatives, friends or neighbours—informal helpers and actual or potential brunt-bearers. Of these 273 people, all but 6 (2%) were able to identify one main carer. 79% of 256 carers interviewed were women, 20% were aged over 75. Less than half these carers had had even a few days' break away from the old person dependent on them during the previous year. Those caring for the most seriously disabled were least

likely to have had a break; 40% of those caring for people
with dementia had not had a holiday of a week or more for
the previous five years. Only 7% of all carers had ever
received respite or relief care to give them a break; even of
those caring for old people with dementia, only 10% had
ever been helped in this way.

Statutory services were not fully reaching many of these
people. Only 34% of 117 severely disabled old people were
being helped by a Community Nurse, 28% by a Home Help
and 20% by visits to a day hospital; as 40% had been visited
by their GP during the previous month, many GPs apparently
failed to refer needy cases to relevant agencies.

Dee Jones concluded:

> It was the consistent and unremitting nature of caring for elderly
> dependants that was particularly stressful to carers. Respite for
> carers further exemplified the Inverse Care Law: the more disabled
> or mentally infirm the dependant the less likely the carer was to
> have breaks or holidays. . . Carers seemed to be faced with the
> stark choice of looking after the dependant with minimal support
> from the community at great cost to themselves or putting them
> into resident accommodation permanently.

Defensive Investment in Community Care

Governments have good reason to be thankful for families
and neighbours who give up large parts of their lives to look
after handicapped children and sick or disabled adults.
According to estimates by Muriel Nissel and Luch Bonnerjea
at the Policy Studies Institute,[9] they saved taxpayers about
£6 billion in 1980. The Equal Opportunities Commission
estimated that about 750,000 people looked after the disabled
elderly at home, of whom three quarters were women,
spending an average of 3.5 to 4 hours a day; the same care
provided by home helps or hospital staff (all very badly
paid) would cost about £3,000 a year for each dependant
person at 1980 prices.

Since the Constant Attendance allowance and other cash
benefits to encourage home care were introduced in the
1970s, there has been at least some official recognition of

the extent of the sacrifices made by families, and above all
by women, to help chronic sick, elderly and handicapped
people in their own homes. 595,000 Constant Attendance,
Severe Disablement and Mobility allowances were paid in
1979-80, totalling £620 million. By 1985-6, 1,185,000
allowances were being paid, totalling £1,130 million. More
people benefited and average value of allowances rose, but
only from 8.7% of average male gross earnings in 1980,
to 11.3% in 1985.[10] NHS spending on community health
services rose from 6.2% of all NHS expenditure in 1980 to
6.5% in 1985; estimated expenditure for 1987 has actually
fallen to 6.4%. From 1978 to 1984, the number of
Community Nurses rose by 8%, but they had to cope with
12% more patients and 26% more people over 65.[11] Spending
on GP and pharmaceutical services, unplanned and unplannable because of independent contractor status, have
risen from 15.7% of NHS spending in 1980 to 17.5% in
1985, and an estimated 17.8% in 1987. The argument that
they are unplannable not because of independent contractor
status but because they are demand-led is not tenable; other
demand-led industries are planned, even though demand can
never be precisely predictable, but GPs remain a law unto
themselves.

In return for these investments in formal and informal
community care, the government obtained a reduction in the
number of hospitals (almost entirely by closing small local
hospitals), and a reduction of 30,500 in the number of
available hospital beds,[11] despite a 10% increase in the
proportion of people aged 75 or more in the general population.[12] DHSS plans for reductions in hospital beds are being
implemented faster than expansion of resources for within-
community care; by 1984, 45% of the planned reduction
in hospital beds had been achieved, but only 17% of planned
day-hospital places and 16% of day-centre places had been
provided.[11]

Community Care: Sentimentalized Exploitation, or Materially Assisted Altruism?

Virtually all social and political groups affirm belief in within-community care, just as they profess their devotion to the family. As unpaid or almost unpaid care by relatives or neighbours is much cheaper than any kind of institutional care, there are powerful material motives for this, but it is also true that most people do want to lead as much of their lives as possible independently in their own homes. Attitudes to the appropriate place for expected death are changing: because more may be done, or may appear to be done, for patients in hospitals today than in the past; because families are smaller and more dispersed; and because fewer women are able or willing to be taken for granted as the natural carers for all their sick, handicapped or dying relatives, and too few men have come forward to take their place.

It is wrong to assume that the present proportion of deaths in the home rather than in hospital is necessarily right. It is difficult to get good evidence on what either patients or their relatives would really prefer, since if they can't have what they like they must like what they have, and bereaved relatives are understandably reluctant retrospectively to criticize management of terminal illness. Only 6% of GPs and 4% of Community Nurses surveyed by Cartwright[6] believed that no expected deaths should be allowed to happen at home, but 14% of bereaved relatives said three months after the death that they would have preferred it to have occurred elsewhere than it did, in hospital if the death was at home, or at home if the death was in hospital, and another 16% were not sure.

The trend is towards death in hospitals rather than the home, and for greater professionalization of care for the sick and handicapped. This can be slowed, halted, or even perhaps reversed by either one of two opposed policies: by policies of sentimentalized exploitation, sustaining obsolete beliefs about the family and the status of women, isolating those who do not comply, and maintaining public opinion in a state of intolerance, blaming the victims of a society organized to give low priority to care of the handicapped, sick and aged; or by policies of materially assisted altruism, with greater investment in material support for carers, and practical steps to encourage men to accept a caring role.

Every study of what actually happens to the chronic sick and elderly testifies to the colossal burdens ungrudgingly borne by the vast majority of relatives, and often of neighbours and friends, and the rarity of refusal by relatives to accept reasonable responsibilities (the definition of 'reasonable' being what critics would accept for themselves). However, doctors, nurses, and even caring relatives and neighbours often blame the effects of bed and staff shortages in geriatric and chronic sick hospitals on the unwillingness of other relatives and neighbours to accept their natural responsibilities. When Cartwright asked GPs the question 'On the whole do you find in this area that most relatives accept reasonable responsibility for home care or do they seek admission to hospital or institution?', 51% thought that 'unwillingness of relatives to look after them' was the main limiting factor on community rather than hospital care, and 25% thought most relatives sought institutional care. Community Nurses were less likely to blame relatives, but still 33% thought unwilling relatives were the main limiting factor, and 9% thought most relatives wanted institutional care. Doctors' opinions were not apparently influenced by the actual proportions of their patients who died at home or in hospital, but those who believed most relatives accepted reasonable responsibility did more home visits than those who did not, and had experienced less difficulty in getting admission when it was needed.

Attempts to find relatives unwilling rather than unable to care for the sick, and without some obvious explanation (for example, that a parent was divorced and estranged, or had problems with alcohol or domestic violence) have all been unsuccessful. A careful study by Prof. Bernard Isaacs of 280 patients admitted from their own homes to a geriatric unit in the East End of Glasgow[13] was typical. It showed that two-thirds were admitted because basic care at home was unobtainable, but the reason for this was that close relatives were either non-existent, were not available through their own ill-health, or were already caring for somebody else. In a few cases personal relations between aged parents and offspring made care impossible, but cases of wilful indifference or neglect by relatives were a factor in less than 1% of admissions.

If communities are driven into a state of seige, their young people demoralized by unemployment or driven away in search for work, their traditions of mutual aid and solidarity expressed through their own trade union and political organizations brought into contempt and personal acquisitiveness and brutal ambition are exalted, real community care, on which all the machinery of the NHS ultimately rests, could collapse. In some inner-city areas it may already have done so.

However, the process of demoralization is always less than frightened outsiders believe. The traditions of solidarity and mutual aid originally used by Lloyd George to initiate construction of a state primary care service are not yet dead, but they are in a damaged state which will not be revived by sentimentalizing ignorance and brutality, past or present. There are, as there have always been, fundamentally conflicting tendencies even within the strong industrial working class culture of mutual support in adversity. On the one hand, organized altruism on a family and local community scale has been a precondition for survival; on the other, it has depended almost entirely on the unpaid labour of women, expected always to make themselves available for months, years, or even lifetimes, regardless of their other ambitions or commitments, or of their previous personal relationship with the patient. If encouragement of community care is not to become a cover for abdication from responsibility for adequate hospitals, the social machinery of home care must be materially supported by more realistic payment for long-term care; legal safeguards for jobs during prolonged absence; better child-care facilities and nursery schools; greater readiness to provide short-term institutional relief; more Home Helps; and a higher proportion of men accepting caring responsibilities in the home, as well as an expanded primary care team.

Community Participation in Defence and Extension of Hospital Care

If communities do still exist, can they be drawn into effective alliance with doctors and other health workers not only to defend the NHS when it is under attack, but also to administer the service and minimize bureaucratic control? Is it possible for their primary care teams to become account-able to them, so that general practice in the NHS can develop as a participative democracy, giving organizational expression to a new reality of care as a form of active health production shared between the team and its population?

Hospital closures have been resisted by community groups led by hospital cleaners, porters, nurses and eventually even by doctors, together with local citizens. Occasionally, as in the Guy's Hospital incident, even Boards of Governors have offered serious resistance to government plans, but as these consist almost entirely of unelected representatives of the business world, this is exceptional. Resistance has sometimes taken non-traditional forms such as work-ins, and there have been many examples of sympathetic action taken by other industrial workers, notably coal-miners, and of mass lobbies of parliament which have certainly influenced govern-ment policies. Such community resistance tends to get good media coverage, most of it favourable, particularly when it has forced government to reveal the ultimate brutality of its policies by sending in the police to forcibly remove elderly patients from hospital wards earmarked for closure, as happened in London in 1982. These local struggles, which have occurred everywhere but most of all in the London area, have been extremely damaging to the government, and to the Conservative Party's cherished image as the natural party of doctors, nurses and socially responsible privilege, though it has to be said that the last Labour government, led by James Callaghan, initiated all these policies of retreat later developed more vigorously by the Conservatives.

The weaknesses of these campaigns have been that they

were defensive, often sentimental and backward-looking, that in the interests of unity in an extremely fragmented workforce it was necessary to overlook serious weaknesses at all levels, particularly the weaknesses of the highest professionals, and above all that they were episodic and not sustainable in the long term. Successful resistance in some hospitals usually meant only that the same closures were imposed in others where resistance was weak. In the long run, Government could always win, though often at heavy political cost. Resistance was built mainly on past loyalties rather than positive plans for the future, and was always vulnerable to the socially divided nature of the hospital workforce, not only the gulf between earnings and expectations of doctors compared with cleaners and laboratory technicians, but also within the 101 grades, degrees and divisions of non-medical hospital workers, each with their own variety of conflicting trade unions, professional associations, and their own fiercely contested rank in the pecking order.[14]

Because closures came first to the oldest, least well-equipped units, their defence did not involve the most innovative centres, though in general medical, nursing and technical staffs at the leading edge of medical science were no less hostile to privatization of care than staffs in hospitals threatened with closure. All too often successful defence looked like preservation of obsolete care at the expense of even slower innovation in the newer hospitals, so that opposition to NHS cuts was divided into those with community-oriented interests who sentimentalized community care and dismissed high technology, and hospital-oriented interests determined to obtain whatever technology was available, ignorant and contemptuous of the possibilities of community care if it were properly resourced. Occasionally whole chunks of new medical science have broken away entirely from the NHS to develop in the private sector, as with Dr Andrew Steptoe's team working on in-vitro fertilization, without any effective protest from anyone, and this could be a serious portent for the future.

Successful resistance, maintained over years rather than

months and personally involving a majority of the public, is possible and will be necessary if hospitals are to resume expansion in those areas of care for which they are most effective. It will have to be built on a new pattern of local democratic control through new institutions, which must include progress at primary care level.

Community Participation at Primary Care Level

The difficulties of creating and maintaining patient-participation groups or Patients' Committees were discussed in the last chapter. The most immediate obstacle is usually the resistance of doctors to the idea in the first place, but even when this is overcome, few communities contain many people with enough time, energy or credulity for yet another committee, tying up yet another evening and probably occasional weekends, generating more paper, more meetings and eventually more subcommittees, and on previous experience unlikely in the long run to sustain more public interest, recruit more workers (rather than talkers) or satisfy more than a fraction of the new expectations first raised. The people in any community who really get things done are always already overworked, and reluctant to join anything unless they are convinced it has practical value and will bring about real changes; they don't want more talking shops.

If we listen to what people talk about in queues, at tea breaks, on the way to and from work, we hear more about their own health and the health of their families than any other topic; there is probably no other subject of greater general interest. To attribute our difficulties in setting up social machinery for participative democracy in the NHS to public indifference must be wrong. There must be some way other than the existing types of Patients' Committee to tap the interest that is certainly there. If there is not, then we must accept that the pace of progress will continue to reflect the attitudes and interests of central power-holders whose own experience of using the NHS by normal pathways is usually remote, and in many cases non-existent.

The general strategy of retreat from public service begun

by the New Conservatives, justified in the broadest terms by the alleged superiority of market decisions over human decisions, always encounters fiercest opposition when translated into concrete and specific local terms. At a local, problem-oriented level at which individual people are directly affected and on which effective action is seen to be possible, the general issues break down into comprehensible parts. Clues to what we need were given by Bagehot, the greatest political theorist the British ruling class ever produced, in his classic *The English Constitution*, written at the historical moment when Disraeli swept his alliance of industrialists, bankers and landed aristocrats into the political gamble of extending the franchise to include their natural enemy, the skilled working man in industry:

> As yet, the few rule by their hold, not over the reason of the multitude, but over their imaginations and their habits; over their fancies as to distant things they do not know at all, over their customs as to near things which they know very well.[15]

For almost 40 years the common people have lived with the NHS as a social right, for most of that time with no more than token charges at the time of use. They have developed deeply-rooted 'customs as to near things which they know very well' regarding access to the service, which are now probably impossible to take away. Access will remain, but access to what? Their imaginations have not changed, or at least they have changed very little, because doctors kept not only their own but the public imagination within the Osler paradigm. Medical science was their property, and criticism of it was their privilege. Patients were wanted only as passive and uncritical consumers, not as fellow-producers.

Both GPs and specialists, and both primary care and hospital nurses, know that the quality of care available is now drifting further and further away from what is scientifically possible, but the community cannot be an effective ally in struggle to rectify this if it is not fully informed and if critical thought is discouraged. If we want effective allies in defending the service, we must learn to

encourage our public not only to hold fast to their right of
free access, but to believe that the service is theirs, that it
ultimately belongs to the people who must be the final
judges of its quality and effectiveness, that it is within the
ambit of 'their customs as to near things which they know
very well'. These customs need expansion, imaginations
and habits must be raised, but this cannot be done without
a frank admission that large groups of patients with common
chronic conditions requiring simple, easily understood, but
regular, conscientious and unhurried ambulant care and
monitoring by familiar, friendly, socially accessible staff,
are not actually getting these things. Some responsibility
for this failure must be accepted by GPs if their demands
for better resources are to be taken seriously.

The diabetics, hypertensives, arthritics, schizophrenics,
asthmatics, epileptics, and otherwise handicapped adults
and children who together with their carers, spouses and
relatives account for a majority of any population if the
word 'family' is defined as those close enough to be
personally concerned about one another, are people with
specific, definable needs, with proven effects on outcomes
if these needs are not met. These patients and their caring
relatives are the realistic base for participative democracy
in the NHS, starting from where we are with the people
we have, beginning with the immediate, practical needs
that are obvious and undeniable to informed patients and
their primary care teams.

These people constitute a potential voting public which
already guarantees a mandate to any government with the
courage to support them; but both mobilization and demands
must be specific, not general, and depend on active search
and patient education at primary care level in each neighbourhood, to define and locate these needs, and measure
precisely the extent to which they are unmet. They require
the kind of information, and the kinds of patient-participation,
implied by the style of primary care team discussed in the
last chapter, with computerized practice information systems
and therefore lists of the names, addresses, and telephone
numbers of each group sharing a specific chronic disorder,

and audited problem-specific clinics which measure the
extent to which needs are met. From these large subsets of
people sharing specific concerns, educated to perceive new
possibilities of what they and their carers could jointly
achieve with better organization, more time, and more labour
(but little more technology), we could begin to develop
indestructible roots of the new popular institutions required
for participative democracy. Their activists would be drawn
not from the relatively narrow circle of people who already
have a wider political concern and confidence that they can
change the world, but from the ranks of mothers with
asthmatic or brain-damaged children, the wives of men with
premature coronary disease, and from hypertensives,
diabetics, and epileptics beginning to accept joint responsibilities for their own care, demanding an effective health
service at all levels rather than an impersonal hit-or-miss
charity.

On such a base, annual reports, annual meetings and
annually elected Patients' Committees would achieve vigorous
and independent life, rather than their present tenuous and
token existence. They would work in association with Local
Authorities and national patients' organizations like the
British Diabetic Association, the Chest Heart & Stroke
Association, and the many other disease-specific national
consumer groups which are already powerful political lobbies.

If such local practice-based patient groups were organized,
it would be difficult to close the cottage hospitals and other
small and cherished local facilities so irritating to tidy-minded
economists and NHS managers. They would have an
intelligible alternative future as local units run in association
with local primary care teams, providing day-hospital and
simple 24-hour nursing facilities for most transient acute
illness, support for chronic disability and handicap, and
terminal care for the majority of patients who do not need
the full technical support facilities of a modern District
Hospital. District Hospitals currently overstretched to accept
all organized follow-up of common chronic conditions such
as diabetes, high blood pressure, obstructive lung diseases
and heart failure, would become easier to defend because

they would be able to give more time to fewer people, returning the routine care of most common illnesses to expanded and improved Primary Care Teams working within guidelines agreed between specialists and generalists.

Limited Demands, Infinite Resources

Patients and their caring families and neighbours, mobilized both to participate in better care and its control by shared discussion of audited progress, are a new and hitherto neglected resource.

Enoch Powell has a gift for lucid epigrammatic conclusions drawn from plausible but unvalidated assumptions. He was the first Minister of Health to assert that infinite demands were bound to collide with finite resources in an NHS free at point of use. Uncritical acceptance of his argument led to a widely quoted Insoluble Equation of medical care:

$$WANTS > NEEDS > RESOURCES$$

The 1944 White Paper which preceded the NHS Act of 1946 foresaw that

> The proposed service must be comprehensive in two senses—first, that it is available to all people and, second, that it covers all necessary forms of health care.

Commenting on this objective, the Report of the Royal Commission on the NHS in 1979 (the Merrison Report) justified retreat, using the Insoluble Equation and a less explicit version of the Enoch Powell argument:

> The impossibility of meeting all demands for health service was not anticipated. Medical, nursing and therapeutic techniques have been developed to levels of sophistication and expense which were not foreseen when the NHS was introduced.[16]

Since 1944, health services have not been unique in developing to unforeseen levels of sophistication and expense. 385 Tornado fighters planned for the RAF in 1977 were estimated to cost slightly more than the entire production of Spitfires before and during World War II, and the cost per ton of comparable warships increased ten to fifteenfold over the same period. If trends prevailing since the 1920s continue, by the year 2036 the entire US military budget will be spent on one aircraft.[17] However, the defence of the realm is still seen as a national responsibility, whatever the changes in costs and technology. The real change in attitudes to NHS funding since 1944 is not technical or economic, but political. In 1944, arms expenditure was justified because we were fighting for a better future for the common people, including a free and comprehensive health service embracing all effective medical science, not just its cheaper parts. The cost and efficiency of measures to save life have changed no more than the cost and efficiency of measures to destroy it. Military research does not depend on generals and admirals standing on street corners with collecting boxes.

The phrase and the equation have been used ever since as self-evident axioms, not only to excuse failure to attain the original objectives of the NHS, but to ridicule the objectives themselves. Is there any real evidence to support them? The influential University of York school of health economists led by Alan Maynard claims to be interested chiefly in micro-economic efficiency within small units of the NHS[18] rather than macro-economic strategies, a view currently shared by most other health economists. In the early 1970s I was invited to a DHSS-sponsored conference at the City of London College, appropriately entitled 'Thinking the un-thinkable'. Keynote speaker was Professor Alan Williams, founder of the York school. As he was speaking to a largely medical audience, his economic arguments had to be simple, so he explained his macro-economic assumptions. On the blackboard he drew the elementary relationship between price and demand for commodities shown in Fig. 9.1.

The demand for any commodity is related to its price. At infinite prices, demand is zero; at zero prices demand is infinite. Therefore in a free health service there is infinite demand. The supply of any commodity must be finite. Therefore there is infinite demand on finite resources in any

Fig. 9.1 National relationship of price and demand according to Prof. A. Williams

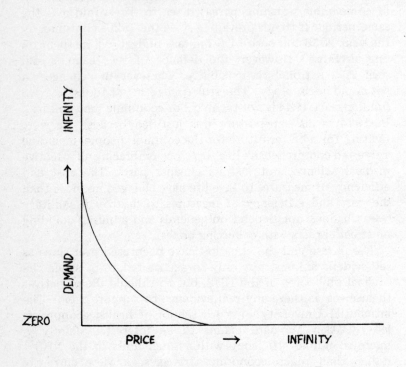

health service free at the time of use, whether paid by taxes or insurance. As for the demands > needs > resources equation, it is taken as axiomatic that consumer wants are greater than patients' needs; GPs, who normally see their patients only when they consult and therefore see what people complain about and not what they endure unaided, rarely disagree.

Once we accept medical care as a commodity, the rest follows. The micro-economists are aware of this, and therefore usually devote a short introductory macro-economic paragraph to explain that the reasons for not regarding medical care as a commodity are sentimental, and imply that all who refuse to accept medical care as a commodity thereby also deny that medical care is an economic unit of any kind. Since all human activities have an economic aspect in that they occupy time which might otherwise be devoted to something else, medical care is no exception. Commodity production is not the only economic form that production can take, but it is the form characteristic of a capitalist economic system. To assert that medical care requires some different form of production requires more independent thought than most people are willing to give it, at least when fixed by the beady eye of an economist, who will in any case ease their consciences by conceding that though medical care must be a commodity whether we like it or not, it is one of a special kind, to be handled with greater sensitivity than boots or cricket bats. They may concede it the special, apparently nonsensical status of impressionist paintings, grand opera or fossil dinosaurs, for which everyone accepts that the market is an ass, but since markets must rule for our own ultimate good as a part of natural law, no one can think of anything better.

Opponents of these arguments have tended to concentrate on the fact that medical care sold as a commodity puts consumers at a disadvantage because they don't have enough information to judge what they are buying. Therefore social justice demands that though medical care remains a commodity, the buying and selling of it is underwritten by the State on the consumer's behalf, and this is supposed to be how the NHS works. This argument applies equally to many other commodities, since as they become more and more technically sophisticated and marketing techniques are used to manipulate demand, fewer consumers are able to make rational choices of any kind, whether they are buying echo-sounders for their yachts or tonsillectomies for their children. It is an ultimately weak defence of the NHS, unless one is prepared to examine the possibility that the stringent consumer protection required to make a reasonably safe medical care market possible is probably required also for an increasing proportion of other commodities essential to life.

A far more effective defence is to question whether

effective medical care is a commodity at all. Of course, there are components of medical care which are commodities. For example prescribed drugs are extremely profitable commodities, which are (in the NHS) ordered by doctors but paid for by the State on the patients' behalf, so that in effect the doctors are the consumers, relatively unrestrained by price, and doctors are the target of promotional efforts by the pharmaceutical industry.

The processes of diagnosis, treatment, and follow-up, however, are not commodities, but joint products of co-operation between care-givers and care-receivers requiring work from both. This productive relationship can be, and has in fact usually been, ignored and concealed precisely in order to maintain market relationships, partly because even when private practice had dwindled to a minuscule proportion of all medical work as it did in the 1960s, it still provided the classical model for professional thought; and partly because having grown up in a capitalist society our imaginations tend always to be limited in this way about all creative work, so that the greatest achievements of mankind, which obviously deny the limits of commodity production and exchange, can only be attributed to genius, freakish behaviour so unique that it requires no explanation and need not fit the machinery of everyday life. Yet in reality the public wants and has a right to expect everyday medical care as free from commercial considerations as the works of Beethoven or Van Gogh.

There are apparent exceptions to this, forms of medical care in which patients really do appear to be almost entirely passive consumers of professional expertise; but these are precisely those medical and surgical crises which are ethically least tolerable as commodities to a public which still retains any feeling at all for social justice. There is no evidence of any public mandate for a commodity market to operate for emergency care even in the USA, let alone Britain.

Moreover as soon as we look at real demands on the NHS, we can see that though large they are not infinite, but defined by ultimately calculable though very complex determinants. Obviously prices attached to particular medical activities must modify their use, the classic case being the effect of charges on prescribed medicines, shown in Fig. 9.2. However, even this simple example shows that many influences other than price determine demand. From 1948 to June 1952, there were no charges for any prescribed drugs or appliances. The number of items prescribed rose steeply, but started to fall a year before the first imposition of charges, and then levelled off. The next rise in charges, in 1956, did coincide with a rapid fall in prescribing, but from then on, out of 10 occasions when new charges were applied, only one (the rise from £0.70 to £1.00 in December 1980) appeared to initiate a fall. Though prescribing was rising rapidly when prescription charges were briefly abolished in February 1965, the rise was less steep after abolition, and prescriptions were actually falling when charges were applied again in June 1968.

What other influences were there on prescribing, other than deterrent charges? Doctors, not patients, are responsible for prescribing. Continued demand does depend on whether patients understand and accept treatment, but no one who actually studies the very complex influences on prescribing and uses of medications[19] could accept so blunt an instrument as prescription charges as a rational means of influencing them. Doctors are influenced by what they learn, for about six years as undergraduates in medical schools where they are taught to be sceptical about the claims of those who make and sell drugs, and then for 30 or 40 years in practice, when more is spent on each doctor for drug promotion by pharmaceutical companies than was spent on training him in the first place.[20] Of course, doctors feel insulted if anyone suggests that their prescribing is influenced by all this, but pharmaceutical companies are not in the habit of throwing money away, and such influence is certainly their intention. A few patients do actively search for medication as other consumers pursue ice-cream or fashion footware, but a large majority do not want to be ill, and avoid both doctors and their prescriptions if they can. The idea that if medical care is free then people will consume it for fun is ludicrous. If water supplied at a fixed charge unrelated to quantity (which, as I write, it still is) has not led people to leave the tap running all day, why should a free health service lead them

Fig. 9.2 NHS prescription charges and items dispensed by chemists and appliance contractors, UK, 1949–86.

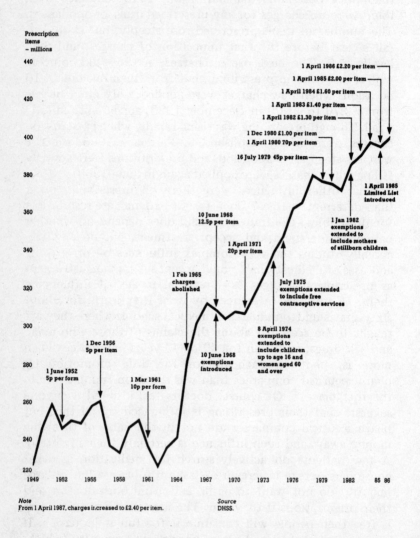

Prescription items – millions

1 April 1986 £2.20 per item
1 April 1985 £2.00 per item
1 April 1984 £1.60 per item
1 April 1983 £1.40 per item
1 April 1982 £1.30 per item
1 Dec 1980 £1.00 per item
1 April 1980 70p per item
16 July 1979 45p per item
1 April 1985 Limited List introduced
1 Jan 1982 exemptions extended to include mothers of stillborn children
10 June 1968 12.5p per item
1 April 1971 20p per item
July 1975 exemptions extended to include free contraceptive services
1 Feb 1965 charges abolished
8 April 1974 exemptions extended to include children up to age 16 and women aged 60 and over
1 Dec 1956 5p per item
10 June 1968 exemptions introduced
1 June 1952 5p per form
1 Mar 1961 10p per form

Note
From 1 April 1987, charges increased to £2.40 per item.

Source
DHSS.

Source: Fig. 4.12, Office of Health Economics Compendium of Statistics, 1987. London: OHE, 1987.

to consult GPs or specialists when they don't think they
need to?

The micro-economists will answer that this is not really
what they mean by infinite demand. What they have in mind
is that when one medical problem is solved, there always
seems to be another to take its place, a fact which they think
Lord Beveridge overlooked when he made his now famous
assumption that a universal free health service would reduce
demand by improving the nation's health. That major and
very costly problems were solved, with great relief for the
service, is not in dispute. There were huge falls in demand,
because of dramatic improvements in health which could not
have occurred at the speed or to the extent they did without
the NHS: respiratory tuberculosis required 25,000 hospital
beds in 1957,[21] but by 1978 the average number in daily use
had fallen to 754;[22] the population in mental hospitals fell
by about two-thirds from 153,000 in 1954 to 67,000 in
1984;[12] and in the first 25 years of the NHS there was a
roughly 10% reduction in the number of hospital beds in
use[23] despite rising standards of care, an ageing population
and an overall population increase of 12%.

Their grand discovery, allegedly overlooked by William
Beveridge and all the liberal Keynesians of the 1940s, is that
medicine never runs out of worthwhile tasks, in which it
appears to resemble every other worthwhile art or science.
Music is not expected to run out of compositions, architecture
is not expected to cease the evolution of building design, so
why should medicine run out of new problems of disease,
death and unhappiness? Medicine must plead guilty to the
charge that like all other worthwhile arts and sciences, there
seems to be no end to it.

Pioneer of this argument was Dr D.S. Lees in his booklet
Health through choice. He maintained that with increasing
prosperity in the 1960s, more money would be made available
for medical care by consumers buying for themselves in a
commodity market, than by taxpayers for the community
at large.[24] Dr Lees now has the satisfaction of seeing his
views generally accepted without ever being subjected to any
objective test. There has never been any evidence from opinion

polls that the general public is unwilling to pay more taxes for a better health service, but approval from a poorly-informed general public is not what the micro-economists have in mind; they are looking to people with enough power and money to sympathize with and understand their kind of accountancy, who will agree that the general public has ever since the war been both promised and given too much for its own good in the way of medical and every other kind of care. They see demand for medical care as infinite because they are infinitely disinclined to meet the social costs of better care for anyone but themselves.

Demands are, with experience, more or less predictable. More importantly, needs are measurable and at a single point in time finite, though certainly complex and greater than present resources can cope with. What should be measured, and how it should be done, was discussed in the last chapter; if we accept that the job can be done (granted sufficient labour), and if we are serious about doing it, primary care teams with listed populations can begin to measure both needs, and the extent to which they are met.

Infinite Resources: The NHS as a Mass Employer

Of course, at any particular time, more of one sort of invest-ment must mean less of another. Even the most wasteful spending on health services is more socially useful than manufacture of weapons, but this is not the most powerful argument against this facile formula for defeatism.

We now have at least three million, more probably four million unemployed people, probably well over a million women who would welcome part-time or full-time work as mature entrants to any industry close to their homes but are not registered as unemployed, and a huge reserve of trained nurses who now do unpaid domestic work. Caring for sick and disabled people is, despite an appalling hsitory of low wages, overwork and inadequate resources, a popular career choice. This reserve of labour is readily available for employ-ment in an extended primary care service.

The reserve of unemployed people living as close to

subsistence level as is possible in a sophisticated modern economy was created deliberately by the first Thatcher government as its principal social and economic weapon to strengthen employers and weaken trade unions. It was the first and most important part of a general strategy aiming to raise the general rate of profit by destroying the conventions of the post-war social settlement, imposing new terms and conditions of investment and employment. Just as a small-scale war in the Falklands turned out to be politically profitable, so did abolition of 'overfull' employment restore the right of management to manage in its traditional auto-cratic style. However, it's easier to start wars and mass unemployment than to stop them. Unemployment went out of control, and the destabilization of society it has caused, in terms of rising crime rates and a growing black economy (though not as yet of organized pressure for political alternatives) are now obvious.

A future government that really wants to abolish un-employment will be able to do so if, and only if, it is willing to give it up as a weapon for social control. Expansion of health services, above all at primary care level, would then be the quickest way to get large numbers of people back into socially useful work. Few difficulties at any level in the NHS arise from shortages of technology or of sophisticated skills. The big problems, for care-givers and care-receivers alike, are not enough people and not enough time. The better health services of the future, though very dependent on rapid technical development, particularly in information techno-logy, will be more rather than less labour-intensive. An expanded voluntary sector, together with trained nurses lapsed from production, would probably become the principal source of recruitment for part-time and full-time community health workers. Though an expanding primary care service with a wider social base would encourage a much bigger voluntary sector—for example, the parents of diabetic, asthmatic or mentally handicapped children—there must be expansion in paid staff, because only paid staff can be fully accountable for work planned and verified against a local population base, and because even volunteers require training, organization and support which only paid staff can be expected to give.

Examples already exist of the sort of expanded employ-ment required. At Sheffield's Birley Moor Health Centre[25] in 1977, 10,000 people were served by 4 GPs, 5 office staff, 3 community nurses, 2 health visitors, 1 midwife, 1 chiropodist and 3 cleaners; 19 staff altogether. By 1987 11,000 people were served by 7 GPs, 3 nurse practitioners, 8 office staff, 3 community nurses, 3 health visitors, 1 mid-wife, 4 community psychiatric nurses, 1 physiotherapist, 1 foot care assistant, 2 occupational health workers, 2 unemployment health workers, 1 dietary nursing assistant, 1 patient liaison worker, 2 employed workers and 2 volunteers on a project for the mentally infirm elderly, 1 Citizens' Advice Bureau worker, 2 patients' librarians and still 3 cleaners; 47 altogether, a 247% increase in staff/ patient ratios in 11 years. Though most GPs do not employ even their full entitlement of reimbursable staff under the 1967 Package Deal, a minority of innovating practices have discovered many important tasks that cannot and should not be done by doctors or even by nurses, but require specialized interpersonal skills over a fairly narrow clinical territory; for example, counsellors who can help people to lose weight, stop smoking, control their alcohol or tranquilizer dependence, manage their children's diabetes, asthma, or sleeping or eating problems. These skills could be taught in day-release courses initially lasting a few weeks rather than months, provided that subsequent work is audited and discussed by the whole team. They require mature, intelligent people, not over-professionalized, who can connect easily with their clients through shared social experience.

Would such expanded teams be effective in improving health, giving earlier and more effective anticipatory care for disease, and easing the burden on our increasingly costly hospital services by more accurate and closely considered referral policies, and by returning to primary care the millions of patients now attending out-patient departments for apparently indefinite follow-up? There are good *a priori* reasons for believing they would, but controlled trials over periods of at least five years are needed to measure the difference in health outcomes between enlarged teams working on this broader front, and smaller teams with a narrower clinical approach.

Must Defeudalization mean Dehumanization?

Whether or not such an expanded team would be good for patients, it would almost certainly be good for the newly recruited care-givers. Incomes would probably not be much better than what most of the unemployed get now on the dole, though travel-to-work costs would be small, removing one common reason for not accepting work offered. Positive effects on health, however, could be substantial. A study by the US Department of Health Education and Welfare published in 1973 showed that the best single predictor of longevity was job satisfaction,[26] and job satisfaction in personal health services is potentially high. Paid employment outside the home has an important preventive and therapeutic effect on depressive illness in mothers with preschool children. If creche facilities and nursery school provision were improved, these women could be one important source of recruitment. Another source could be disabled and handicapped people of all kinds. Personal experience of illness or handicap is an important asset in care-givers, which could encourage greater patient input into production of medical care, more effective for care-receivers and more satisfying to care-providers.

Years ago it was assumed that the NHS, the largest single employer in the UK with over one million employees, should set an example as an employer of disabled and handicapped people. Hospitals had a long tradition of providing badly paid but secure sheltered employment for many people uncompetitive in the job market. People were taken on for a lifetime of service, so that high morale and docile acceptance of an almost feudal hierarchy of command could be maintained despite wages at or below subsistence level. The low-wage structure and feudal hierarchies of the old hospital tradition were bound to change, and in 1969 they did, not because consultants and Hospital Governors discovered that it was impossible for a hospital porter to live on a wage of £16 or a ward cleaner on £12 a week, but because hitherto docile health service unions were driven to militancy. In 1967 there was just one strike in the NHS involving 500 staff for one day, an average of 0.69 days lost per 1,000 staff compared with 100.00 days per employee for the UK as a whole. In 1973 there were 18 strikes involving 59,000 staff for 298,000 days, and average of 353.5 days per 1,000 staff compared with 324.4 for the UK.[16]

In 1983, the DHSS axed the root of benign paternalism; circular HC83(18) ordered all Health Authorities to put all cleaning, laundry and catering out to competitive tender. Subsequent circulars forbade protection of existing pay and conditions. As lowest tenders were normally accepted without regard to existing tenure, quality of service or job satisfaction, hospital workers were forced to submit in-house tenders for their own jobs at lower wages. The DHSS claims it has saved £73 million by contracting-out of services, and £48 million of this has come from in-house tenders—workers who 'voluntarily' reduce wages, hours, and staffing levels in order to keep any jobs at all. These reductions not only reduce the already very low incomes of hospital workers, but also reduce standards of work. Reviewing evidence from monitoring of work of private contractors in public services, the Labour Research Department estimated that the standard of services such as cleaning and catering had fallen by an average one-quarter to one-third.[27]

What was once a secure, long-service occupation in which personal relationships and collective morale were important is now a casualized occupation without job satisfaction and with a high labour turnover. The aim is profit, not service, and loyalty of employers to their workforce or of the workforce to patients is now a thing of the past, at least so far as management is concerned. About 35,000 hospital workers live in tied hospital accommodation, and may lose their homes with their jobs; when private contractors took over catering at Northwick Park Hospital in Harrow, the Queen

Elizabeth Hospital in Birmingham, and Farnham Road
Hospital in Surrey, workers were evicted from their homes,
and this was only prevented at St. Mary's Hospital in
Paddington by militant unionists who occupied the houses
and organized a public campaign. Up to 1986, there had been
a gross loss of 17,500 jobs from the NHS, and a net loss
(after allowing for staff employed by the private agencies)
of 5,500 jobs; further gross and net losses of about the same
size are planned from future privatization.

Since building of new hospitals and scrapping of old ones
began in the 1960s, management of the NHS has increasingly
been modelled on management of industry. For industry in
a capitalist society, production of bricks, boots and all other
commodities is not an end in itself, but a particular means
to the universal end of all economic activity; the realization
of a maximum return on capital—profit. Any company which
fails to follow this ruthless policy will quickly find it has
been eaten by another which does. Though this is not yet
the objective of the NHS (though nothing is now unthinkable) its principal administrators, now drawn from private
industry rather than the civil service, as well as most members
of its governing boards, have found a close equivalent—
savings. In practice, the NHS is not organized to maximize
output in terms of real and measurable improvements in
health, reductions in age-standardized death rates or the
prevalence of measured disabilities, but to minimize costs.
Since all public service costs are seen as potentially reducible
tax burdens, this is, in a way, still an indirect search for
profit, so everyone can feel comfortable with what might
otherwise appear a useless endeavour. The women who lost
their jobs when hospital cleaning and catering contracts go
out to tender, who have only taken such hard and badly
paid work because they can't manage without the money,
will so far as possible claim whatever other social benefits
are available to pay the rent and feed the children, and most
of the savings for the health service will be lost as increased
costs for unemployment and supplementary benefits. The
women who remain, trying to cope with more work done by
fewer people, will no longer have the time to chat to patients

and listen to their troubles, which nurses are now, and doctors long ago became, much too skilled, precious and overworked to do. And the large multinational firms which all over Europe and North America recruit the easily-exploited migrant labour most profitable for this work do very well indeed. The NHS, which should be our principal growth industry for friendliness, fellowship, generosity and compassion, will be dragged into the same trough as everything else, for these qualities turn out to have been tolerable only within the deferential hierarchy of medical masters, patient serfs and lady-nurses-in-waiting, when medical care was all faith and no substance; human relationships are not affordable within a science-based service which is both effective and properly paid.

Unless there is a fundamental change in social direction throughout the NHS, in hospitals as well as in community services and primary care, the idea of the NHS as a source both of expanded, labour-intensive service employment, and of happier and healthier working relationships, is absurd. Above all, health workers at all levels must have the time to talk to people and listen to them—in fact, have time to do their work as they were trained to do it; not only to cope, but to care.

Community as a Precondition for Health and its Loss as a Cause of Mortality

The society which denies society, the state which claims only to hold the ring while every man fights every man, according to rules written by and for which men, limited only by what the rest will tolerate, still claims to look after its casualties. The gladiatorial life may be a rotten business, but it is, after all, wonderfully productive of the sophisticated gadgets required to make the contestants think they are alive in such intolerable conditions. If we can learn to move with the times, enjoy a life in which everyone and everything is for sale, and even the biggest millionaires have a sporting chance of losing and being eaten by their rivals, we may perhaps be able to keep ourselves amused for the 80 years or so we have on this earth.

There is now a large body of scientific work measuring the damage to health which results from such an alienated society, in which everyone must either be a winner or a loser. Its most obvious application is to mental or emotional illness. There is compelling evidence from rigorous and detailed studies of random samples of women with young children that depression, in the fairly exact sense claimed by psychiatrists, is essentially a social disorder caused by isolation and a lack of confiding adult relationships, treatable by correcting these deficiencies.[28] After a lifetime of careful, cautious work in epidemiological social psychiatry, George Brown[29] reached this important conclusion:

> I believe that depression is essentially a social phenomenon. . . I would not make the same claim for schizophrenia, though its onset and course are also greatly influenced by social factors. Society and depression are more fundamentally linked. I can envisage societies where depression is absent and others where the majority suffer from depression. While this is science fiction something not too unlike it has been documented. At least a quarter of working-class women with children living in London suffer from a depressive disorder which, if they were to present themselves at an out-patient clinic, psychiatrists would accept as clinical depression, while women with children living in crofting households in the Outer Hebrides are practically free of depression no matter what their social class. . . I know of no compelling reason to believe that the many bodily correlates of depression such as those revealed by work on bioamines are any more than the *result* of social and psychological factors.

Like other people, in unconscious practice if not conscious theory, most doctors most of the time remain Cartesian dualists, seeing mind as an independent inhabitant of the brain, rather than as its function. Of all organs, the brain is dominant, the central control system for rapid response to environmental change; the brain is therefore *always* involved to some extent in any disorder affecting any organ, and so is its function, the mind. Both by doctors and by the laity, disorders are in practice still considered as *either* physical *or* psychological. Within the Osler paradigm it is not easy to conceive of purely social causes of physical disease, that is to say, physical disorder precipitated by disordered social function. Unless some intermediate agent can be found, such as nicotine, alcohol or dietary deficiency, gross social disorders such as isolation, lovelessness, worklessness, egotism, loss of trust, loss of respect, loss of creative function or belief in some world-historical perspective giving meaning and purpose to life, are all unacceptable and incomprehensible as contributory causes of disease.

The first general review I know of this important field was by John Cassel in his Wade Hampton Frost lecture to the American Public Health Association in 1975.[30] A wide range of causes of death tend to be associated with unstable or marginalized status with deprivation of meaningful social contact, including tuberculosis,[31] schizophrenia,[32,33] multiple accidents[34] and suicide.[35] Though often associated with poverty, this hypothesized general effect on host resistance to a wide range of diseases and causes of death is probably independent of this: both upward and downward social movement are associated with increased disease rates[36] and with mortality from coronary heart disease[37] and stroke;[38] so is loss of a spouse, at all ages and in all social groups and classes.[39-42]

The more general concept of host resistance impaired by loss of meaningful social contact, leading to increased vulnerability to a wide range of environmental risks with several final common pathways of outcome, has been tested prospectively by Lisa Berkman and Leonard Syme in the Alameda County studies in California.[43] Their study population was 6,928 adults, 86% of a stratified random sample of households. In 1965 these people answered questions about the number of friends and relatives they felt close to, how often they saw them, and their membership of churches and other formal or informal social groups, and 96% of them were followed up nine years later in 1974. In the age-range 30–69 at entry, there were 371 deaths. Comparing people with most social ties with those who were most isolated, and standardizing for age, isolated men were 2.3, and isolated women 2.8 times as likely to die during the 9-year follow-up. Statistically, these differences were highly significant (p. = .001). There was no evidence that the effect depended on illness at entry, and it applied to all the main causes of death. The effect was statistically independent of all other known risk factors for premature death, including health status at entry, socioeconomic status, smoking, obesity, alcohol consumption, exercise, and use of preventive health services.

Community or the lack of it, the extent to which people have a non-adversarial relationship with others to support them through difficulties, perhaps biochemical, dietary, virological, bacteriological, oncological and genetic difficulties as well as the more obvious life crises, may determine outcomes no less than the many other powerful causal factors for disease with which we are familiar. This is as much an area for controlled observation and experimental science (and just as absurd an area for mysticism and unfalsifiable speculation) as the details of biochemical transmission of nerve impulses or the actions of enzymes at cell surfaces. Man has only gone through roughly 10,000 generations since his line branched from the other apes. More than any other animal we are adaptable, omnivorous and omnipotential, capable of all crimes but also of all heroisms. Our rate of evolution has been uniquely accelerated by our capacity for non-genetic inheritance, which depends on giving—not selling—useful knowledge to our descendants. For most of that time, survival of individuals has depended on survival of groups, and survival of groups has depended most of all on that particular kind of far-sighted species-loyalty we call altruism. So much so that even when collective crime becomes state policy, criminal behaviour on the lines of 007, Rambo and other monsters is recognized as counter-productive; military murder has to be romanticized into selflessness even if the purpose and consequence is little better than piracy. Is it therefore not likely that there is, in terms of disordered physiology, some serious discordance between our social need for good fellowship, and our social reality, the society of winners and losers, the war of every man against every man?

Mistrust of Grand Causes

Outside the public health field, clinicians are instinctively hostile to generalized explanations of causes of disease, and of the grand social remedies that follow from these, partly because these explanations are usually speculative, simplistic, and ignore the lifetimes of painstaking work required to test them, but also because they lie outside their own fields of action and competence as defined by the Osler paradigm. Their entire personal and historical experience confirms their view that the way to solve big apparently insoluble problems is to break them down into little ones, at least some of which may be soluble. Because doctors learn their trade in museums of advanced pathology, they look at the causal chains that lead to end-stage disease at its penultimate point, seeing most clearly the few, often complex and technically demanding, corrective options still open to them. The simpler alternative options that might have existed at an earlier stage are no longer there, and these doctors of advanced pathology have little experience of dealing with them in their only appropriate setting, outside hospitals, within the community.

But even clinicians working in the community tend to have essentially the same attitude to causation, and therefore to treatment. They can, though with some difficulty, redefine Oslerian hospital medicine in terms of primary personal care, acting at a personal level on a different set of options appropriate to earlier stages of disease, but they will still, because they are clinicians and *only* clinicians, fail to recognize pervasive causes of disease which are actually affecting the whole population in varying degrees, precisely because they are so pervasive. The causes are too big to be recognized. Instead, they perceive the effects, and are mainly concerned (as the patient is also) with the questions 'Why her, why him, why me?'. The problem is seen purely in terms of individual susceptibility.

For example there is now an unmanageably vast research literature on the effects of personality and emotional behaviour on susceptibility to coronary heart disease originating from the work of Rosenman and Friedman in

California.[44] They hypothesized that men with aggressive, competitive, ambitious personalities, who drove themselves hard against the clock, were more susceptible to coronary heart disease than men who were more easy-going. Early work in the USA tended to confirm this, at least for white middle-class middle-aged men, though attempts to replicate it in the UK have generally not been successful,[45] and even in the USA tests of the hypothesis have tended to give tantalizing but inconsistent results,[46] suggesting that though the hypothesis contains a truth within it, its formulation is faulty; the question is not being asked in a sociologically meaningful way.[47] The most interesting point, however, is the way in which specialists in this field seem uniquely preoccupied not with changing a form of society which produces this apparently lethal distortion in personality, exalting it and offering it every kind of material reward, but with identifying those most damaged by it and perhaps offering them some personal advice about how to compete without being competitive. High-risk subjects are advised to adopt 'drills' which disrupt the pattern of aggression and positively reinforce corrective behaviours such as going for a walk in the park, browsing in bookshops, or having non-working lunch hours, not wearing a watch, or spreading out work schedules to a more leisurely pace.[48] There is some evidence that in patients who have already survived a heart attack, such remedial training does help to prevent a second one,[49] but all these measures presuppose that the high-risk subject has control of his pattern of work and working environment, an absurd assumption for most employed people.

The obvious alternative is to remove the cause. If there is a maniac in the town centre spraying passers-by with a machine gun, a shop selling flak suits might do good business, but the answer would surely be to call the police and have the man arrested. There are two reasons why this solution does not appeal to most doctors. First, they say that though the evidence of a causal connection may be suggestive, it falls short of proof. Certainly the evidence against socially encouraged type A behaviour is much less convincing than

the evidence against cigarette smoking as the main cause of
lung cancer in the 1950s, when the most eminent British
and US statisticians were both vigorous opponents of the
theory, so convinced of their rightness that they both
accepted substantial fees from the tobacco companies. I
doubt if this is the main reason why British doctors, at least,
are doubtful about tackling social causes. Even if proof is
incomplete, many will agree that a less competitive, more
tolerant, more sharing society in less of a hurry to get
everything finished the day before yesterday would be a help
to us all in so many ways that possible benefits in reduced
heart disease might be relatively insignificant compared with
other social gains. There is less belief in the UK than the USA
that what's best for business must always be what's best for
the country and most of the people who live in it, though
perhaps there is much the same cynicism about alternatives.

The second reason is more important. Social causes may
be, probably are, important as causes of coronary heart
disease and probably many other diseases, and individual care
and advice probably do have less potential for measurable
benefit to the population; but it's not our job. Somebody
has to offer personalized advice and preventive monitoring,
and somebody has to do the best they can to limit or reverse
heart damage when prevention fails. If we don't do it,
nobody else will. The socially and politically conscious
doctor will answer that this is not enough; if doctors are
convinced that a major cause of ill-health exists in society
which could be remedied, whether it is the national economy
which might be changed by political action, or a dangerous
local failure to segregate pedestrian from powered road
traffic, they should be out there with other socially and
politically conscious citizens, holding up their banners,
offering their petition sheets, running their sponsored miles,
pestering their Members of Parliament, attending the ward
meetings of their chosen parties, or even creeping out in the
middle of the night to paint slogans on old colliery workings.

I happen to be a socially and politically conscious doctor,
and I have done all those things, but I am far from convinced
that they were ever more important or effective than my

medical work. Only occasionally have they grown directly out of it and been a completely natural part of it; most of the time they have been a bolt-on option, and the machinery of local general practice would have continued much the same with or without my overtly political activity. If social factors influence the behaviour of disease on a community-wide scale, GPs and other primary care workers must concern themselves with them as a normal and central part of their work, not as a fringe option to be added by some doctors and ignored by others. GPs are paid to meet personally presented demand, not to search for needs or to concern themselves with the health of their registered populations. They have organized themselves to adapt passively to the shape of demand thrown up spontaneously by pressures of the symptom and work-absence markets, which although cash-free is still much the same old balance of supply and demand.

Effective action on community-wide causes of ill-health is too important, and already has too much consensus support, to leave to tiny groups of activists prepared to undertake agitational work, and in any case this is no way to run a railway; we are not talking about political symbolism, but the real care of real people, an important job which at present is simply not being done. If at least one GP in every group had the paid time and in-service training to take responsibility for monitoring local health and organizing the local community to act on its own behalf, we would quickly discover readiness to recognize and act on causes, rather than confine attention to effects. Of course, we would only be at the beginning, and would have to learn as we went. Most of the big ideas about causation will turn out to be wrong, but if we don't start acting we shall never find out.

Concepts of Disease

Like other workers, doctors are comfortable with what they know, and mistrust philosophical approaches which threaten or discard old ideas without assurance of something better. They are also fond of their skills; they may be willing to

improve or add to them, but they naturally resent being
told they are obsolete or redundant.

In 1952 the medical scientist Sir George Pickering[50] was
the first to perceive what should already have been an obvious
truth, that levels of blood pressure were continuously
distributed through the general population, were related to
a continuously distributed risk of heart disease and stroke,
and therefore that separation of people into two qualitatively
distinct groups, one 'hypertensive' and the other 'normo-
tensive', was an artefact arising from attitudes in professional
observers rather than from biological evidence. Virtually the
whole medical Establishment closed ranks against the idea,
and Lord Robert Platt continued to fight on its behalf till
he died 26 years later, though with somewhat diminishing
fervour as his supporters thinned through age and defection.
At some point Pickering's heresy became official wisdom, it's
difficult to say when because rather than concede a knockout,
most of his opponents quietly ducked out of the ring. The
truth of what he was saying about high blood pressure
became obvious, but the general issues he raised about the
nature of disease, and his most important conclusions about
the nature of decision-making in its treatment, are still
ignored.

In his beautiful and perceptive essay on the Platt-
Pickering contest, John Swales[51] traced its origins to the
conflicting traditions of personal clinical care and bedside
teaching personified by Platt, and of clinical and laboratory
science represented by Pickering. He thought a similar
conflict of experience underlay the more muted differences
between Sir John Ryle, the first British professor of social
medicine, and Pickering's mentor, Sir Thomas Lewis, who
founded the first department of clinical science in the UK,
at University College Hospital. Ryle believed that methodical
observation of the natural history of disease in real people
was central to the medical tradition, and the most fruitful
area for research; his most influential book was called *The
natural history of disease.* Platt, Swales believes, was in the
same tradition. His ten years in private practice before he
devoted himself entirely to teaching consultancy and the

presidency of the Royal College of Physicians gave him the time and personal contact between doctor and patient for his communication skills to be fully developed, on which all clinical skills ultimately depend; putting his final thoughts after a lifetime at the top of British medicine, Platt had this to say in his valedictory Harveian Oration:[51]

> Clinical science has shown an unfortunate tendency to follow only the methods of physical science, which try to prove everything by contrived experiments to the neglect of discovery by deliberate and relevant observation and the kind of evolutionary or if you like teleological thinking necessary to the study of biology.

Pickering, on the other hand, though a first-class clinician, was above all an experimental scientist. To me, the accusation that British clinical scientists are in general any less sensitive to the complexities of individual patients, or any less capable of sustained observation over large numbers of cases, is unsupported by experience. That they are frequently insensitive to the feelings and opinions of patients is certainly true, but unfortunately that is equally true of all doctors; the clinical scientists are no worse in this respect than the rest of us, and often better. 'There is a rabble even among the gentry', and it can usually be roused against all who base their work chiefly on laboratory science.

Swales believes these traditions will continue in inevitable but on the whole fruitful and gentlemanly conflict; 'The naturalist and the scientist have always made uneasy bedfellows in British medicine.' This seems to me to miss the essence of the conflict, which is not between bedside and laboratory science, but between the experience of consultant physicians who make uncontrolled observations on moderately large numbers of patients whose relation to any known population is a matter of guesswork, and the experience of medical scientists whose techniques are too detailed, too costly, and occasionally too hazardous to be applied to more than a few patients, but who are by their scientific training educated to accept the inherent difficulties of applying the conclusions of experiments on small numbers to whole populations. It is no accident that it was Pickering, the supposedly remote and impractical clinical scientist, who used the techniques of epidemiology to test his hypotheses on a large representative population; Pickering was the more imaginative naturalist, and opened the door to an exciting new chapter in medicine which Platt was unable to recognize.

Ordinary doctors, certainly all GPs, were bystanders in that controversy, but its pivot was really their central concern. About 150 times each week GPs have to categorize a patient as normal or abnormal, well or diseased, however absurd this absolute distinction may appear, because that is how the Osler paradigm works, and that is what they have been taught. In a better-fed, better-housed society, fewer patients have gross end-stage disease, more have earlier, quantitative rather than qualitative departures from—from what? From normal? From the average? What if, as all the evidence suggests, the entire distribution of blood pressure, and therefore the average level of blood pressure, is too high compared with entire populations living under different conditions, which do not suffer from diseases consequent upon high blood pressure?

In the old days it was simple. The patient complained of a symptom traditionally attributed to high blood pressure, say headache or shortness of breath. You measured blood pressure once, and if the systolic pressure was over 140 or the diastolic pressure was over 90, the patient had the disease 'hypertension', with a treatment, antihypertensive drugs. Now, thanks to the machinations of clinical scientists, where there was certainty, there is doubt. Knowing that neither headache nor shortness of breath are likely to be caused by high blood pressure or cured by its control, GPs still measure it, both to reassure the patient, and because every person's blood pressure must be known if serious but non-symptomatic high blood pressure is to be fully ascertained and treated. Knowing that blood pressure is extremely variable, they measure it not once but (for example) three times over as many days, with perhaps the following result: 146/92, 134/86, 152/104. They can no longer attribute the symptoms to high blood pressure, so a longer interview is necessary to explore other possibilities. It is no longer possible to put all patients either in a white box labelled 'normal' or a black box labelled 'disease'; there now has to be a third, grey box labelled 'we don't know'. In my clinic patients now measure their own blood pressure 28 times before we take a decision on starting what may be a lifetime of treatment. Our decisions are based on the average of these 28 readings, on evidence of other risk factors for stroke and coronary heart disease, and on the results of randomized controlled trials in the UK and Australia which involved more than 40,000 patient-years of treatment.

The Platt earth provided a sure and stable foundation for achieving not very much; naturally so, since as Pickering pointed out we only had to know how to count to two (normal or abnormal). Pickering and his quantified doubt began to introduce the ideas and methods of science to daily practice, not just the products of science unscientifically used. Unlike the hospital specialists, GPs have the resources for this; not the technical resources (which are not very demanding) but the human resources. In my practice I have 1,700 beds, a lot more than any hospital specialist, and they are in a real community where real people live real lives. On such a population base there is no limit to what could eventually be achieved, joining the techniques of experimental medical science with those of epidemiology and of participative democracy in a new streetwise synthesis; medical science with a human face. The research problems of hypertension will probably continue to pile up an increasing confusion of conflicting and uninterpretable facts until this is done.[52]

If all conditions susceptible to medical treatment were, like high blood pressure, quantitative deviations within a continuous distribution, rather than qualitative transformations like a stroke or a fractured femur, the entire concept of disease would disintegrate. In fact, diseases involving major organ damage do fit reasonably well into the old idea of diseases as something which people either have or have not got. These can be listed as a sort of bestiary, with their names, modes of recognition, and the best ways to shoot them without killing the patient. The concept presupposes that the disease exists as an entity separate from the patient, a sort of obligatory parasite which cannot exist without a human host, but is sufficiently independent to be a potential target. To attack this concept as an imperfect, incomplete reflection of biological reality is stupid; all scientific concepts are imperfect reflections of reality, and the real question is, is there some other concept which is less imperfect and more useful? The answer to that depends on the nature of the human material we are dealing with. In primary care in an advanced industrialized society, it seems to me that the disease concept applies well to advanced organ damage, but certainly not to the quantified and reversible deviations from health which precede them, eventually contribute one of several precipitating causes of death, and which will increasingly become the heart of clinical practice outside hospitals.

The new concept we need is anticipatory care of health rather than treatment of disease. It differs from the old in two ways. First, it deals with quantified points on a continuous distribution of risk for events (diseases) which have not yet occurred and are not causing symptoms severe enough to ensure that people will present as patients. It can, of course, be applied to obviously sick as well as to apparently healthy people. A man of 35 with insulin-dependent diabetes and a blood pressure of 154/98 unquestionably has a disease (insulin-dependent diabetes) which makes him qualitatively different from other people, and will if untreated quickly cause intolerable symptoms (thirst, weight loss, and eventually fatal ketoacidotic coma). Population screening is not needed to identify him; he will come soon enough once the disease has got going. His moderately raised blood pressure is entirely different, and cannot usefully be regarded as a disease; if it is not treated it is likely in a diabetic to cause irreversible kidney damage, with dialysis, transplant or death from kidney failure perhaps 10 or 15 years later, but it is not currently causing any symptoms, in fact he is likely to feel a little less well on antihypertensive treatment than without it. Whereas the outcome of untreated insulin-dependent diabetes is certain death within a few months or perhaps years, the outcome of untreated high blood pressure in this range, even in a diabetic, is based on probabilities, not certainties. He needs both disease care within the old Osler paradigm, and anticipatory care of his remaining health in the new paradigm.

Secondly, anticipatory care differs from the old paradigm in that it drops the pretence that any disorders, illnesses, diseases, or injuries can ever be truthfully defined without a social component, sometimes large, sometimes small, but always present in some degree. At a certain biological age, placed chronologically around 85 years, death becomes a normal event biologically, but social attitudes to this have to be taken into account and cannot in practice be disregarded in medical decisions. The question is not usually serious with well-defined disease states causing gross symptoms, but for quantified deviations from health such as high blood pressure, obesity, airways obstruction, depression, period pains, non-insulin-dependent diabetes, high blood cholesterol, alcohol and tobacco addiction or chronic back pain, the points at which medical interventions begin have important social consequences which must be taken into account in deciding whether to intervene in that poorly-defined frontier between health and disease so detested by hospital specialists, who naturally prefer a well-defined beast at which to aim their sophisticated weapons, but which is home ground for the GP. All medical decisions, follow-up with potential problems of dependence, prescription of potentially hazardous drugs, legitimized absence from work or changes in division of labour within the family, referral to hospital specialists entering a pipeline from which it may be difficult to escape, surgery, radiotherapy, chemotherapy, even the decision to do nothing but wait and see, all have social implications which should be taken into account.

Clinicians usually have the illusion that they already do all this, but this view is not supported by any evidence. Within the Osler paradigm, they regard 'diseases' such as high blood pressure, obesity or airways obstruction as independent wholly biological entities, requiring specific treatments for their control. Social factors are taken into account only in order to obtain compliance from the patient in accepting that treatment. Yet the controlled scientific evidence on which any rational treatment should be based is social as well as biological in nature. The Australian blood pressure trial[53] showed that 13,000 patient-years of treatment were required to save 5 lives with antihypertensive drugs in people with diastolic blood pressures in the range 95–110; there were 6 deaths in people randomized to treatment and 11 in the equal number of untreated controls. The Medical Research Council mild hypertension trial[54] found that about one in five of men treated with the most commonly-used anti-hypertensive drugs became impotent, a problem reversible by stopping the drug, but only if the (previously unknown) association was recognized. In return for extremely small gains in strokes prevented (and no gain at all in preventing all causes of death put together, which were the same in both groups in both these trials) a substantial price was paid in impaired social function. Obviously, wherever we are dealing with continuously distributed risks, choice of a threshold for diagnosis or for treatment (which in practice become inter-changeable terms if one always implies the other) must depend on weighing all the available evidence for and against intervention, giving full weight to social as well as biological factors.

The Restabilization of Society

The argument has moved a long way from its starting point, the necessity of community and its present endangered state. I have tried to show that effective clinical medicine is not possible without a community dimension: because the community provides most of the informal care on which professional care outside hospitals has to depend, and because the practice of medicine cannot be scientific unless it is conceived of, planned and researched in relation to the needs of real, non-institutional, unreferred populations.

There are familiar arguments, from both the traditional Right and the traditional Left, which agree that society is, and always has been, going to the dogs. In 1912, BMA president Sir James Barr[55] predicted that health insurance 'would impair the independence, increase the sickness, and hasten the degeneracy of a spoonfed race'. In 1979 a retired coal miner, asked if he thought things were getting better, replied 'Oh ah, things are getting better, it's only people are getting bloody worse'.[56] There is a lot of support for both these opinions among all classes of society, and though the clichés differ, the thought is essentially the same.

There is enough truth in both perceptions for all of us with sustained experience of real work in real communities to feel some sympathy at least some of the time with both these cries of despair; but the world has been going to the dogs for so many thousands of years, in which we have achieved such obvious moral as well as material advances, that we have to recognize them as the snarls of tired and bitter old men which, though understandable, are of no help to anyone. A certain minimum credulity and optimism about the future of the human race is not only a fundamental requirement for humane science, but also justified by the balance of historical evidence. Community is under attack, as it has always been, by powerful people who think they can do better for themselves by climbing on the backs of their fellows, and by weak people clinging to their coat-tails, but to suggest that it is down on a count of nine and that all we can do is curse the world's fate is a betrayal of the cumulative struggle of 10,000 previous generations both to survive, and to make some permanent gain for civilization against piracy; as many or more people are working and speaking up for community today, as at any time in the past.

One of the functions of medical care has always been to stabilize society. The negative aspect of this has been obvious; doctors have largely replaced parsons as respectable and respected agents of the ruling class, policing the social insurance system in much the same way as clergy once kept the keys of heaven and hell. Yet it is also true that in a world packed with dynamite, some social peace has to be preserved even for necessary and inevitable conflicts between classes and ideologies to continue without destroying civilization itself, whatever opinions we hold about the ways in which it should be socially transformed. As Marx and Engels wrote in 1847, fundamental class conflicts throughout history have ultimately 'ended either in a revolutionary reconstitution of society, or in the common ruin of the contending classes'.[57] A primary care system based on participative democracy within relatively small units of population, the communities in which people actually live, could be an important obstacle to the de-civilization of society, whatever its motives or cause, as well as a starting point for community of a new kind.

The economic and political system we live in, the assumptions it leads to about what is possible, the limits to popular imagination, have not changed fundamentally since Bagehot wrote in 1867; but the quantitative changes in production of every kind of material and intellectual wealth, actual and potential, are colossal. The capitalist system, which cannot exist without continually revolutionizing techniques of production in search of lower labour costs and higher returns on investment, or without expanding to seek cheaper labour wherever it can be found, is compelled continually to destabilize itself. Nothing and no one is ever allowed to stay still, or even to proceed more calmly and peacefully in search of a better life; relax for one moment and whole industries are gobbled up, to reappear wherever there are poorer, more desperate but for the time being more profitable people. The gap between how the world lives and how it could live gets wider and more obvious every day.

We need a transformation of the ways in which we think about society and community, about medical professionalism, about health services, about how they should be financed from the social product, and about how central and peripheral leadership and initiative should be integrated. A social base for such a transformation exists, real though presently dispersed. How it might be mobilized is the subject of the final chapter.

NOTES

1. Rees, T.L., *The origin and destination of migrants to and from the South Wales valleys with particular reference to the Upper Afan*

valley, Cardiff: Department of Town Planning, University of Wales Institute of Technology, 1976.

2. 'Families in the future. Study Commission on the Family', London: SCF, 3 Park Road, London NW1, 1983.

3. Jones, A.G., Jones, D.A., *Termination of pregnancy in Wales 1969-72*, Cardiff: Welsh Office, 1973.

4. 'The role of regional policy in South Wales: with particular reference to valley communities', *Home Office/West Glamorgan CDP Research Team working paper no. 7*, Cardiff: Department of Town Planning, University of Wales Institute of Technology, 1974.

5. Parker, G., *With due care and attention: a review of research on informal care*, London: Family Policy Studies Centre, 1985.

6. Cartwright, A., Hockey, L., Anderson, J.L., *Life before death*, London: Routledge & Kegan Paul, 1973.

7. Wilkes, E., 'Where to die', *British Medical Journal 1973*; i:32-3.

8. Jones, D.A., Vetter, N.J., 'Formal and informal support received by carers of elderly dependants', *British Medical Journal 1985*; 291:643-5.

9. Nissel, M., Bonnerjea, L., *Family care of the handicapped elderly: who pays?*, London: Policy Studies Institute, 1 Castle Lane, SW1E 6DR, 1982.

10. Central Statistical Office. Social Trends 17. London: HMSO, 1987.

11. Radical Statistics Health Group, *Facing the figures: what is really happening to the NHS*, London: RSHG, c/o British Society for Social Responsibility in Science, 25 Horsell Road, N5 1XL, 1987.

12. Office of Health Economics, Compendium of health statistics, 6th edition. London: OHE, 1987.

13. Isaacs, B., 'Geriatric patients: do their families care?', *British Medical Journal 1971*: 4:282-6.

14. Neale, J., *Memoirs of a callous picket: working for the NHS*, London: Pluto Press, 1983. Jonathan Neale's book now out of print, should be required reading for every medical student, doctor, and everyone else working in the NHS. The only wrong thing about it is the title, which is misleading. In fact, it is a beautifully written, balanced, well informed and careful account of the almost incomprehensibly complex world of labour in hospitals, and never gives in to the rancour and divisive recrimination endemic among so many opiners on medical care.

15. Bagehot, W., *The English constitution*. First published 1867. London: Fontana, 1963.

16. 'Report of the Royal Commission on the National Health Service' (Merrison Report), Cmnd 7615. London: HMSO, 1979, p. 10.

17. Smith, D., *The defence of the realm in the 1980s*, London: Croom Helm, 1980, p. 156.

18. Maynard, A., 'In discussion', pp. 24-5, following, 'Economic Directives', pp. 12-19, in Zander, L. (ed.), *Change: the challenge for the future*, London: Royal College of General Practitioners, 1984.

19. Dunnel, K., Cartwright, A., *Medicine takers, prescribers, and hoarders*, London: Routledge & Kegan Paul, 1972.

20. Abel-Smith, B., *Value for money in health service*, p. 83. London: Heinemann, 1976.
21. 'A review of the medical services in Great Britain', (Porritt Report), London: Social Assay, 1962.
22. *Hospital In-patient Enquiry 1978*, London: HMSO, 1981.
23. Godber, G., *The health service: past, present and future*, p. 38. (Heath Clark lectures), London: Athlone Press, 1975.
24. Lees, D.S., *Health through choice: an economic study of the British National Health Service*, Hobart Paper no. 14, London: Institute of Economic Affairs, 1961.
25. Birley Moor Health Centre, 'Report to Joint management meeting 17 March 1987'. This centre has pioneered not only excellent neighbourhood care, but also a unique emphasis on occupational health, including management of problems of mass unemployment.
26. 'Work in America', Department of Health Education & Welfare, Washington: US Government Printing Office, 1973.
27. *Privatisation: paying the price*, London: Labour Research Department, 1987.
28. Brown, G.W., Bhrolchain, M.N., Harris, T.O., 'Social class and psychiatric disturbance among women in an urban population', *Sociology 1975*; 9:225-54.
29. Brown, G.W., 'Depression: a sociological view', pp. 225-34 in Tuckett, D., Kaufert, J.M. (eds.), *Basic readings in medical sociology*, London: Tavistock Publications, 1978.
30. Cassel, J., 'The contribution of the social environment to host resistance', *American Journal of Epidemiology 1976*; 104:107-123.
31. Holmes, T., 'Multidiscipline studies of tuberculosis'. In Sparer, P.J. (ed.), *Personality, stress and tuberculosis*, Chapter 6, New York: International Universities Press, 1956.
32. Dunham, H.W., 'Social structure and mental disorders: competing hypotheses of explanation', *Milbank Memorial Fund Quarterly 1961*; 39:259-311.
33. Mishler, E.G., Scotch, N.A., 'Sociocultural factors in the epidemiology of schizophrenia: a review', *Psychiatry 1963*; 26:315-51.
34. Tillman, W.A., Hobbs, G.E., 'The accident-prone automobile driver: a study of the psychiatric and social background', *American Journal of Psychiatry 1949*; 106:321.
35. Durkheim, E., *Suicide: a study in sociology*, London: Routledge & Kegan Paul, 1952.
36. Christenson, W.N., Hinkle, L.E., 'Differences in illness and in prognostic signs in two groups of young men', *Journal of the American Medical Association 1961*; 177:247-253.
37. Marmot, M.G., Syme, S.L., 'Acculturation and coronary heart disease', *American Journal of Epidemiology 1976*; 104:225-47.
38. Nesser, W.B., Tyroler, H.A., Cassel, J.C., 'Social disorganisation and stroke mortality in the black populations of North Carolina', *American Journal of Epidemiology 1971*; 93:166-75.
39. Kraus, A., Lilienfeld, A., 'Some epidemiologic aspects of the high mortality rate in the young widowed group', *Journal of Chronic Disease 1959*; 10:207-17.
40. Maddison, D., Viola, A., 'The health of widows in the year follow-

ing bereavement', *Journal of Psychosomatic Research 1968*; 12:297-306.

41. Parkes, C.M., Benjamin, B., Fitzgerald, R.G., 'Broken heart: a statistical study of increased mortality among widowers', *British Medical Journal 1969*; i:740-3.

42. Rees, W.P., Lutkins, S.G., 'Mortality of bereavement', *British Medical Journal 1967*; iv:13-16.

43. Berkman, L.F., Syme, S.L., 'Social networks, host resistance, and mortality: a nine-year follow-up of Alameda County residents', *American Journal of Epidemiology 1979*; 109:186-204.

44. Rosenman, R.H., Brand, R.J., Sholtz, R.I., Friedman, M., 'Multivariate prediction of coronary heart disease during 8.5 year follow-up in the Western Collaborative Group study', *American Journal of Cardiology 1976*; 37:902-10.

45. Johnston, D.W., Cook, D.G., Shaper, A.G., 'Type A behaviour and ischaemic heart disease in middle aged British men', *British Medical Journal 1987*; 295:86-9.

46. Sensky, T., 'Refining thinking on type A behaviour and coronary heart disease', *British Medical Journal 1987*; 295:69-70.

47. Cohen, J.B., 'The influence of culture on coronary-prone behaviour', Chapter 14, pp. 191-8 in Dembroski, T.M., Weiss, S.M., Shields, J.L. et al (eds.), *Coronary-prone behavior*, New York: Springer Verlag, 1978.

48. Friedman, M., Rosenman, R.H., *Type A behaviour and your heart*, New York: Knopf, 1974.

49. Friedman, M., Thoresen, C.E., Gill, J.J. et al., 'Alteration in type A behavior and reduction in cardiac recurrences in postmyocardial infarction patients', *American Heart Journal 1984*; 108:237-48.

50. Pickering, G.W., 'The natural history of hypertension', *British Medical Bulletin 1952*; 8:305-9.

51. Swales, J.D., *Platt versus Pickering: an episode in recent medical history*, London: Keynes Press, 1985.

52. Julius, S., Weder, A.B., Egan, B.M., 'Pathophysiology of early hypertension: implications for epidemiologic research', chapter in Gross, F., Strasser, T. (eds.), *Mild Hypertension: recent advances*, pp. 219-236. New York: Raven Press, 1983.

53. Management Committee, Australian National Blood Pressure Study. 'The Australian therapeutic trial in mild hypertension', *Lancet 1980*; i:121.

54. Medical Research Council Working Party. 'MRC trial of treatment of mild hypertension: principal results'. *British Medical Journal 1985*; 291:97.

55. Gilbert, B.B., *British Social Policy 1914-1939*, London: Batsford, 1966.

56. Seabrook, J., *What went wrong? Working people and the ideals of the Labour movement*, p. 31, London: Gollancz, 1979.

57. Marx, K., Engels, F., *Manifesto of the Communist Party 1847*.

Chapter 10
A NEW SOCIAL ALLIANCE

This book has sought to develop six features of medical professionalism, alternative to those of the Osler paradigm:

1. Where Osler sought association with medical science, while forced to retain the customs of secrecy and mutual deception of pre-scientific hope because (through the placebo effect) they were still more generally effective than science, we must accept the full implications of experimental science in daily practice, for both groups and individuals, practising an open style of medicine which admits to ourselves, our colleagues, and our patients what we don't yet know and what we haven't yet done.

2. Where Osler saw original science as a rare and superior activity developed only within laboratories, and clinical innovation as confined to a few hundred beds in teaching hospitals, applied uncritically by GPs as best they could in the entirely different conditions outside, we must learn to apply scientific principles imaginatively to the health care of millions of people as they actually live and work.

3. Where Osler handled disease as an entity qualitatively distinct from health, we must learn to deal with measurable, continuously distributed variables in which disease (requiring active remedial intervention) is difficult or even impossible to separate from health (requiring active conservation).

4. Where Osler's doctors, though usually unable to inter-

315

vene usefully to change the course of illness, were masters of their pseudo-industry as unquestioned as bishops and cardinals, we must accept that effective medical care, and even more the effective conservation of health, requires an enormous range of skills other than those of doctors, including skills of other medical, nursing and health professionals who have been systematically subordinated to and exploited by us and our predecessors, and that our own skills will survive only if they can be shown to be useful.

5. Where Osler could treat patients as passive consumers of care which doctors devised and nurses implemented, but patients unquestioningly endured, we must accept patients as colleagues in a jointly designed and performed production, in which they will nearly always have to do most of the work.

6. Where Osler sought his peer models and patrons among aristocratic gentlemen and the gentrified robber-barons of the first megacorporations, we must look to a more dependable alliance with the ordinary people we serve.

These six features have a single common theme, which Osler implicitly accepted but never articulated, because society in the first decade of the 20th Century appeared to be permanent, and professionalism seemed likely to share that permanence if it remained uncritical. All medical acts are social acts within a changing, people-made story, all medical services are social services with a history, and a social and historical view of human biology is at the centre of effective medical science.

The whole of medicine ultimately serves practical human ends; to be consistent with science, it must serve whole populations according to their needs rather than be merely available to individual demanders or purchasers of care, whether as a state-subsidized or freely marketed commodity. This means that the practice of medicine, and the professionalism derived from it, are related to the distribution of wealth and power in society, to its history and culture, and to the priorities that result from these, and medicine is thus inescapably a political subject.

It also means that medical practice has itself an effect on society. This effect may be particularly important today, when medical care pursues its objectives in a fundamentally different way from other forms of production, to some extent at least contradicting an otherwise commercial society. Doctors will not be able to influence or understand what is happening to their profession or to medical science, nor will they be able to make their own potential contribution to a more civil, less dangerous and damaging society, unless they recognize that they have political choices; that an important part of future history is in their hands, and theirs alone, giving them a civilizing power they must not abdicate in a world now too dangerous for neutrality.

In real politics (choices about what kind of world we want to live in, not about where individual politicians try to get themselves) medical care is moving from the periphery to the centre. We have already entered an era when unless democracy becomes truly participative we may lose what we have gained, achieved not passively through evolution of some natural law of spontaneous social ascent, but always through active work and open criticism. Doctors and laity who have hitherto ignored new developments in medical practice and relied on assumptions based on the Osler paradigm, developed from the now almost exhausted alliance between well-dressed but illusory care and infant medical science, have to face a new set of choices.

Can Doctors Become a Progressive Rather Than a Conservative Social Force?

According to polls cited in the medical press, 47% of British doctors voted Conservative in the 1987 election, a mere 7% for Labour. I have been unable to find data for the medical vote for earlier elections, but figures for all higher professions including medicine showed 15% for Labour in 1945, falling to 10% in 1950 and 6% in 1951.[1] This suggests that collapse of medical opposition to the NHS in 1948 and consolidation of general professional support for it by the 1960s[2] were not translated into medical votes for Labour. The real effect of the popularity of 'socialized medicine' was on the Conservative Party, which first dropped its opposition to the NHS, and then claimed credit for its invention, eventually agreeing a virtually bipartisan policy with the Labour Party, except for ritual disputes about prescription charges.

In traditional terms, doctors have generally been too rich and secure to be attracted to any kind of socialist belief. Ever since World War II British doctors have enjoyed higher incomes and greater job security than any other profession, including ministers and members of parliament. In Western Europe in 1982, average annual net earnings for GPs from insurance-based or NHS-type systems before tax ranged from £40,000 in Denmark to £14,000 in Italy and the Irish Republic, with the UK ranking sixth out of 10 nations at £29,000.[3] This does not take into account substantial additional earnings in many of these countries from private practice (negligible in UK general practice) or NHS index-linked pensions which are envied by doctors abroad. Using an older set of figures, Klein[4] estimated the ratios of all doctors' incomes to average per capita income for all occupations as follows:

German Federal Republic	8.5:1
France	7.0:1
USA	6.7:1
Sweden	4.6:1
UK	4.5:1

Doctors are drawn overwhelmingly from privileged backgrounds. This trend has increased over the past 20 years, and is still increasing now. Even in the 1960s, 40% of British medical students came from professional families (3% of the population). Though only 29% of school leavers with three or more A-level passes are privately educated, they get 57% of medical school places.[5,6]

British doctors may on average be less affluent than their European, US or White Commonwealth colleagues, but they have a narrower range of income (fewer are either millionaires or poor), better pensions, and total job security once they achieve an ultimate career post as a consultant or GP. Compared with other people in Britain who work for a living they are rich; not promising material for traditional socialist parties. This question has been interestingly discussed recently by Steve Watkins, with a particularly useful analysis of medical professional organizations in relation to the political Left, though not a lot about GPs.[7]

Proletarianization of Doctors?

Nevertheless, in the USA, where medical millionaires are said to be commonplace, a serious case has been made for what McKinlay and Arches call the proletarianization of physicians, in a paper which deserves careful reading,[8] together with important modifying comment by Chernomas.[9] They present a rigorously argued case that in the USA, citadel of medical autonomy, there is a trend, uneven and incomplete but growing rapidly, for previously self-employed independent medical entrepreneurs to be first drawn, then driven into large groups under commercial management, of which the archetype is the Health Maintenance Organisation (HMO). These are directed at the most profitable sections of the public rather than the poor, bureaucratized enterprises controlled by investors rather than doctors, aimed at maximizing commodity-production of care and corporate profit, rather than either improved health for patients or greater job-satisfaction or personal income for doctors. The means of medical production are becoming too costly and too complex for doctors to own and control on their own, a process much accelerated by medical competition, which inflates the technical and minimizes the communicative components of care. Like other skilled technicians in modern society, doctors are therefore forced to become workers dependent on the sale of their labour-power to employers rich enough to own and control the means of producing a commodity which becomes more profitable as it becomes more (often unnecessarily) technically sophisticated.

In Marxist terms, objective social class position depends not on income or prestige, but on the social relations of production. According to this analysis, the open or latent conflict of interest lies not between rich and poor, but between those who live by owning the machinery of production, and those who live by working it for the owners. On this view, doctors who live by offering their skills for hire by others who own the machinery without which those skills cannot be expressed, rather than by doing their own work with their own tools, are workers employed for someone else's profit, however fiercely they may cling to their traditional status as independent professionals. In this sense, the proletarianization of US doctors is now proceeding with some speed, and could become an important factor in their future socialization and political stance, though to most people this requires imagination bordering on fantasy.

This applies much less to British doctors, at least to GPs. The assimilation of the medical profession to the needs of the State occurred earlier and more completely in Britain than in any other fully developed country, in particular contrast with the USA, where it was delayed by exceptionally powerful professional resistance. Assimilation to the needs of the State protected the British medical profession from the market, and thus paradoxically defended medical autonomy both from internal competition and from external commercial pressures. In the USA, successful professional resistance to assimilation to the needs of the State left medical entrepreneurs more vulnerable to commercialization on a larger scale, ideologically as well as economically, and the market was also potentially more profitable and easily exploited; Americans not only had more money, but were also culturally accustomed to part with it for medical care, a habit British patients have now almost lost. It is difficult to be indignant about the commercialism of medical megacorporations if you have already accepted that physicians are essentially businessmen. The British medical ideology has preserved stronger elements of social duty, which may now to an important extent resist commercial pressures. More importantly, perhaps, it has left British GPs in charge of their own work. For both good and ill, they have been able to suit themselves, and as the New Conservative State makes its first tentative moves to return GPs to the market place, they will resist.

Assimilation of doctors to the needs of capitalist production has in all countries begun later than for other trades and professions. This has generally been attributed to uniquely fierce resistance by the medical profession; but all occupational groups, starting with the peasant forced from his strip of land to make way for the squire's sheep, have always resisted loss of control of their means of production as long as they could, so this alone is not an adequate explanation. A more important factor has been the illusory nature of most medical care until about 1935, and much of it since. While so much medical activity depended on personal transactions between doctors and patients both of whose main functions were to maintain hope and maximize the placebo effect, doctors depended very little on their machinery, all of which could be carried in a little black bag and used in their front parlours, but very much on their personalities, which they alone could control. Now that medical care depends on costly buildings, machinery and supporting staffs which have to be shared with many other health workers, medical personality has become just one of many instruments available to investors in search of new fields for profit, and except in personal psychiatry, no longer provides sufficient machinery for effective or convincing production of medical care.

Paul Starr[10] points out that US doctors have, by their obstinate hostility to employment of any kind by the State and their insistence on independent entrepreneurial status, rendered themselves uniquely vulnerable to the process of proletarianization, though he does not use this confusing but logically precise term. Unassimilated to State service, they are wide open to take-over by megacorporations. The aim of capitalist production is to maximize profit through sale of commodities in the best markets; if medical care is the commodity, improvements in health are only a byproduct of such sales, will not minimize overall costs (because any commodity justifies itself by its sale, whether or not it is effective) and will aim at those in greatest need only to the

extent that the State underwrites the cost. Now that medical
care is potentially effective and real, rather than a relatively
cheap but ineffective gesture of compassion, the State is
only too willing to abdicate responsibility and hand over to
the market. Under an administration eager to demolish even
such partial elements of State service as the American Medical
Association has allowed to exist, doctors are being driven
into a situation in which they will cease to control the
purpose or quality of their work, which ultimately threatens
the independence both of the profession and of medical
science.[11,12]

The process has been described by Freeman[13] in the *New
England Journal of Medicine* in 1985. He sees the weakening
grip of gentlemanly medical professionalism naively and
uncritically, but has been forced to question assumptions
hitherto unchallenged within the medical Establishment:

> With health care costs for the United States approaching 11% of the
> gross national product, the current reformation of health care policy
> is being molded by a quest to relate the costs of production to the
> prices of services and then to reduce the production costs. The
> apparent shift in health care policy is one that moves us from a
> scientific to an industrial orientation. In the past the financing for
> health care at all levels was designed to support the development and
> application of scientific principles and knowledge. Physicians viewed
> their patients from the perspective of scientists and humanists,
> whose task it was to diagnose in detail the problems of patients and
> to treat them with the best that medical skill and technology have to
> offer. The issue of quality eclipsed that of quantity. After all, the
> physicians who designed the health care system were trained as
> scientists, not economists or business people.
>
> However, business people are becoming the most important
> influence in the redesign of the health care system. . . This new
> party on the scene is pressing for a thorough redesign of the delivery
> system. Its orientation is to become actively involved in the business
> of health care—that is, to relate the price of the product to the cost
> of production, as in the industrial model.

The US industrial model of general practice is the Health
Maintenance Organisation, the HMO, and this is the model
which attracts both the New Conservative politicians, and a
few of the more ambitious medical politicians who advised

the government as the Green and White Papers on primary care were prepared. HMOs have been well described by Linda Marks in her excellent King's Fund discussion paper on primary care:[14]

> In Health Maintenance Organisations, a rapidly expanding sector of US health care, professionals act within a clear management framework and management control is exercised over a whole range of care. Procedures are codified; standards are set in relation to criteria for hospital admission, management of inpatients (length of stay, drug regimens, investigations) and the use of ambulance services; and protocols are devised for the management of common disorders such as hypertension. Styles of communication (with patients and other colleagues) may be monitored. A relatively high proportion of patients will be seen by 'allied personnel'.

HMOs in the USA have developed rapidly among the affluent middle class, and something very like them could be encouraged in the UK as the top level of a two-tiered service in the highly competitive, consumerist society actively pursued by the New Conservatives, and more or less acquiesced in by the dominant elements in the Labour, Liberal and Social-Democratic Parties. Though cheaper than the previous US model, demand-led fee-for-service care by independent medical entrepreneurs paid for through private health insurance, HMOs are still far too costly for low earners or the indigent. The norms used for clinical protocols tend to be legalistic rather than realistic, reflecting the aggressive tradition in US medicine which has always overstated the value of medical interventions and thereby raised the legal penalties of failure; a good example is the almost universal US practice of medication for high blood pressure from a threshold of diastolic 90 mmHg, compared with about 100 mmHg in Britain, although controlled trials probably justify this only from about 110 mmHg, certainly not more than 100 mmHg.[15] From the doctors' point of view, however, the main consequence of HMOs is that they lost control over their work. The doctors lose the possibility of becoming creative craftsmen, and their patients lose the possibility of becoming colleagues. Patients and doctors are at last compelled to leave the informal, pre-industrial world where imagination, though rare enough, was still possible, to enter a new world of medical conveyor belts organized by a board of management geared not to improved health, but the generation of profit. This world will certainly be scientistic, but as a substrate for the development of medical science as understood in this book, it is likely to be a far more hostile environment than its alternative, neighbourhood care with local control, with needs measured by health burdens rather than available incomes, and outputs measured in health outcomes rather than medical procedures.

Starving the NHS to Feed the Private Sector

Because British doctors accepted employment by the State, the immediate threat most of them face is not that they become cogs in a capitalist machine, but that they have somehow to meet rising public expectations with resources which are already declining in relation to traditional needs (because of an ageing population), apart from the new requirements of advancing medical science. They are employed in a deteriorating public service grudgingly funded by a government committed to reducing public spending by every available means.

Those who cannot tolerate this must either act to change it, which means looking for entirely new social allies, or move to the private sector. Private practice will increasingly provide employment for some specialists, but their privileges will not include exercise of the highest medical skills, since these must by definition be available equally to all who need them. If they are not, their skills will ultimately be distorted and damaged, whether doctors realize this or not, just as any tool is changed by the material on which it is used. They will follow the same path as their US colleagues; the private sector will, however tricked out with gadgetry, not be independent practice but just another branch of a multinational megacorporate business.

If present staffing levels of the NHS are not raised, roughly half the students now entering UK medical schools will never have a career post in the public service.[16] Britain has only 13.6 practising doctors per 10,000 population, compared with 19.2 in the German Federal Republic, 17.1 in Sweden, 16.7 in the USA, 16.4 in Canada, and 15.2 in Australia; but the UK government aims to reduce the number of UK doctors in the NHS to 11.9 per 10,000,[17,18] a staff cut of 16% over the next 10 years. Over this period our medical schools will be educating 70% more doctors. As a *Lancet* editorial concluded,

> How can Government justify the training of 70% more medical students than can find career posts in the NHS while accepting that the projected NHS staffing establishment is about half that to be expected in a developed country? It is difficult to escape one of two conclusions: either the Government has no knowledge of or control over what is happening; or half the students are intended for a vastly expanded private sector.

True medical unemployment for British graduates is as yet nothing like the problem in Spain, Italy and Portugal, for example, where entry to medical schools has been unrelated to planned requirements for medical manpower, because the aim has for the past 150 years been to provide careers for entrepreneur doctors rather than to staff a public service. However, two generations of British doctors have come to assume that the Welfare State will guarantee employment for any doctor willing to do useful work; this guarantee has now disappeared. Demotion of the NHS to universally under-funded mediocrity, with our reputation as an innovating world medical power reduced to fleecing rich Arabs in Harley Street, could quickly destroy the loyalty of most doctors to the Conservative Party, and force them to look in new directions for their social allies. For example, consultants in Reading paid for whole-page advertisements in local newspapers to tell the public about the breakdown of NHS hospital services. Actions of this kind, unthinkable even five years ago, are becoming commonplace.

Doctors and the Future of Science

The same argument applies to a wide range of other skilled occupations which though nominally professional and independent, now consist almost entirely of salaried workers without real control of the nature, purpose, or outcome of their work. To be a physicist, chemist, geologist, metallurgist, agronomist, biologist or graduate engineer today means to be employed either in private industry, or at some level of education or government service. The best incomes are always in private industry, work elsewhere is done either for job-satisfaction or because nothing else is available. Until the advent of applied nuclear physics, science was generally an academic activity with usually remote applications to production and the needs of the State, and its independence from the market and military and industrial secrecy was generally respected. Since the war, academic independence in the sciences has retreated to a point where half of all British scientific research is on weapons development, compared with 33% in France and 10% in the German Federal Republic. State funding of universities has become conditional on readiness to put scientific skills at the service of the State and of private industry. University departments have been forced increasingly to depend on direct commercial investment in their research in return for new knowledge which becomes the property of the investor, rather than the common knowledge of mankind. If present Government policies continue, by 1990 there will have been a 30% cut in Government support for universities in real terms since 1980; these figures come from a presidential address to the BMA in 1986 by Sir Christopher Booth, director of the M.R.C. Clinical Research Centre, revealingly entitled 'Better a commitment to health and research than to missiles'.[19]

In the USA, megacorporate industry has not only penetrated the universities, but seduced leading scientists from pursuit of knowledge for the world to pursuit of another million dollars for themselves. Molecular biologists now found their own companies and become millionaires, their discoveries just one more commodity in the market.[20]

Scientists are becoming, as Brecht's Galileo predicted, 'a race of intelligent dwarfs who can be hired for anything'.[21]

Forward to the Jungle?

British doctors, in hospital and in general practice, are now in a bewildered and uneasy state. The only thing they can be sure about is that nothing is for sure. Future society is beginning to look very unpleasant, even to people who make a great deal of money out of things as they are, and might make even more in a more entrepreneurial service. Granted total professional dominance, despite their initial hostility to the NHS, doctors found it and its parent society pleasant places to live and work. Now that dominance and apparent autonomy are coming to an end, they are at last beginning to be made accountable, not to the patients they serve, but to a State chiefly concerned to evade responsibilities formerly taken for granted, or to corporations whose shareholders must be satisfied if they are not to be eaten by more ruthless competitors. Accountability is not in terms of lives saved or improved, but of cash saved or profits made.

More doctors today than at any time in the past are becoming open to political alternatives, though as yet they have hardly been offered one. They are looking for a way out, and are beginning to realize that it can't be backwards; private general practice on the old model is no longer feasible for more than at most 5% of the population. The only credible choices are between accountability for cash to an increasingly centralized and authoritarian State presently governing in the interests of megacorporate multinational companies, together with some more elegant care for a privileged minority on the HMO model, or accountability for performance to local populations within the devolved, peripheralized State authority advocated in this book; but whereas accountability to centralized authority is already well advanced for the hospital services, is beginning for general practice, and will come by default if we do nothing, accountability to local populations and a peripheralized State machine can be won only through active mass education and united action by all grades of health workers, and these have scarcely begun.

Is the Welfare State Reversible?

In 1986 Professor Therborn of Nijmegen[22] marshalled evidence that so long as democracy prevailed, the welfare state was an irreversible institution in all advanced capitalist countries. Even the USA and Japan devoted over half their public expenditures to welfare purposes by 1981. Since he wrote, however, his own country, the Netherlands, has entered a crisis of welfarism centred particularly on the health service. Dutch health services have developed in ways which are indefensibly wasteful and extravagant; referrals by GPs to specialists are so high (more than twice as high as in the UK), initiated so casually and on what UK GPs would regard as such trivial indications,[23] that half the population is now being referred for some kind of specialist care each year. Even more perhaps than in the UK, if and when doctors become accountable for the effectiveness and efficiency of their work, they will find wide areas that are incompatible with social conscience. Inevitably, full advantage will be taken of this to attack the principle of a free and universal public service. Major faults in health services, education, and social services of all kinds, denied by trade unions and professional organizations too weighed down by defensive armour to be capable of imaginative counter-attack, leave huge gaps in the ideological defences of the Welfare State.

Therborn seems to leave out of account the possibility that the Welfare State may not be wound up, but privatized. Though the USA spends about four times as much per head on medical care as the UK, it is spent through a fragmented, fully entrepreneurial, fee-paid service which to British eyes appears to be a non-system. Unless we can develop a new social alliance to extend medical professionalism in new ways, if the NHS can be run profitably and more cheaply by entrepreneurs, only increasingly bankrupt and un- convincing traditions will delay passive privatization by apparently inevitable processes of decay in public and growth in private services. More than sentimental outrage will be necessary to preserve the Welfare State in the health sector. Though journalists can use them to make better copy, health services are not more important to a civilized society than either education or full employment. If these other features of society can be sacrificed to greed, so can our health services, though the softening-up process may be more difficult. Nations which can seriously contemplate privatization of prisons will consider anything, if it seems to make sense in cash terms.

Neither the Welfare State as a whole, nor the NHS in particular, can be defended just as they stand. The stamp of elitist authority imposed on them by social history as a precondition for their birth is now more than ever a liability, which must be overcome if the medical profession is to secure more dependable sponsorship from a broader social base. Above all, we have to overcome the profound divisions between health workers which have inevitably developed in an industry in which all but the doctors have always been expected to survive on subsistence wages, and in which even job security is now a thing of the past.

The Doctor-bashing Tradition

Each time the medical profession opposed legislative reforms of health services which made them accessible to more people in need, it forfeited more of the political respect and confidence of the public. People are not sorry for the poor doctors, any more than they are sorry for the poor farmers; in practical politics, there are no poor doctors or poor farmers, and no protests by the BMA or the National Farmers' Union will change that popular impression.

The NHS, above all in its hospitals but on a smaller scale in each general practice team, is an upstairs-downstairs world of grotesquely unequal wealth and power, riven with traditions of snobbery and servility, in which health workers at all levels fight one another for whatever shreds of status they can get after the top doctors have helped themselves.[24] Doctors have, with few exceptions, stood aside from the struggles of other health workers for subsistence wages and elementary job security. Coal miners, not doctors, took effective action in 1982 to support the nurses in their battles for a living wage.

It is therefore difficult for other health workers to see doctors as even potential allies, and easy for anyone without any more positive policy to sound militant by raising a flag against medical oppression. Progressive doctors are mostly too ashamed of this record of collective arrogance and indifference to argue, and try to distance themselves from their colleagues in the hope that they may be accepted as honourable exceptions.

Of course, many doctors are rich enough to be little capitalists and landlords, and many GPs are still very bad employers, taking full advantage of the job-satisfaction which still ties some receptionists to work for around £1 an hour without a written contract, and more or less un-limited overtime without pay. However, to dismiss the whole profession on these grounds as potential allies would be as ridiculous as if porters or ward cleaners were to dismiss nurses on the grounds that they also tend often to be arrogant or condescending in their attitudes to less glamorous and even more badly paid and insecure occupations in the health service; no doubt these are attitudes some nurses pick up from doctors, because doctors dominate the culture of hospitals and the health service, so that one way or another medical attitudes are mirrored from top to bottom of all their many divided and divisive hierarchies.

In the great demonstrations of the London unions around the time of the dock strike of 1886 and the socialist revival, the top hats and white kid gloves of the printing compositors were in the front ranks; the 'gentlemen comps'. They were probably better off than most London GPs in those days; but unlike doctors trapped in the social assumptions of the Osler paradigm, they identified their own interests with those of other working men, and the need for unity was understood both by these elegant aristocrats of labour, and by dockers trying to escape from an animal existence through a guaranteed sixpence an hour. No doubt much might have

been said (and was said, privately) about the smug respectability of the gentlemen comps, but it would not have been
helpful to a cause more serious than these sectional differences. Doctors certainly deserve criticism, but they also
deserve some credit for producing more evidence about their
own failings than any other occupational group I can think
of. The unity of health workers is difficult, but it can and
must be achieved because without it all of us will lose the
NHS as a comprehensive service available to all according to
need, although it has generally been a rotten employer and
its attitude to staff relations has been feudal. Where we are
going to is more important than where we have come from.

Enlightened protagonists of primary care get tired of
opposing the obstinate vanity of medical professions in
nearly all countries, which insist both on occupying the
middle of the road to health, and on moving along it at a
pace determined not by public needs and scientific advance,
but by the personal preferences of their weakest colleagues,
and all of this at prohibitive prices. Understandably, plans
for primary care, from the World Health Organization to
the Cumberlege Report, tend to bypass the doctors as an
irrelevance to health. Though doctors are only a subset of
all health workers, they are a necessary subset, just as health
workers are not the only people who determine the state
of the public health, but are nevertheless vital to its
maintenance. No movement for better health is really likely
to succeed without them, nor will the medical profession
itself usefully survive if it does not learn to accept a less
arrogant role.

From Where We Are, With the People We Have

If the medical profession wishes to survive as a large body of
workers privileged to apply medical science to all who need
it, it must learn to accept new social allies; and if those new
allies are to have any hope of attaining power in government,
they must learn to accept the doctors, in both cases not as
they are, but as they can become. Despite the immense
cultural difficulties in doing so, the British working class has

got to redefine itself to include people who have lived,
thought, and felt differently from industrial workers, who
are for the most part ignorant of social relationships within
heavy industry and manufacturing, but who are now coming
into collision with a section of the ruling class which has
deserted a large part of its traditional social base, as well as
its more thoughtful peers. People have to be allowed and
encouraged to change.

Ideal people, who think and behave in all respects as we
hope people will one day behave in some future better
society, at present scarcely exist. If they are to be found
anywhere, they are in coal-mining communities like the one
I have lived and worked in for the last 26 years. Even in
such communities, these people of the future are rare;
serious plans must be based on the real people we have,
produced by the society we have. It's a damaging society,
that's why we want its structure to change; so why be
surprised that it produces damaged people like ourselves,
capable of heroism but also of weakness and self-seeking?

We have to make a start from where we are with the
people we have. The NHS contains elements of a future
more equitable, stable, happier society on which we can
build. In the minds of the people it remains a successful
demonstration of the superiority of service for need over
commodity production for profit. Imaginatively extended,
at primary care level it could be an important new vehicle
for development of the social machinery of participative
democracy, and of the new attitudes to measured evidence
needed for a society in which every cook not only really
does learn to rule the State, but also learns to make up her
mind about road safety, the hazards of nuclear power, or
what to do and what not to do about her high blood pressure
or her period pains, on the basis of evidence. If we want to
survive, we must enter a new age of Popular Science, not
awestruck by incomprehensible technology, but with the
immediate scepticism and ultimate faith of real science.

The Social Function of Medical Science

The Osler paradigm secured a credible and profitable association with science at a time when effective medical science
scarcely existed. Both Osler himself and his successors who
led the profession were aware of this gap between the hopes
of patients and the reality which doctors could deliver, and
strove always to reduce it. At the leading edge of practice
particularly, this has been the most potent force in medical
professionalism. That is to say, in any open conflict between
the needs of medical science and other less worthy professional ambitions, science has had to come first, because
public faith in the profession has depended on the assumption
that no other outcome is possible; which is why such conflicts
have generally been concealed not only from the public but
from professional consciousness.

Medical science is now advancing at exponential speed, a
fact which will be rammed home by the arrival during the
next few years of practical techniques resulting from fundamental discoveries in molecular biology. These will for the
most part not be effectively or economically applicable to
symptomatic illness within episodic consultations; to be
used efficiently, they will require personal continuity, team
care within the community, close in every way to how and
where people live and work, with patients fully able to share
in decisions about their lives, which even more than now will
depend on intelligent assessment of conflicting probabilities
rather than dogmatic positive assertions. There is no way
that these new functions can be accommodated within the
old Osler paradigm; either we shall develop a new kind of
primary doctor able to incorporate the best of the old
within a new, wider, more imaginative but also more planned,
measured, and quantified mode of care, or GPs will lose
social efficiency by splitting into two groups, one responding
to demands within the old paradigm but in large profit-
oriented organizations over which they will have no control,
the other seeking for needs without doctors, in organizations
for primary care which would have to re-invent the wheel,
and turn other health workers into the new kind of doctor

we really need.

Medical science has potentially acquired a new and important social function at a new social level. Traditionally, of all highly educated men and women, family doctors have been closest to real communities of ordinary people, representing scholarship and learning to a scientifically more or less uneducated public. Much of this may have been sentimental hokum, but not all of it. The science and scholarship this represented originally tended to contain both negative and positive elements. Negatively, the doctor merged scientific with social authority in a generally authoritarian, intimidating, and dogmatic approach, dressed in a waistcoat and smelling of carbolic. Far from reflecting the power of Medical Science, this authority was designed to conceal its weakness, to bridge the gap between hopes and realities and to reinforce the placebo effect. The positive elements, on the other hand, were the connection with innovative science (the doctor who kept up with professional literature, and occasionally used a scientific imagination to apply it to local circumstances), naturalist curiosity, and occasional frank admissions of ignorance, which meant a lot when they came from an educated man because they implied the constructive doubt central to scientific thought. When Sir James Mackenzie, the greatest general practitioner Britain ever produced, took up his unhappy appointment as a consultant at the London Hospital Medical College, his contemporaries heard a new and characteristic phrase: 'I do not know. . . I wonder, I do not know. . .'

This combination of continuous critical revision, objective measurement, evaluation of evidence and constructive doubt, linked with rocklike faith in the urgency and reality of social progress, defines a truly scientific approach to the world. If this approach could be brought to community level, if it were in everyday use by primary care teams and the populations they serve, we might gain some more solid ground on which to halt the retreat and begin again to build a better society of participative democracy.

Mass Experience of Quantified Doubt

We already have the necessary beginnings of this. Ever since thalidomide, all of us, doctors and patients alike, have known that *all* medication which can do good can also in some circumstances, not always predictable, do harm. For example, more than 30 years after it was clearly proved, more doctors and more patients are beginning to understand that blood pressure is a continuously distributed, graded risk, so that any division between normal and abnormal must represent a practically rather than biologically determined decision, namely the point beyond which medical intervention is more likely to help than to harm the patient, based on the best evidence we have from controlled trials. Gradually it is becoming understood that many other important reversible indicators of future ill health can, like high blood pressure, no longer be effectively handled with the crude yes–no system of disease labelling we have learned in the Osler paradigm; airways obstruction, obesity, alcohol and nicotine damage, non-insulin-dependent diabetes, and a steadily growing list of other kinds of chronic damage are becoming wholly or partly amenable to quantified measurement with appropriately quantified treatment, balancing probable gains against possible risks.

This kind of medical care will demand doctors who read original work in scientific journals, with sufficient independent judgement and confidence to apply them in the always unique conditions of their own locality, and to think beyond the generally primitive, episodic level of medical thought transmitted in teaching hospitals. It will require nurses who not only insist on having a protocol to work to, but also recognize that protocols should be based on evidence, and that as new evidence becomes available, protocols must change; nurses must therefore also read and ultimately contribute to original scientific literature, and think and act for themselves; and therefore the professional distinctions between doctors and nurses must diminish and their training should overlap. And it will require patients who can begin to cope with the limited but threatening uncertainties of real medical care and the science of organized doubt, rather than the bland reassurance of medical pretence and its scientistic technical certainties.

There has already been more change in this direction than most people realize. In the early 1970s the Medical Research Council needed to recruit 18,000 patients to a trial of the effectiveness of drugs in preventing stroke, heart attacks and other complications of moderately raised blood pressure. The only way to get so many subjects was through GPs. Recruiting 176 practices to the trial, 600,000 people were screened and 18,000 followed in the trial, demonstrating for the first time anywhere in the world that data of high quality could be collected on a large scale, whether from searching records, from interviews, from blood samples, from electrocardiographic tracings, or other clinical or laboratory procedures, from ordinary group practices with a research nurse attached. This General Practice Research Framework has now expanded to 300 group practices covering about 3 million people, and is now undertaking a variety of multicentre research studies which would be impossible with smaller populations, or without the access and continuity made possible by association with general practice. Obviously work on this scale must have an effect on the attitudes to consultation and consequent tasks of both health workers and the populations they serve.

Medicine has always been unique among sciences in that it has had to act without adequate data (another way in which it resembles politics); or at least appear to act, which in this context comes to the same thing, because doctors have had to believe in what they were doing. Medicine has never been able to observe nature undisturbed, or to contrive simple experiments with the freedom available to physicists, chemists, or non-human biologists, because it was dealing with distressed human material. In the past all this was a serious weakness, and made medicine the least scientific, least quantified of sciences, most heavily contaminated with a humbug particularly hard to eradicate, because the placebo effect, supported by a little token technology, was generally more useful and effective than serious attempts at scientific clinical medicine. The placebo effect imparts and sustains hope; hope, and even more, hopelessness, have physiological consequences; there is nothing inherently unscientific about the placebo effect, the fault lies in our attitude to it. Most of all, this was the case in general practice, the area of clinical medicine most remote from laboratory medical science and most exposed to patient pressure for something (anything) to be done. In general practice it was even more difficult than in hospitals to observe without acting, or to recognize good outcomes as results of the natural history of illness rather than medical intervention.

Though the culture of general practice remains less scientistic than the culture of specialist practice in hospitals, the real situation is now potentially reversed. Scientific work in hospitals is limited in a fundamental way by the self-selection of sick people whose health breakdown seems serious enough to justify the disruption of their lives involved in hospital referral or admission, and their separation from a still unknown total population. The position of a hospital-based doctor as a medical scientist resembles that of a botanist offered a dead branch fallen from a tree, and asked to determine its cause of death without any opportunity to examine the surviving stump; except that the botanist would at least be aware of this limitation, whereas the division of labour and diagnostic resources between doctors working in hospitals and in the community makes it difficult for specialists surrounded by scientistic machinery to perceive opportunities for scientific work outside, with less machinery, but with access to whole populations. The number of GPs who read and contribute to serious medical scientific literature has increased rapidly over the past 30 years, particularly during the last decade. Innovation in truly scientific, population-based practice is now beginning to occur on a large scale, though in a minority of practices and still limited by the structure and traditions of practice, and by dwindling DHSS leadership and material support since 1979. The key, of course, is organized contact with the whole population at risk; without this, GPs content to deal only with presented demand are no better than hospital specialists, and much worse in that they are less well organized, staffed and equipped, and more isolated from peer criticism.

The basic scientific development of various parts of medicine will continue to occur mainly in hospitals and laboratories, perhaps even more so in this new age of molecular biology. The validation and therefore the development of the practice of medicine *as a whole*, however, will be established for the first time in primary care. GPs and all the members of primary care teams will become, as many already are, peripheral scientists. They have not only their registered populations, the unique and essential human material for this, but also all the previously inconceivable data and information-handling power of microcomputers, photocopiers and telefax, which will give the smallest peripheral unit intellectual resources which thirty years ago would have required a national university library and an army of office workers.

Just as every GP was, in the Osler paradigm, an outpost of established social authority, every health centre could now become an outpost of popular science. But our opportunities are greater even than that; each such outpost of science is in intimate daily contact with all of the people. With such a basic social unit we have an already functioning growing point for popularized science and a new kind of participative democracy, in a mature, literate and industrialized society.

Primary Care Centres as Growing Points for Participative Democracy

Practices which accept responsibility for the health care of their registered populations, as well as for responding to demands for diagnosis and treatment of disease and other problems already recognizable by patients, should review their work and report their findings back to their populations. How this is done seems to me to be not very important. It could be a comprehensive annual report (hopefully not too overloaded with statistics) or it could just be evidence from a random sample of records about one particular problem such as unwanted pregnancies, uptake of cervical smears or prevention of maturity-onset diabetes by control of obesity; the point is that the information should be based on an audit of real, randomly-sampled material, with discussion of the problems of omission rather than meaningless boasts about how many patients have been seen, how many smears have been taken and so on, without relation to the numbers at risk. Unless we know what ought to have been done, we cannot evaluate what has been done. Writing of medical records in 1971, the material evidence on which all measures of the quality of medical care have to be based, Lawrence Weed[24] wrote:

> We should continually remind ourselves that not to think quantitatively about the needs of all of the people has qualitative implications for most of the people.

Public discussion of the problems revealed by such a report would help people to gain confidence in themselves, not only patients but the primary care team. In recognizing the reality of the problems facing both the team and the population it serves, and the initially huge gaps in performance on both sides which must be remedied, we can at last stop pretending we are all perfect and get down to effective work. Of course work of this kind would present difficulties, but they would be new difficulties of growth, openness and inexperience, rather than the old difficulties of defensive pomposity, secrecy, jealously guarded job demarcations and stagnation.

A future government that is serious about not just maintaining the NHS but imaginatively improving and extending it as one part of a more general commitment to a fundamentally different and more wholesome society, would give resources and legislative recognition to such developments. The exact forms of this recognition are not important now. What is important is that a number of working models should be available from which to choose, adapted to the specific problems and opportunities of a wide variety of neighbourhoods.

The forward march of Medicine is not halted, nor, for long, is the forward march of Labour; their paths must and will converge. De-industrialized Britain needs growth industries. In their widest sense, health care and education are potentially our biggest employers, and so they should be, in a truly civilized state. We need a larger, more imaginative, more generous society than the one we have now to make room for them, but it will also be a more sceptical society, forcing us to build with less haste, but more solidity.

Brecht showed Galileo as a passionate intellectual, who understood that his work depended on teamwork with intelligent working men, lens-grinders and instrument makers, but sponsored by men with gold and the power it gives, their intelligence reduced to cunning by long misuse in self-service. The pope, a scholar and therefore a reluctant enemy of science, must be persuaded by his chief inquisitor to snuff out this first candle of quantified, measured, sceptical curiosity about the world, deferring to no authority but the evidence of experiment:

> The inquisitor: They say it is their mathematical tables and not the spirit of denial and doubt. But it is not their tables. A horrible unrest has come into the world. It is this unrest in their own brains which these men impose upon the motionless earth. They cry, 'the figures compel us!' But whence come these figures? They come from doubt, as everyone knows. These men doubt everything. Are we to establish human society on doubt, and no longer on faith?

Questions are more important than answers, what we have yet to do is more important than what we've done. As we climb our ladder of knowledge we can see ever wider frontiers of ignorance. The human race and all its worthwhile tasks are growing. We can and must establish human society on measured doubt; that is our faith.

NOTES

1. Burnham, J., *The middle class vote*, London: Faber & Faber, 1954.
2. Mechanic, D., Faich, R., 'Doctors in revolt'. In Weinberg, I. (ed.), *English society*, New York: Atherton Press, 1968.
3. Reynolds, B., 'Where to find the good life in the EEC and still be

a GP', *Medeconomics 1982*; 3:52-3.
4. Klein, R., 'International perspectives on the NHS', *British Medical Journal 1977*; iv:1492.
5. 'Report of the Royal Commission on Medical Education', (Todd Report), London: HMSO, 1968.
6. Donnan, S.P.B., 'British medical undergraduates in 1975: a student survey in 1975 compared with 1966', *Medical Education 1976*; 10:341-7.
7. Watkins, S., *Medicine and Labour: the politics of a profession*, London: Lawrence & Wishart, 1987.
8. McKinlay, J.B., Arches, J., 'Towards the proletarianization of physicians', *International Journal of Health Services 1985*; 15:161-93.
9. Chernomas, R., 'An economic basis for the proletarianization of physicians', *International Journal of Health Services 1986*; 16:669-74.
10. Starr, P., *The social transformation of medicine*, New York: Basic Books, 1982.
11. Relman, A.S., 'The new medical-industrial complex', *New England Journal of Medicine 1980*; 303:963-70.
12. Ginzberg, E., 'The destabilisation of health care', *New England Journal of Medicine 1986*; 315:757-61.
13. Freeman, S.A., 'Megacorporate health care: a choice for the future', *New England Journal of Medicine 1985*; 312:579-82.
14. Marks, L., *Primary health care on the agenda? A discussion document*. Primary Health Care Group, King's Fund Centre for Health Services Development, London, 1987.
15. Hart, J.T., *Hypertension: community control of high blood pressure*, 2nd ed., London: Churchill Livingstone, 1987.
16. Editorial, 'Medical student numbers and medical manpower', *Lancet 1987*; i:723-4.
17. DHSS consultative document. 'Hospital medical staffing: achieving a balance', London: HMSO, 1986.
18. Nussey, S.S., Pilkington, T.R.E., Saunders, K.B., 'Where will this month's medical school intake go?', *Lancet 1986*; ii:977.
19. Booth, C., 'Better a commitment to health and research than to missiles', *British Medical Journal 1986*; 293:23-6.
20. Kenney, M., *Biotechnology: the university-industrial complex*, New Haven: Yale University Press, 1986.
21. Brecht, B., *The life of Galileo*, London: Eyre Methuen, 1963.
22. Therborn, G., Roebroek, J., 'The irreversible Welfare State: its recent maturation, its encounter with the economic crisis, and its future prospects', *International Journal of Health Services 1986*; 16:319-38.
23. Hull, F.M., Westerman, R.F., 'Referral to medical outpatients department at teaching hospitals in Birmingham and Amsterdam', *British Medical Journal 1986*; 293:311-14.
24. Weed, L.L., 'Quality control and the medical record', *Archives of Internal Medicine 1971*; 127:101.

INDEX